Lifelong Motor Development

fourth edition

Lifelong Motor Development

Carl P. Gabbard
Texas A&M University

PEARSON

Benjamin
Cummings

San Francisco   Boston   New York
Cape Town   Hong Kong   London   Madrid   Mexico City
Montreal   Munich   Paris   Singapore   Sydney   Tokyo   Toronto

Publisher: Daryl Fox
Acquisitions Editor: Deirdre McGill
Development Manager: Claire Brassert
Project Editor: Susan Malloy
Assistant Editor: Christina Pierson
Marketing Manager: Sandra Lindelof
Production Editor: Steven Anderson
Project Coordination and Composition: The Left Coast Group, Inc.
Copy Editor: Deborah Kopka
Proofreader: Joan Wai
Photo Research: Brian Donnelly, Cypress Integrated Systems
Cover Designer: Yvo Riezebos
Manufacturing Buyer: Stacey Weinberger
Cover Printer: Phoenix Color
Text Printer: R.R. Donnelley

Cover Photo: © Martin Barraud/Getty Images

Credits can be found on page 469.

ISBN 0-8053-2849-1

Library of Congress Cataloging-in-Publication Data
Gabbard, Carl, 1948–
    Lifelong motor development / Carl P. Gabbard.—4th ed.
        p. ; cm.
Includes bibliographical references and index.
    ISBN 0-8053-2849-1 (hdc.)
    1. Motor ability. 2. Human growth.
    [DNLM: 1. Human Development. 2. Motor Activity—physiology. WS 103
G112L 2004] I. Title.

    QP301.G24 2004
    612'.04--dc21

                                        2003004328

PEARSON

Benjamin
Cummings

www.aw.com/bc

1 2 3 4 5 6 7—RRDV—07 06 05 04 03

This book is dedicated with deep affection to Luke,
my beloved grandson,
who has helped me reaffirm
why I chose and continue to love
my profession and life itself.

Contents

To the Student   xv
Preface   xvii

part one   *An Overview of Lifelong Human Development   1*

1   *Introduction to the Developmental Perspective   3*

The Primary Determinants of Motor Behavior   6
General Terminology   6
  Prerequisite Terms   6
  Motor Development Terms   8
Significant Observations (Assumptions) about Development   9
Periods of Life-Span Development   13
The Developmental Continuum   14
Research in Motor Development   17
  Why Study Motor Development?   17
  Methods of Study   18
Theoretical Views   22
  Contributing Views   23
  Environmental Context Theory   25
  Biological Systems Theory   29
Careers in Motor Development   31
  Summary   32
  Think about It   33
  Suggested Readings   33
  WebLinks   34

part two   *Biological Growth and Development   35*

2   *Heredity and Neurological Changes   36*

Heredity   37
Neurological Changes   39
  Basic Structure and Function   39
  Early Developmental Changes   46
  Neurological Changes with Aging   60
  Summary   62
  Think about It   63
  Suggested Readings   64
  WebLinks   64

3 *Physical Growth Changes 65*

An Overview of Physical Growth and Development 66
Prenatal Development 68
The Pubescent (Adolescent) Growth Spurt 70
Changes in Body Proportions and Physique 74
Body Proportions 74
Physique 81
Changes with Aging 82
Structural Development 82
Height 82
Skeletal Growth 86
Changes with Aging 89
Body Mass 91
Body Weight 91
Body Composition 92
Changes with Aging 101
Maturity Estimates 102
Morphological Age 102
Dental Age 103
Sexual Age 103
Skeletal Age 103
Maturity Variations 106
Implications for Motor Performance 108
Summary 109
Think about It 111
Suggested Readings 112
WebLinks 112

4 *Physiological Changes 113*

Cardiorespiratory Development 114
Basic Structure and Function 114
Early Growth and Development 115
Aerobic Power 118
Anaerobic Power 119
Heart Rate 121
Cardiac Output and Stroke Volume 123
Vital Capacity and Pulmonary Ventilation 123
Blood Characteristics 124
Blood Volume 124
Red Blood Cells Content 125
Blood Pressure 125
Basal Metabolic Rate 126
Muscular Strength 127

Flexibility   130
Changes with Aging   133
    Change in Cardiorespiratory Function   133
    Change in Basal Metabolic Rate   134
    Change in Muscular Strength   134
    Change in Flexibility   135
       Summary   138
       Think about It   139
       Suggested Readings   139
       WebLinks   140

5   *Factors Affecting Growth and Development   141*

Prenatal Development   142
    Principles of Teratogenic Effects   142
    Internal (Maternal) Factors   143
    External (Environmental) Factors   145
Nutrition and Physical Activity during Postnatal Development   149
    Nutrition   150
    Physical Activity   151
Glands and Hormonal Activity   159
    Pituitary Gland   159
    Thyroid Gland   161
    Pancreas   161
    Adrenal Glands   162
    Other Glandular Functions   162
       Summary   163
       Think about It   164
       Suggested Readings   164
       WebLinks   164

part three   *Perception and Information Processing   167*

6   *Perceptual Development   169*

Visual Perception   172
    The Visual Process   172
    Developmental Change in Visual Structures   173
    Developmental Change in Visual Functions   173
Kinesthetic Perception   184
    Structure and Function of the Kinesthetic System   184
    Development of Kinesthetic Perception   185

Auditory Perception   193
Structure and Function of the Auditory System   194
Development of Auditory Perception   194
Tactile Perception   195
Perceptual Integration   196
Visual-Kinesthetic Integration   197
Visual-Auditory Integration   198
Auditory-Kinesthetic Integration   198
Changes with Aging   199
Visual Perception   199
Auditory Perception   200
Kinesthetic Perception   200
Gibson's Ecological Perspective   202
Movement-Based Approaches   204
Summary   206
Think about It   207
Suggested Readings   207
WebLinks   207

7   *Information Processing and Motor Control   209*

Attention   211
Alertness   211
Divided Attention   212
Selective Attention   213
Memory   215
Memory Structures   215
Memory Abilities   217
Processing Speed and Movement Time   222
Programming   224
Schema Theory   226
Developmental Theories of Motor Control   227
Changes with Aging   232
Attention   232
Working (Short-Term) Memory   232
Long-Term Memory   233
Metamemory and Knowledge   233
Processing Speed and Movement Time   234
Programming   235
Summary   236
Think about It   237
Suggested Readings   238
WebLinks   238

part four   *Motor Behavior across the Life Span*   *239*

8 *Early Movement Behavior*   *242*

Reflexive Behavior   244
Importance of Reflexes in Infant Development   244
Types of Reflexes   246
Theoretical Views of Reflex Behavior and Voluntary Movement   257
Spontaneous Movements (Stereotypies)   259
Rudimentary Behavior   261
Postural Control   262
Rudimentary Locomotion   265
Manual Control   273
Motor Asymmetries   279
   Summary   282
   Think about It   283
   Suggested Readings   283
   WebLinks   283

9 *Motor Behavior during Early Childhood*   *284*

Fundamental Motor Skill Development   286
Basic Terminology   286
Methods for Studying Change   287
Movement Patterns (Process Characteristics)   289
Running   289
Jumping   293
Hopping   298
Galloping, Sliding, and Skipping   299
Throwing   301
Catching   304
Striking   310
Kicking   313
Ball Bouncing and Dribbling   316
Climbing   318
Fine Motor Manipulative Behavior   320
Finger Differentiation   320
Construction and Self-Help Skills   322
Drawing and Writing   322
Bimanual Control   325
Functional (Motor) Asymmetries   326
Handedness   327
Footedness   328
Eye Preference   329
   Summary   330
   Think about It   331
   Suggested Readings   331
   WebLinks   331

10 *Motor Behavior during Later Childhood and Adolescence* *332*

Bases for Age- and Gender-Related Quantitative (Product) Motor Performance Changes **334**
Quantitative (Product) Changes in Motor Performance **338**
Running Speed 338
Throwing 340
Jumping 342
Kicking 343
Catching 344
Striking with an Implement 345
Hopping 345
Ball Bouncing and Dribbling 346
Balance 347
Motor Skill Refinement **347**
Youth Sport Participation 347
School Physical Education 352
Summary *353*
Think about It *354*
Suggested Readings *354*
WebLinks *354*

11 *Motor Behavior in the Adult Years* *356*

Peak Motor Performance **358**
Growth and Physiological Function 358
Motor Performance Characteristics 361
Considerations of Race 364
Regression **365**
Biological Theories of Advanced Aging 365
Biological Regression and Motor Performance 368
Changing Movement Patterns 377
Physical Activity and Longevity **381**
Summary *383*
Think about It *383*
Suggested Readings *384*
WebLinks *384*

part five   *Assessment*   *387*

12   *Assessment*   *388*

Basic Terminology of Assessment   **390**
Purposes of Assessment   **391**
Considerations for Proper Assessment   **393**
Assessment Instruments   **394**
   Newborn Assessment   395
   Infant Assessment   398
   Assessment of (up to) School-Age Populations   403
   Process-Oriented (Fundamental Movement) Assessment Instruments   407
   Other Commonly Used Instruments   411
   Tests for Older Persons   413
     Summary   *416*
     Think about It   *417*
     Suggested Readings   *417*
     WebLinks   *418*

part six   *Sociocultural Influences on Motor Development*   *419*

13   *Sociocultural Influences on Motor Development*   *420*

Basic Terminology of Socialization   **421**
Socializing Processes and Agents   **422**
Primary Influences during Childhood and Adolescence   **424**
   The Family   425
   Peer Relations   427
   Coaches and Teachers   430
   Gender-Role Expectations and Stereotyping   431
   Self-Esteem   432
   Possible Influences of Race   434
Primary Influences during Adulthood   **435**
     Summary   *438*
     Think about It   *439*
     Suggested Readings   *439*
     WebLinks   *440*

References   441

Index   455

Credits   469

To the Student

Once again I want to address you in this special section, because I realize not all students are overwhelmed at the notion of reading the preface of a college text. The fourth edition of *Lifelong Motor Development* is a study in one of the most fascinating and relevant subjects you will encounter. What could be more interesting than understanding human behavior across the life span—a look back and, perhaps more intriguing, a glance at days to come? This text is a window into the dynamics of one of our most natural, joyful, and important behaviors—movement! You are about to begin a fascinating journey through the study of motor behavior and the marvelous machine that controls it from its prenatal beginnings to older adulthood. Let the journey of a lifetime begin!

What endless questions vex the thought,
of whence and whither, when and how

—Sir Richard Burton, *Kasidah*

CARL GABBARD

P.S.: Reading the preface may lend some insight into how your instructor may use this text.

Preface

In the tradition of the previous versions, the fourth edition of *Lifelong Motor Development* is published with the goal of being the most comprehensive, up-to-date, science-based text of its kind. More than 50% of the citations are new. Because of its diversity of subject matter and unique provision of chapter objectives, this text is appropriate for beginning and advanced students. The essence of *Lifelong Motor Development* is grounded in science and includes the latest theory and research related to our understanding of physical growth and motor behavior across the life span.

As in past editions, this version includes the popular conceptual model of the developmental continuum that depicts the phases of lifelong motor behavior. This framework is descriptive and integrates much of the material presented in the text. To complement the model, this edition provides a much-improved guide to address perhaps the most relevant issue in contemporary motor development: the study of how individuals acquire coordinated movement, or, the study of *perception to action*. This is an examination of the agents for change that underlie motor behavior. The author's personal framework for presenting this approach is the *developmental systems perspective* that advocates that development is the product of dynamic interacting processes between the various biological and environmental systems. The fourth edition of *Lifelong Motor Development* provides a framework for studying these systems in the context of human motor development.

No book of science can be fully appreciated unless it is user-friendly. Overall, this edition is more concise, provides more accurate illustrations, and better stimulates students to enjoy and think critically about the subject matter. It is also more sensitive to coverage of gender issues and use of gender appropriate language.

Additional Changes to the Fourth Edition

Additional changes to the fourth edition include the following:
- Updates and new research highlights from interesting studies of brain research, dynamic systems, embodiment (motor and cognition

relationships), affordance theory, information processing (motor programming), aging, and others.
- Improved life-span coverage with expansion of material on adult development and aging that is not found in most developmental texts.
- Expanded coverage of youth sports.
- More *Think About It* critical thinking questions in the margins to stimulate reflection on previous material and experience.
- Inclusion of chapter *WebLinks*.
- New motor assessments based on a dynamic systems perspective.
- Updated growth charts.
- More application using examples to illustrate research findings and theoretical ideas.

■ Basic Organization

Lifelong Motor Development presents a topical and chronological approach to the study of human motor development. Although there are good arguments for using either format entirely, the intent is to provide the student with a multidimensional perspective. The topical sections offer a rich feel for the interrelatedness of the lifelong developmental process. On the other hand, conceptualizing life-span development within a framework for study and placement of significant events necessitates a time-related continuum. This text provides such a developmental framework; however, it is based on the premise that while change may appear phasic (stagelike), its underlying processes are continuous. It is the continuous nature of development that requires topical discussions.

The basic organization of the text is not different from the previous edition. For first-time users (in brief), *Lifelong Motor Development* is divided into six parts. Part One consists of a single chapter that presents a multidisciplinary overview of lifelong human development with emphasis on basic developmental principles, terms, issues, and theoretical approaches. Also provided is a conceptual model of the phases of motor behavior used as the framework for the material presented in Part Four, "Motor Behavior across the Life Span." Part Two is devoted to topical discussions on the body of information related to lifelong biological growth and development. Chapters 2, 3, and 4 provide information on the various hereditary, neurological, and physical characteristics that, together with experience, form the bases for motor behavior across the life span. Chapter 5 deals with factors and conditions that may affect the course of biological growth and development.

Chapters 6 and 7 (Part Three) present comprehensive topical discussions of lifelong perceptual development and information-processing characteristics, including the latest theory on perception to action. The chapters in Part Four (8 through 11) provide a chronological (phase model) description of motor behavior characteristics across the life span. Coverage begins with early movement behavior (chapter 8). It extends through early childhood (chapter 9), later childhood and adolescence (chapter 10), and finally to motor behavior during the adult years that is characterized by peak performance and with older age, regression (chapter 11).

Part Five (chapter 12) offers a broad perspective on the diversity of motor assessment techniques and discusses the considerations for selecting and implementing a wide variety of assessment instruments. Part Six (chapter 13) presents a discussion of the influence and importance of sociocultural factors on motor development from a lifelong perspective.

■ *Pedagogical Features*

An important goal in creating this text was to make it a *teachable* resource with an *effective learning system*. Each of the six parts of the text begins with an overview of its content. Included in the introduction of each chapter are *chapter objectives* and *key terms*. The objectives reflect the conceptual framework used by identifying the important facts, topics, and concepts to be covered. Marginal notations are provided to aid the reader in identifying text material related to chapter objectives. Consistent feedback from users suggests that these characteristics are quite useful in developing (customizing) course materials. For example, in some instances instructors may wish to designate selected (rather than all) chapter objectives for course coverage. This can be especially useful for advanced studies of motor development.

Think about It questions are found in the margins of each chapter with the intent of stimulating critical thinking and active involvement with the subject matter. Like the objectives, they can be used for a variety of instructional purposes.

Key terms appear in boldfaced type in the text and pinpoint the words of greatest importance to understanding the broader concepts of each chapter; these and other significant terms are highlighted throughout. A chapter *Summary*, list of *Think about It questions, Suggested Readings*, and *WebLinks* are presented at the end of each chapter. Supplements available with the fourth edition of *Lifelong Motor Development* include an Instructor's Manual with Test Bank and Transparency Masters and a PowerPoint presentation CD with lecture outlines and key figures and tables from the text.

And finally, a much desired outcome of the fourth edition of *Lifelong Motor Development* is that the reader will feel the excitement associated with studying and understanding human motor development from a life-span perspective.

Acknowledgments

The fourth edition of *Lifelong Motor Development* is the outcome of much more than my efforts. I am most grateful for the continuous and diligent efforts of the scientific community in providing the knowledge base. Much of the inspiration for creating the fourth edition came from comments from current users, colleagues, and students. Many thanks to the following reviewers: R. R. Apache, University of Nevada, Las Vegas; Martin Block, University of Virginia; Stephen Langendorfer, Bowling Green State University; Scott Modell, California State University, Sacramento; Lynda Reeves, Minnesota State University, Mankato; James Reid, University of Tennesee, Martin; Marco Santello, Arizona State University; Judy Schultz, Washington State University; Martin Short, University of North Dakota; Cynthia Williams, Winston-Salem State University; Jin Yan, California State University, Hayward. Thanks also to third edition reviewers: Robert Kraft, University of Delaware; Nancy Halliday, Hofstra University; and Steve Chepu, Springfield College.

With this edition, I also owe a special debt of gratitude to Benjamin Cummings, specifically Christina Pierson, Daryl Fox, Deirdre McGill, Susan Malloy, and Sandra Lindelof, for their support and dedication in making this edition the very best text in lifelong motor development.

An Overview of Lifelong Human Development

PART ONE presents an overview of lifelong human and motor development. Because developmental psychology is the basic body of knowledge from which an understanding of growth and motor behavior is derived and appreciated, much of this section focuses on its fundamentals. Basic developmental principles, terms, and theoretical approaches and issues are provided to aid the reader in forming an eclectic perspective of human development and motor behavior across the life span.

Along with the basic elements of developmental psychology, chapter 1 provides the initial introduction to the ways in which motor development parallels other human experience across the life span. Highlighting this section is a conceptual model of the developmental continuum of life-span motor behavior. This model provides a basis (conceptual framework) for describing and integrating much of the material presented in subsequent chapters.

Complementing the continuum, the reader is provided information that addresses one of the

chapter

1   Introduction to the
    Developmental Perspective

most important issues in contemporary motor development: What factors underlie change across the life span? This includes biological changes such as those observed in older adults and explanations for how individuals acquire coordinated movement, the study of *Perception* → *Action*.

1 Introduction to the Developmental Perspective

OBJECTIVES

Upon completion of this chapter, you should be able to

1.1 Explain the *developmental systems perspective* and describe its relationship to motor development.

1.2 Define the term motor development and describe its association with the life-span perspective.

1.3 Discuss the multidisciplinary approach to studying motor development.

1.4 Briefly describe the five major goals of the developmental specialist.

1.5 Describe the primary determinants of motor development and behavior.

1.6 Define the general terms that are unique to the fields of human and motor development.

1.7 Discuss and support the major observations (assumptions) associated with human development.

1.8 Outline the periods of life-span development.

1.9 Illustrate and briefly describe the developmental continuum for life-span motor behavior.

1.10 Discuss the purpose and identify the primary strategies used in conducting research in the scientific study of life-span development.

1.11 Name and describe the major theoretical views on human development.

KEY TERMS

developmental systems perspective

change

motor development

life-span perspective

multidisciplinary approach

heredity

maturation

environmental contexts

affordances

growth

development

motor behavior

cephalocaudal development

proximodistal development

aging

continuity

discontinuity

stages

phase

critical period

sensitive period

plasticity

periods of life-span development

developmental continuum

cohort effects

developmental contextualism

ecological systems theory

Gibson's ecological perspective

ecological task analysis model

information-processing view

developmental biodynamics

eclectic theoretical perspective

Objective 1.1

As a general philosophy for the study of lifelong human and motor development, this text supports and is firmly grounded in the **developmental systems perspective** (e.g., Gottlieb, 1992; Lerner, 2002; Lewis, 2000). This approach advocates the notion that human development is *the product of changing relations between the developing person and his or her changing multilevel environmental contexts.* A person is a dynamic, self-organizing unit consisting of several systems (e.g., neurological, muscular, skeletal, and cognitive) with multilevels within each system. Examples of environmental contexts, known as ecological systems, include the home, school, and culture, and social influences within (e.g., family, peers, and coaches). The interpretation of human development emphasizes the reciprocal interactions between all our biological characteristics and the environment. Prominent theories that complement the systems approach and add to our understanding of lifelong motor development are the focus in this and subsequent chapters.

The study of virtually any aspect of lifelong human development is inquiry into **change.** For change to be labeled developmental, it must have a successive character. For example, changes seen at a later time are at least influenced in part by the changes that occurred earlier. In essence, the study of development implies systematic and successive changes over time.

Objective 1.2 ➤ Lifelong motor development is a vital part of the field of *human development* over the life span. In general terms, **motor development** is the study of movement behavior and the associated biological changes in human movement across the life span. From another perspective it may be viewed as the process of change in motor behavior resulting from the interaction of biological systems and the environment.

Basic to a comprehensive understanding of this field of specialization is knowledge related to the characteristics and principles of *growth* (change in size), *development* (change in level of functioning), and *motor behavior* (performance). Traditionally this area of inquiry was studied by developmental psychologists primarily interested in the childhood stages of development. In more recent years, however, the scope of motor development has been extended in recognition that the developmental process is continuous and observable from conception to the final stage in human life. This **life-span perspective** is based on the theory that the developmental process extends beyond puberty and young adulthood. Significant physiological and motor behavior changes occur during older adulthood and are important to our understanding of the full scope of human development. Hughes and Noppe state, "To examine only isolated segments of the life span is equivalent to studying isolated scenes from a film or play" (1991, 6).

Objective 1.3 ➤ Along with the promising trend to view motor development from a *life-span perspective* has emerged the practice of studying behavioral change using an integrated **multidisciplinary approach.** That is, it is generally accepted that behavior in any domain (cognitive, affective, and psychomotor) is the product of many influences. To have a fuller understanding of human development, one should consider the full range of possible influences. Perhaps the strongest support for this point of view has been seen among those individuals interested in child development from a total development perspective; professionals from such fields as developmental psychology, exercise physiology, medicine, biomechanics, and sociology have provided data adding to our understanding of total human development and behavior.

THINK ABOUT IT

Why is it important to have a general understanding of human development in order to gain insight into lifelong motor behavior?

Objective 1.4 ➤ Developmental psychologists and motor development specialists seek to accomplish five major goals: (a) to determine the common and characteristic changes in behavior, function, and appearance across the life span; (b) to establish when these changes occur; (c) to describe what causes these changes; (d) to determine whether change can be predicted; and (e) to find out whether these changes are individual or universal.

An excellent commentary by Thelen (2000) offers a contemporary discussion of the description and history of motor development (see Suggested Readings). Thelen and other prominent researchers repeatedly emphasize how research in motor development has evolved from being satisfied with describing general changes (e.g., crawl, walk, and run), to identifying the biological and environmental processes that underlie these changes.

The Primary Determinants of Motor Behavior

Objective 1.5 ➤ At this point in the discussion a relevant question is "what determines motor development?" More specifically, what factors influence growth, development, and motor performance across the life span? Figure 1.1 illustrates the interrelated nature of human development as supported by the developmental systems view—that is, how one's biological characteristics (heredity, maturation, and self-organizing properties) interact with environmental contexts (ecological systems and affordances) to determine, in large part, motor development and behavior at any given point in time. Each of these terms will be defined in the following pages.

■ *Figure 1.1*

The determinants of motor behavior

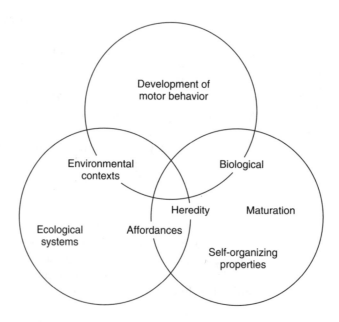

General Terminology

Objective 1.6 ➤ As with any specialized field of science or education, motor development has established its own terminology and adopted words from related disciplines. The study of motor development cuts across several disciplines and subareas within the study of movement behavior and therefore uses a considerable amount of the general terminology of these related fields. Familiarity with this terminology will be important in developing a clear understanding of the developmental perspective.

Prerequisite Terms

Heredity refers to a set of qualities that are fixed at birth and account for many individual traits and characteristics. The cells of normal humans possess 46 chromosomes arranged in 23 pairs. These chromosomes are made up of thousands of genes that influence such traits as eye and hair color, personality, intelligence, height, muscle fiber type, and general body build. Although these traits are strongly influenced by genetic structure, they may be modified by environmental factors.

The term **maturation** is often used interchangeably with the words *growth* and *development*. Maturation, however, is a more distinctive process that actually refers to the qualitative functional changes that occur with age. In essence, it is the timetable of developmental events. Primarily innate (i.e., genetically determined) and mostly resistant to external influences, maturation is a fixed order of progression; the time intervals may vary but the sequence of appearance of characteristics generally does not. The development of locomotion, for example, follows a consistent order (sit, walk, and run) and an approximate age of appearance. Other relevant terms are:

Environmental contexts are the circumstances, objects, or conditions by which one is surrounded. A key term related to this general descriptor is **affordances.** Affordances are opportunities for action that objects, events, or places in the environment provide, such as toys, stairs in the home, and a swimming pool. These affordances provide the stimulus for motor development.

Experience refers to conditions within the environment that may alter or modify various developmental characteristics through the learning process.

Learning is the relatively permanent change in performance that results from practice or past experience.

Readiness is the combination of maturation and experience that prepares an individual to acquire a skill or understanding.

Adaptation is the process of altering one's behaviors to interact effectively with the environment. The term is often used to describe the complex interplay between the individual and the environment. The developmental aspects of maturation and the individual's experience interweave to create behavior.

Motor Development Terms

As previously mentioned, *motor development* is both a process and scientific field of study. As a process, it may be viewed as the lifelong changes in motor behavior resulting from the ongoing interaction between biological processes and the environment. The study of motor development focuses on the biological changes associated with movement behavior across the human life span. More specifically it is the study of lifelong growth, development, and motor behavior (performance).

Growth, often used interchangeably with *development* and *maturation*, refers to observable changes in quantity; in this context, growth represents an increase in body size. Although maturation may be a factor in the growth process, environmental factors may also contribute.

Development is a term that can be applied to several human behaviors. Basically, development refers to the process of change in the individual's level of functioning. Those changes may be either quantitative or qualitative in nature. Development is a product of growth as well as of heredity, maturation, and experience.

Motor behavior is the product of biological characteristics and environmental influence and refers to observable changes in the learning and performance of a particular movement or motor skill.

In its purest sense, the term *motor* refers to the underlying biological and mechanical factors that influence movement (or observable action), even though the terms *movement* and *motor* are frequently used interchangeably. As noted earlier, motor (or movement) performance is influenced by several integrated factors. Learning, integrated with growth and basic developmental factors, is a primary influence.

Learning was earlier defined as a relatively permanent change in performance resulting from practice or past experience. Although learning cannot be observed directly, it can be inferred from a person's motor performance. The term *motor learning* refers to a relatively permanent change in the performance of a motor skill, also resulting from practice or experience. Another term used frequently in the movement literature is *motor control*, referring to the area of study concerned primarily with the underlying processes involved in movement and how various movements are controlled. The focus of motor control study is on understanding specific neural, physical, and behavioral aspects of human movement.

Cephalocaudal and *proximodistal* are general terms used to describe the predictable sequences of growth and motor control. **Cephalocaudal development** is growth that proceeds longitudinally from the head to the feet. Complementing this physical growth is a gradual progression of increased muscular control, moving first from the muscles of the head and neck to the trunk and then to the legs and feet. **Proximodistal development** is growth that proceeds from the center of the body to its periphery—that is, growth and motor control occur in the trunk region and shoulders before the wrists, hands, and fingers. These developmental trends are typically observed in young children who exhibit greater coordination in the upper torso than in their legs and feet (cephalocaudal). Similarly, children will exhibit gross shoulder movements in their first attempts to draw, long before their ability to make fine motor cursive forms is developed.

The scope of motor development includes the study of biological change over the life span; therefore the term *aging* has relevance to our understanding of the developmental process. **Aging** has been characterized as the deteriorated capacity to regulate the internal environment (e.g., cellular, molecular, and organismic structures), resulting in a reduced probability of survival. It may also be thought of as the process of growing old regardless of chronological age.

■ *Significant Observations (Assumptions) about Development*

Objective 1.7 ➤ Now that we have defined the field and talked briefly about primary goals, let's consider some basic assumptions. The following observations concerning human development have direct implications for the study of lifelong motor behavior and guide the general orientation of this text. In past years, and perhaps to some extent today, these points are considered somewhat controversial. However, while the degree of impact for each may be debatable, their presence in the developmental process is evident. Arguably, the most dramatic of observations is the *interactive* and *dynamic* roles that nature (biology) and nurture (environment) play in development. This assumption is described in the latter part of this section and represents the pervading theme in this text.

1. *Human development is a continual and cumulative process from conception through older adulthood.* The only thing that is constant is change. Although development appears and may be described as stagelike at times, its bases are underlined by **continuity** of specific processes. Puberty, for example, though it appears to be an abrupt, discontinuous event, is actually a gradual process occurring over several years. Changes such as this are based on quantitative improvements. For example, as hormonal, neural, and muscle components gradually increase, various functional abilities may then appear such as menarche, walking, exhibiting strength, and coordination. With aging, the various systems steadily transform through periods of maturing and regression of function. Added to this is the daily effect of experience with our environment.

At times, theorists prefer to describe development as distinct stages in the life span. This is referred to as the **discontinuity** view. For

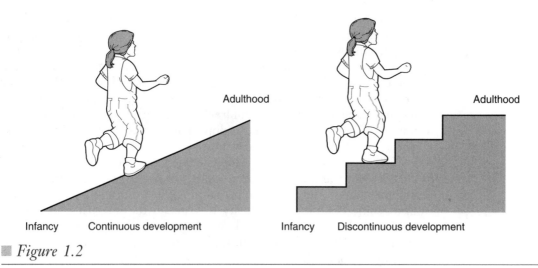

Adulthood   Adulthood

Infancy   Continuous development   Infancy   Discontinuous development

▇ *Figure 1.2*

Development is frequently described by continuity and discontinuity views

example, Piaget and Erikson describe development in terms of **stages,** or periods, when common developmental milestones for each of us occur. This concept suggests qualitative differences in how individuals behave (e.g., think, move, and feel) at certain periods in their lives. Underlying this view, it appears that development undergoes rapid changes as one stage ends and a new one begins, which is then seemingly followed by a relatively stable period with minimal transition. Figure 1.2 illustrates the continuity (a) and discontinuity (b) views of development.

As readers of developmental literature, you will come across other terms in this and other texts that have meanings similar to the concept stage, such as *sequence* and *phase.* However, in this context, a **phase** (or sequence) may also describe qualitative transitions over time that generally are not strictly affixed to specific age levels. The basic premise is that a specific behavior may be accomplished at varying age levels but generally in the developmental order identified. A phase underscores the relatively continual-overlapping characteristics of development. An example of this is illustrated in following pages that present the developmental continuum for motor behavior.

From a research (rather than descriptive) perspective, the problem appears to be one of identifying which developmental processes are controlled by continuous underlying constructs or mechanisms (continuity) and which processes are influenced only when experiential events or environmental forces interact with the individual (discontinuity). From a contemporary motor behavior perspective, Thelen and Ulrich, in reference to dynamical systems theory, emphasize that one of the primary challenges of this line of research is to "account for discontinuities in performance arising from processes that are themselves continuous" (1991, 2).

2. *The study of human development is a holistic process.* To understand lifelong motor behavior fully, we need an eclectic theoretical perspective—that is, a view of the developmental process that emphasizes the significant interrelationships among the physical, cognitive, and psychosocial aspects of behavior. This also takes into account the significant impact that environment can have on development. Its importance is such that it warrants separate consideration.

3. *Environmental context plays a major role in development.* To understand motor behavior at any point in the life span, one must consider the impact of such things as the individual's history, culture, and opportunities for practice (affordances). Environmental context provides the nurturing effect that interacts with human biology (nature) to produce behavior.

4. *There are critical and sensitive periods in development.* A **critical period** refers to an optimal time for the emergence of certain developmental processes and behaviors. Such periods have been described in relation to, for example, emotional bonding with a parent and nutrition needs at specific times during early childhood. Recent research in early brain development complements this concept by suggesting that there are windows of opportunity in which neural networking (brain wiring) is optimal, based to some extent on environmental stimulation. (This topic will be discussed in greater detail in chapter 2.) These findings suggest that the general window of opportunity for critical wiring of movement is through the first 5 to 6 years of life, which has significant implications for early movement experiences and motor development programming. For example, suppose there is an optimal period between 4 and 8 months of age for the infant to acquire basic reach-grasp skills. If this assumption is correct, infants who do not have an opportunity to learn the skill during that critical period may never be as proficient as if they had acquired it during the optimal time period.

However, it also should be noted that humans have the astonishing ability to display considerable resilience to adverse conditions. For example, some children born into low socioeconomic conditions with lack of proper nutrition, education, and enrichment experiences achieve significant successes in their lives.

Although similar, a **sensitive period** reflects a time in the life span when individuals may be especially "sensitive" to specific influences. An example is possible exposure to teratogens, which are agents such as drugs, stress, and alcohol that can cause fetal malformation. The embryonic and fetal periods have been reported as especially sensitive to teratogens.

5. *Development is aided by positive stimulation.* An excellent example of this is in reference to recent research in early brain development.

Scientists have found that to achieve the precision of adult neural circuit patterning, the brain must be stimulated. Deprived of a stimulating environment, a child's brain may suffer. Complementing these observations are comments that are rather common among leading researchers in the field, such as "experience is the chief architect of the brain" (Perry, 1997, 55) and "early experiences can completely change the way a person turns out" (Chugani, 1996, 56). Fortunately, for the field of motor development, research also shows that physical activity as a form of stimulation has significant developmental effects on the brain; this applies to older persons as well (Greenough, 1996; Kempermann & Gage, 1999). This is just one example in the life span of how stimulation affects development. Other strong cases for support have been shown for the effects of exercise on muscle and bone development.

6. *There is much plasticity in human development.* Humans have a dramatic capacity for change **(plasticity)** in response to positive or negative life experiences at virtually all periods in the life span. This is especially evident with biological characteristics such as neural and bone development. In essence, some structures have the amazing ability to reorganize themselves, thus being somewhat plastic (flexible). Refer to the examples regarding critical and sensitive periods in development that link plasticity to positive and negative experiences such as injury and deprivation (Diamond, 1988).

7. *Motor skill development is a multifaceted, dynamic phenomenon.* A central theme in contemporary motor development research is the idea that development of movement abilities is not tied predominantly to a predetermined (genetic) process that emerges simply as one matures. Becoming motorically skillful is generally a process that reflects the interaction of certain biological traits, environmental influences, and task constraints. An assumption complementing this perspective is that individuals acquire certain skills and behaviors based on the unique dynamics of their self-organizing *properties* and *affordances* provided by the environment. Current views of motor development strongly emphasize the roles of exploration and selection in finding solutions to new task demands (Bertenthal & Clifton, 1998; Thelen, 2000).

8. *With advanced aging, it is inevitable that most abilities will regress.* Certain aspects of advanced aging, such as the decline in vision and hearing, loss of muscular strength, and general psychomotor slowing are undesirable and inevitable. One of the exciting possibilities of development, however, is that certain undesirable aspects may be reversed or modified to be less detrimental in their effects. Scientists are becoming increasingly confident that someday even purely biological deterioration may be reversed by techniques developed through research and a better understanding of the mechanisms underlying the aging process.

Aging takes its toll on almost every facet of physiological function, but the quality of life among individuals can be extremely variable.

As noted earlier, the guiding assumption and pervading theme of this text is that *biology and environmental context play vital interactive roles in development.* Human development stems from the dynamics of biological and environmental systems. This relationship provides the resources for individuals to achieve their potential, since the interplay of these factors is unique to each person. In the past, focus appeared to be more on the issue of nature versus nurture and which has the most influence on development. A common example of this is whether children naturally crawl at 6 months and walk at 12 months because of what they have learned from the environment or because of some unfolding biological process. These are the types of questions on which theories are based. However, after considerable discussion and research, the only possible conclusion is that both nature and nurture contribute to all behavior traits and the extent of their contribution cannot be specified for any trait. Therefore, it is understanding the interplay of the two factors that is more meaningful.

Periods of Life-Span Development

Objective 1.8 ➤ Closely associated with the life-span approach to studying the various aspects of motor development are designated **periods** (stages) **of life-span development** representing approximate chronological age behavior. The following stages compose the framework for addressing each aspect of motor development.

Prenatal (conception to birth) This is where the story of human development begins. The *prenatal period* is one of immense physical change that begins with genetic transmission and continues through a number of cellular and structural variations. Development of the embryo and fetus are genetically predetermined, but there are several environmental influences on prenatal development. Significant stages of growth and development within this period are the *embryonic* period (up to 8 weeks) and the *fetal* period (8 weeks to birth).

Infancy (from birth to 2 years) The first month of *infancy* is known as the *neonate* period. This period of development has become a popular area for specialized study because of the possibilities for observing initial motor responses and infant survival characteristics. Infancy is a time of extensive dependency on adults. It also marks the beginning of many motor and psychological activities such as language, symbolic thought, and sensorimotor coordination.

Childhood (from 2 to 12 years)   Due to the large number of developmental milestones reached during this period, *childhood* is divided into two stages:

1. *Early childhood (from 2 to 6 years).* This period corresponds roughly to the time in which the child prepares for and enters school. It represents a significant stage in the development of fundamental motor skills, perceptual-movement awareness, and the ability to care for oneself.
2. *Later childhood (from 6 to 12 years).* Sometimes called the elementary school years, this is a period of fundamental motor skill refinement and the mastery of certain academic skills. Physical growth slows substantially, and thought processes are usually more concrete than in the adolescent period.

Adolescence (from 12 to 18 years)   The term *adolescence* comes from the Latin verb *adolescere,* which means "to grow into maturity." With this period begin the physical changes relating to one of the major landmarks in human development: puberty. Some of the dramatic changes associated with adolescence are accelerated growth in height and weight, the appearance of secondary sex characteristics, the ability to reproduce, and deepening of the voice. This is also a period in which the degree of logical and abstract thought increases, as well as a concern about identity and independence.

Adulthood (18 years and older)   The period of *adulthood* has traditionally been subdivided into three stages:

1. Young adulthood (from 18 to 40 years)
2. Middle-age (from 40 to 60 years)
3. Older adulthood (60 years and older)

With the increased interest in the physiological and motor behavior changes that take place with aging, a greater focus merged on the characteristics of adults who are from 30 to 70 and older.

The Developmental Continuum

Objective 1.9   ➤ Figure 1.3 illustrates the **developmental continuum** of life-span motor behavior by depicting the relationship of behavior to specific age-related stages and phases. The notion of a phase in this context is the relatively continual/overlapping characteristics of human development. Developmental stages are included to complement the overlapping relationship as related to motor behavior characteristics normally associated with chronological age categories. The general premise underlying this model reflects the primary assumption that development

▦ *Figure 1.3*

▦ *Figure 1.3*

The continuum depicts the phases and stages of lifelong motor development

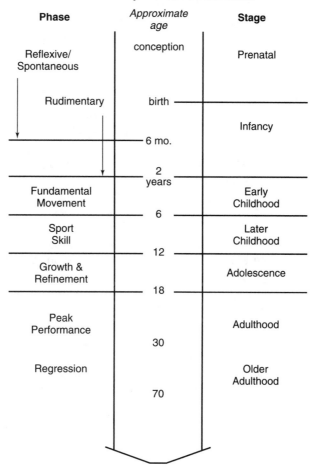

The Developmental Continuum

involves continuous and cumulative change from conception to older adulthood.

More detailed discussions related to characteristic behaviors associated with each of the phases will follow in later sections of this text. The following is a brief overview of the categories of motor behavior across the life span.

Reflexive/spontaneous movement phase. The *reflexive/spontaneous movement phase* is that span of motor behavior that begins at about the third fetal month and continues on after birth into the first year of life. Movements at this phase mirror the relative immaturity of the nervous system. As the system matures, reflexes (involuntary motor responses) and spontaneous movements (stereotypic rhythmic patterns of motion that appear in the absence of any known stimuli) are gradually phased out as voluntary control increases.

Rudimentary phase. The *rudimentary phase* corresponds with the stage of infancy (from birth to 2 years). Rudimentary behavior is voluntary movement in its first form. These movements are determined to a large extent by maturation and appear in a somewhat predictable sequence. Motor control generally develops in a cephalocaudal/proximodistal order and is characterized by such behaviors as crawling, creeping, walking, and voluntary grasping.

Fundamental movement phase. The *fundamental movement phase* is acknowledged as a major milestone of early childhood (from 2 to 6 years) and of life-span motor development. Considered an outgrowth of rudimentary behavior, this phase witnesses the appearance of a number of fundamental movement abilities: perceptual-motor awareness (e.g., body awareness and balance); locomotor skills (e.g., running and jumping); nonlocomotor skills (e.g., twisting/turning and stretching/bending); and manipulative skills (e.g., throwing and kicking). These abilities establish the foundation for efficient and more complex human movement in later phases of development. More than 30 characteristic movement skill abilities that emerge during the early childhood period have been identified.

Sport skill phase. The motor skills and movement awareness abilities the child acquires during the fundamental movement phase gradually become more refined and, in many instances, adapted to sport and recreational activities in the *sport skill phase.* The primary stimulus during this phase is the individual's increased interest in sport skill events and the ability to learn and practice these movements.

Growth and refinement phase. Growth may occur during all periods of development, but perhaps the most significant motor behavior change is seen at the time of puberty and the accompanying growth spurt that generally marks the first stage of adolescence. This is the *growth and refinement phase.* As the levels of hormones rise in the body, changes in muscle and skeletal growth provide a new dimension within which acquired motor skills can be asserted. During the later stages of adolescence, sex differences (mainly favoring males with regard to physical size) become more apparent due primarily to the increased amount of androgen hormones.

Peak performance. Most sources have identified the time of *peak performance* (peak physiological function and maximal motor performance) to be between 25 and 30 years of age. As a general rule, females tend to mature at the lower end of the range (from 22 to 25) and males at the upper end of the range (from 28 to 30 years). This is especially evident in three of the most influential factors in motor performance: strength, cardiorespiratory function, and processing speed.

Regression. Although considerable variation among individuals is apparent after 30 years of age, most physiological and neurological factors decline at a rate of about 0.75% to 1% a year (McArdle et al., 2001; Wilmore & Costill, 1999). During this phase the phenomenon known as *psychomotor slowing* (primarily in speeded tasks) appears, and the earlier developmental process of differentiation begins to reverse, which results in similar performance characteristics among the very young and the older adult. The *regression* of motor behavior is generally characterized by decreases in cardiovascular capacity, muscle strength and endurance, neural function, flexibility, and increases in body fat. Though exercise training has not been shown to retard the aging process, it does allow the individual to perform at a higher level.

■ *Research in Motor Development*

Objective 1.10 ➤ The study of motor development has emerged as a full-fledged scientific endeavor only in recent years. Although researchers and the medical profession have been concerned with motor development as long ago as the days of Hippocrates, little scientifically designed inquiry was conducted until the 1930s. During that period, psychologists such as Bayley, Shirley, Gesell, Ames, and McGraw interested primarily in child development began to establish the database upon which the life-span perspective was later formed. Motor development specialists then began to contribute to the literature led by the pioneering efforts of such individuals as Wild, Espenschade, Eckert, Rarick, Glassow, Halverson, and Roberton.

Today researchers across several disciplines are actively involved in the scientific study of growth and motor behavior across the developmental continuum. The science of motor development is supported by millions of dollars in research funds annually, and the results of that research are disseminated through numerous highly respected technical journals and instructional periodicals. Through the efforts of researchers in basic inquiry, educators and parents gain information with which to implement effective educational programs and understand the characteristics of human behavior. An excellent article by Thelen (2000) discusses in some detail the evolution and status of motor development as a field of scientific inquiry (see Suggested Readings).

Why Study Motor Development?

The importance of studying motor development is tied closely to our need to understand the diverse nature of life and self. From conception until death, physical growth and motor behavior are an integral part of human development. To fully understand human behavior, we need to gather knowledge of all the determinants of existence. Some important reasons for studying motor development are summarized in the following statements:

1. To interact effectively with other individuals we need to be aware of what they can and cannot do—motorically, cognitively, and socially.

2. If we understand what constitutes the normal range of motor development, we can better understand and guide individuals who may be developing abnormally.

3. We can use our understanding of motor development to improve health and optimize motor performance.

4. Our understanding of motor development contributes to a more comprehensive body of knowledge that, in turn, enables us to better understand ourselves.

Methods of Study

In the quest to understand motor behavior across the life span is the goal of explaining *change*. We change with age, but we do not change because we get older. Instead, we change because we are affected by the dynamics of the body and environmental influences that occur as we age. So, how can researchers identify the factors related to change? They do this through scientific methods of study.

As mentioned, the study of motor development has evolved into a legitimate and contributing field of research. It is important to have knowledge of the way researchers gather their data for drawing conclusions about the way motor development takes place. Although a discussion of the numerous experimental and statistical techniques is beyond the scope of this text, it helps to have a general understanding of those research designs and data collection methods used most frequently.

Investigators use the scientific method to answer questions about human development. For example, the investigator first formulates a hypothesis, which is a hunch, guess, or prediction about some aspect of motor development. The hypothesis (or research question) is then tested by collecting evidence in the form of data and analyzing the information to determine whether it supports or rejects the original assumption. In most cases, the study is repeated with different subjects to further confirm the original findings.

In addition to the study of individuals of similar age (e.g., 5-year-olds), a special interest of developmentalists is investigations that focus on the relation of increasing age to some other variable. The primary types of research designs used to address this interest are cross-sectional, longitudinal, microgenetic, and sequential.

Cross-Sectional Design   The vast majority of research studies in motor development have a *cross-sectional design*. Investigators observe age differences by selecting individuals that represent different age groups and measuring their behaviors. In the cross-sectional study, subjects are chosen carefully so individuals in the different age samples are as nearly alike as possible in all ways other than age. The primary value of this design is that it permits a developmental change to be detected in a fairly

Using the scientific method, researchers record kinematics (angle and velocity of movements) during infant reaching

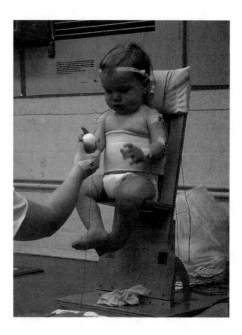

short period of time. However, it has its limitations. Researchers cannot be certain that the behavioral differences are due to age, because all individuals grow up under different circumstances such as education, nutrition, and habits of physical activity. These circumstances are referred to as **cohort effects.**

Longitudinal Design   One of the most popular and perhaps the most reliable type of design is the *longitudinal design.* In this method, data are collected on the same individual over an extended period of time, usually across several years. One strength of this design is that development is observed directly and not implied, as with the cross-sectional and cross-cultural methods. It may be one of the best designs, but the method has weaknesses. Over a long period of time, subjects may move away, testing personnel may change, and the cost of the study in time and money may be a problem. Repeated testing of the same subjects may also be a problem. The individual's performance may improve with repeated test sessions because of increasing familiarity with the task (the "practice effect") rather than because of increased maturity. The shorter the span of time and the fewer the number of measurement sessions, the easier it is to conduct a longitudinal study. Figure 1.5 on page 20 compares cross-sectional and longitudinal designs.

Microgenetic Design   A unique modification of the longitudinal approach is the *microgenetic design* (Siegler & Crowley, 1991). With this

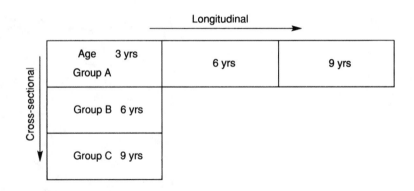

■ *Figure 1.5*

Cross-sectional and longitudinal designs

approach, change is tracked over a series of sessions from the time it begins until it stabilizes, as subjects master an expected or novel task. This method can be quite effective for observing behavior that emerges over a relatively short period of time, such as specific reflexes and initial infant reaching. It offers the potential for unique insight into the developmental process.

Sequential Design   The *sequential design* offers some improvement over the longitudinal and cross-sectional strategies. This method includes elements from each of the other two designs in that it allows the researcher to study several different-aged samples over a period of years. An advantage of the design is that subjects with different characteristics (e.g., age and background) can be compared at the same chronological age to identify existing behavioral differences. Another is that a study of this type can be conducted in a relatively short span of time. Table 1.1 presents a summary of developmental research design characteristics.

Regardless of the design used, data must be collected. Systematic observation is perhaps the most popular method for collecting data, and it is the basic tool of any science. If researchers wish to focus on naturally occurring spontaneous behavior in a natural setting (e.g., at home, at play, and at school), the method is known as *naturalistic observation. Structured observation* requires the researcher to manipulate the environment in some way, as is the case when the study is conducted in a laboratory setting or in a familiar environment in which new elements are presented. Known as the *experimental method*, it is the most powerful design for explaining change by cause and effect.

In other techniques the individual is questioned directly. The *case history* provides an in-depth analysis of background information on the individual. The *interview* generally does not provide as much background information, but it is especially valuable if the goal is to obtain a lot of information in a short period of time. In the interview, researchers actively probe the individual's ideas, feelings, and motives; the data come

■ TABLE 1.1
_____

Strengths and Limitations of Developmental Research Designs

Design	Description	Strengths	Limitations
Cross-sectional	Observe subjects of different ages at one point in time	Detects change in short period of time	Differences may be distorted because of cohort effect
Longitudinal	Observe subjects repeatedly at different ages	Shows individual differences in development and relationships between early and later events and behaviors	Age-related changes may be distorted because of biased sampling, subject dropout, and cohort effects; lengthy and expensive
Microgenetic	Track change from the time it begins until it stabilizes as subjects master a novel or an everyday task	Offers unique insights into the processes of development	Requires frequent observation of subjects' behaviors; the time required for change is difficult to anticipate
Sequential	Follow groups of subjects born in different years over time	Permits both longitudinal and cross-sectional comparisons; reveals existence of cohort effects	May have the same problems as longitudinal and cross-sectional designs

THINK ABOUT IT

In addressing the limitation of correlation research, how many different explanations are there for the observation that children who watch more television have more body fat?

in the form of words rather than observed actions, as is also true of the case history. The *survey* (questionnaire) is similar to the interview except the researcher seeks written responses to a series of questions.

Information gathered in this manner, or in combination with direct measurement of some type, is often analyzed using a *correlational method*. The goal is to describe the strength of relationship between factors. For example, are children who watch more TV (parent survey) fatter (as measured by skinfold or bodyweight)? Obviously, a limitation of this method is that it does not determine cause-and-effect factors.

One of the most commonly used methods of collecting information about motor development is through the use of *standardized tests*. These tests are widely available and offer researchers a source of objective data. The chapter (12) on assessment includes a detailed discussion of motor development tests and makes recommendations for their use.

To design an investigation that conforms to the scientific method, the researcher must make a series of choices. Experts agree there is no single appropriate investigative method. The choice should depend on the research question under investigation, the available resources, and the investigator's judgment.

Theoretical Views

Objective 1.11 ➤ In the field of developmental psychology, theories are used to describe various patterns of behavior and to explain why those behaviors occur. From this perspective, a *theory* may be defined as a set of concepts and propositions that allows the theorist to organize, describe, and explain some aspect of behavior. To gather a comprehensive and meaningful understanding of motor development, it is essential to know something about the way individuals learn and react to their environment. Theories that have earned respect for describing some aspect of behavior enrich our knowledge of the complexities of human development.

In the early years of developmental psychology much of the information reported, especially on motor development, was of a descriptive nature. That is, researchers viewed and explained development through a systematic cataloging of growth norms and age-related behaviors. One of the primary views was that maturation (i.e., maturational theory) rather than learning (or the environment) was the main impetus for developmental change. In recent years, contemporary views of development have taken a much more comprehensive and explanatory perspective of developmental change. These theories consider the environmental *context* in which development occurs and try to explain the *mechanisms* and *processes* accounting for change (growth, development, and behavior), thus attempting to provide a more comprehensive explanation of the dynamic interaction between the organism and its environment.

As noted in the chapter introduction, as a general philosophical view of human and motor development, this text supports the *developmental systems perspective*. This approach underscores the dynamic interaction between the multilevel biological and environmental systems (figure 1.1), that is, the changing relationship between the developing person and his or her changing environmental contexts. The discussion that follows provides a brief description of the prominent theories that fit this perspective; they are grouped for convenience as *Environmental Context Theory* and *Biological Systems Theory*. This is not to say that select theories do not recognize the importance of other domains, since most contemporary models do and it is their primary contribution to this discussion that justified the grouping. Each theory provides information that helps us understand the complex mechanisms, processes, and factors involved in life span changes in motor development. These theories will be described in greater detail in relevant sections of the text.

Before the discussion of the theories most directly relevant to the determinants of motor development and the developmental systems perspective, a brief mention of three other *contributing views* is warranted. Although these approaches may seem more indirect to our focus, each continues (as is the case here) to be used to explain specific aspects of the developmental process with relevance to motor development.

In addition, no dialogue of life-span development would be complete without comment on theories of advanced aging. Although most treatises on this subject focus on the biological aspects of advanced aging, evidence also suggests that an individual's longevity and quality of life are influenced by social factors. Selected theories are described in chapter 11 with the discussion of regression. Chapter 13 will discuss some views on how an individual's perspective on aging and social experiences may influence the aging process. It is hoped that with this information, the reader will develop a better understanding of the aging process as influenced by nature and nurture.

Contributing Views

Maturation View   Gesell's *maturation theory* played a significant role in the evolution of the study of child development during the 1930s and 1940s. Gesell was a pioneer of systematic observation; his timetables detailing when most children achieve certain developmental milestones are still widely used today. Basically Gesell's theory contends that development is the result of inherited factors and requires no stimulation from the external environment. The maturational view of development emphasizes the emergence of patterns of development of organic systems, physical structures, and motor capabilities under the influence of genetic forces. Gesell believed that growth of the intellect and of the motor functions was tied closely to growth of the nervous system, a perspective that underlies our fundamental understanding of phylogenetic and ontogenetic motor behavior. Unless certain neurological and biological characteristics are sufficiently developed (matured), it may be futile to practice certain phylogenetic skills. On the other hand, learning and experience (practice) are necessary for the existence of ontogenetic behavior. For example, maturational theory is illustrated in those developmental charts that show how human locomotion develops in the infant from rolling to walking.

Although maturation plays an important role in early development, there is a strong argument that Gesell's view does not give enough importance to learning and the self-organizing properties of the person, therefore making it difficult to study developmental processes.

Learning-Behavioral View   Bandura (1986, 2000) is one of the main architects of contemporary arguments associated with observational learning and social learning theory. *Observational learning* contends that virtually all of what individuals (children) learn comes from observing others. Bandura suggests that through observational learning (also called *modeling* or imitation), we cognitively represent the behavior of others and then are likely to adopt this behavior ourselves. For example, a boy may adopt the competitive manner of his father (as seen while golfing) and display such behavior when observed with the boy's peers. Positive behaviors may also be adopted, for example, after observing peers or family members participating in healthy physical activity. For an excellent review of research on children's modeling of motor skills refer to Weiss, et al., (1993).

THINK ABOUT IT

Think of a few major role models in your life and describe how they have affected your development, in general and with regard to motor development.

The application of behavioral learning theory plus cognitive processes to the development of learning is known as *social learning theory*. This view emphasizes behavior, the environment, and cognition as key factors in development, with each factor influencing the other factors. According to this theory, because we think, we are able to foresee probable consequences of our actions (and alter our behavior). Therefore the individual has the ability to control behavior and, if desired, accept or resist environmental influence. Expectations are an important variable in this model.

Both the behavioralist and social learning views may be criticized for lack of elaboration on the biological determinants of children's development, especially the fact that children mature at different rates.

Cognitive-Developmental View Of the theories of cognitive development, Jean Piaget's efforts have perhaps had the single greatest effect on modern developmental psychology. Piaget (1963, 1985) believed that the individual discovers solutions to problems primarily through interaction with the environment. According to *Piaget's theory of cognitive development*, the child is not a passive recipient of events (as most behaviorists propose), but, rather, the child seeks out experiences. Piaget's studies focused on the structure of cognitive thought and its orderly sequence of development. Though Piaget did not deny the significance of maturation in development of the intellect, he did not view all of development as the unfolding of biological processes as maturational theory contends. Piaget instead viewed the developmental process as the interaction of biological maturation and environmental (the more contemporary term is *contextual*) experience. The researcher believed that an innate force drives children to actively pursue cognitive *equilibrium* (balance).

According to Piaget, cognitive structures are developed as the result of organization and adaptation. *Organization* is the building of simple perceptual and cognitive processes into higher-order mental structures. *Adaptation* is the process of continuing change that takes place as a result of the individual's interaction with the environment. To explain the process of adaptation, Piaget uses the terms *schema, assimilation,* and *accommodation*. A *schema* is the basic unit of an organized pattern of behavior (cognitive structure) or of representations of actions or concepts. A schema may be used just as it was originally programmed into memory, or it may be altered in some way to meet the demands of a changing environment. The process of *assimilation* is at work when individuals deal with the environment through their current schema. *Accommodation* refers to the modifying process that takes place when the structure of basic schema is changed to meet the demands of the environment, such as in the performance of a novel task. Thus, adaptation is the balance between assimilation and accommodation, which provides a temporary state of equilibrium. The notion of the organization of similar cognitive functions into schema was formalized into schema theory (Schmidt, 1975, 1977) to become one of the foremost explanations of the way motor skills are acquired.

One of Piaget's lasting contributions to developmental psychology was the notion of stages. Piaget's broad distinctions among four basic periods of development from infancy through adolescence continue to be used. Piaget proposed that these particular periods of cognitive development are based on qualitative, structural changes that have a fixed order and cannot be skipped.

Many of Piaget's writings make references to movement activities and the importance of play. Piaget believed that through play (both structured and free), the child has the opportunity to test novel physical, cognitive, emotional, and social behaviors that cannot otherwise be accommodated in the real world. Once the behaviors are tested through play, they become part of memory; hence, from a cognitive perspective, play is a medium for intellectual development. In general, several of Piaget's ideas are mentioned with credibility in contemporary dynamic systems theory literature (e.g., Thelen, 2000; Thelen & Smith, 1994; Van Geert, 1998). Perhaps most notable is the use of the classic Piagetian task, A-not-B error, that will be described in chapter 6. This task has been used to test the notion that movement is not separate from cognitive processes. This is an issue that has drawn considerable interest in recent years among developmentalists.

Environmental Context Theory

A term and theory closely linked to the developmental systems perspective and this determinant of motor development is **developmental contextualism.** Lerner (2002), one of the originators, describes this view as part of the more general developmental systems perspective. As a bases for behavior and developmental change, both focus on the integrative dynamic relationship between the developing person and the changing context within which he or she lives. However, while the developmental systems model is more comprehensive, with equal attention paid to the contributions of biological and environmental systems, contextualism gives more attention to how context influences personal development.

Three prominent theories that provide considerable insight into this determinant of motor development are *Bronfenbrenner's Ecological Systems Theory*, *Gibson's Ecological Perspective*, and the *Ecological Task Analysis (Constraints) Model*. The first provides an excellent framework for studying and understanding the various multilevel ecological systems; Gibson's model gives insight into an important question in motor development:

How do individuals perceive and act on the environment in the form of *affordances?* The third perspective incorporates the characteristics of the person (biological factors) and the environment, and introduces the importance of a third factor, the task.

Ecological Systems Theory   One of the most extensive models of the contextual approach is the **ecological systems theory** proposed by Bronfenbrenner (1986, 2000). This perspective emphasizes the broad range of situations and contexts individuals may encounter. These characteristics continue to be affected and modified by the individual's contextual surroundings. Bronfenbrenner describes the settings or environments (contexts) in which individuals develop as five distinct systems: the microsystem, mesosystem, exosystem, macrosystem, and chronosystem (see figure 1.6).

In brief, the *microsystem* is the setting in which the individual lives; the contexts include the person's family, peers, school, and neighborhood. The *mesosystem* is concerned with the interrelationships among the various settings within the microsystem; for example, the relationship of family to school experiences, or family to the community. When experiences in another social setting in which the individual does not have an active role influence what the individual experiences in an immediate context, the setting is the *exosystem*. An example of this is city government (parks), which is responsible for the quality of play and recreational opportunities. The *macrosystem* involves the culture in which the individual exists. In many instances, behavior patterns, beliefs, and other products of a particular group are passed from generation to generation. In many cultures, sport and dance are an integral part of the setting, thus providing the individual with the refinement of such behaviors. The final contextual influence is the *chronosystem*, which involves the patterning of environmental events and transitions over the life span, that is, the sociohistorical contexts. For example, females of today are much more likely to participate in athletic endeavors than they were 40 years ago.

THINK ABOUT IT

How have your environmental surroundings influenced the person you are today, in general and with regard to physical being and motor skills?

Gibson's Ecological Perspective   As noted earlier, **Gibson's ecological perspective** provides insight into an important question in motor development: How do individuals perceive and act on information in the environment? Proposed by Eleanor and James Gibson (1979, 2001), this view contends that infants, for example, can directly perceive information in the environment and act with a reasonable response. This is in contrast to the traditional constructivist notion suggesting that past experience is critical in order to act on information in a meaningful manner.

In the Gibsonian perspective, perceiving is experiencing. The infant is an active explorer in this process where perception and motor action are coupled (Thelen, 2000). That is, we cannot study perception

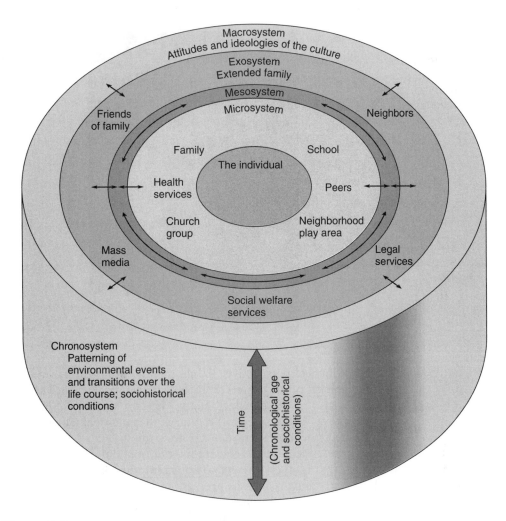

Macrosystem
Attitudes and ideologies of the culture

Exosystem
Extended family

Mesosystem

Microsystem

Friends of family

Neighbors

Family

School

The individual

Health services

Peers

Church group

Neighborhood play area

Mass media

Legal services

Social welfare services

Chronosystem
Patterning of environmental events and transitions over the life course; sociohistorical conditions

Time
(Chronological age and sociohistorical conditions)

■ *Figure 1.6*

Bronfenbrenner's ecological theory of development

independent of movement. The environment provides affordances (e.g., toys and stairs) that invite and challenge the child to perceive and act on information (see Figure 1.7 on page 28). The notion of affordances emphasizes that there is an ecological fit between the individual and the situation. This theory will be discussed in greater detail in chapter 6 (Perception) as we begin to examine the Perception → Action process.

Ecological Task Analysis (Constraints) Model The **ecological task analysis (ETA) model** (Burton & Davis, 1992) is as an excellent approach to observing and studying motor behavior across the life span

▪ *Figure 1.7*

Affordances chal-
lenge the infant to
act on the environ-
ment and develop
skills

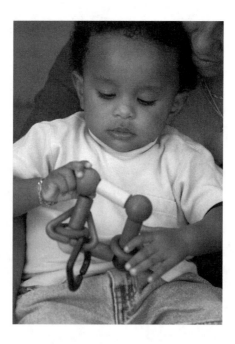

from an ecological perspective. While incorporating the developmental systems elements of the *performer* (biological factors) and the *environment*, emphasis is also given to a third factor, the *task*, as part of the environmental context. The underlying notion is that the qualitative and quantitative aspects of movement emerge from these factors. Newell (1986) described these elements as constraints that may influence developmental change; that is, they interact to constrain the control of motor tasks.

This general approach has been adopted in a wide range of life span research. To illustrate, in her work with age-related changes in posture and movement (e.g., walking, reaching, and lifting objects), Woollacott states that "an inevitable accompaniment of the aging process for many older adults is a restriction in their ability to move independently within the *context* of constantly changing task demands and environmental *contexts*" (1993, 56). In essence, though these individuals can manage (walk) independently within their home environment, when presented with a different set of contextual factors such as standing on a moving bus, walking up and down stairs, or moving across unfamiliar surfaces, their level of mobility may be significantly hindered. This same general scenario is applicable to the infant learning to walk. In these examples, postural (a biological factor) and task constraints would apply.

For the young infant, the constraint of posture also underscores the ability to reach for objects while in the prone and sitting positions. Although the term *constraints* may be somewhat misleading, since it implies a limiting factor, it should also be viewed as a potential affordance to motor behavior.

Biological Systems Theory

The following theories—*information processing* (programming) and the three perspectives appropriately grouped as *developmental biodynamics* (Lockman & Thelen, 1993; Thelen, 2000)—complement the developmental systems perspective by providing unique insight into the mechanisms and processes involved in the development of coordinated movement. In brief, as the individual perceives information and desires to act with a motor response, voluntary movement requires the formulation of a motor program (a plan of action). This plan includes control of the perceptual and motor systems. The theories discussed here and in chapter 7 address the control processes involved and their developmental unfolding.

Information-Processing View Since its introduction in the 1970s, the **information-processing view** has been one of the dominant approaches in the field of cognitive psychology and motor behavior (Bjorklund & Rosenbaum, 2000; Siegler, 2001). The information-processing approach depicts the mind as a system through which information flows. Scientists who support this approach have drawn close analogies between the human mind and a computer. That is, the brain and central nervous system are the *hardware* and the mental processes (such as attention, perception, memory, and problem solving) are the *software*. Like computers, human minds have a limited capacity for processing information. With development, changes in the capacities of cognitive structures, including critical strategies, occur. The primary challenge for researchers is to provide an understanding of how individuals' thinking changes as they develop across the life span. Richard Schmidt, one of the leading scientists in the field of motor behavior, notes that the information-processing perspective studies movement from the point of view of the human as a processor of information; it focuses on storage (memory), coding, retrieval, and programming, with the result of production of an outcome (movement). Unlike Piaget, many information processing theorists insist that cognitive development is not stagelike; instead, mental programs develop gradually over time and involve quantitative rather than qualitative change.

Developmental Biodynamics One of the most exciting and promising approaches to the comprehensive study of motor development emerged in the 1990s. Sparked by advances in the neurosciences, biomechanics, and behavioral sciences, **developmental biodynamics** represents an interdisciplinary attempt to integrate promising theories and findings related to the behavioral study of *perception* and *action* (Bertenthal & Clifton, 1998; Lockman & Thelen, 1993; Thelen, 2000). In essence, the primary attempt is to describe and explain the intimate connection between the brain and body. This approach represents a vast improvement from the more traditional maturational approach, which described change in a descriptive series of developmental milestones. Although this approach is just beginning to address the challenges associated with a developmental synthesis of the brain-body phenomenon, researchers have already made significant contributions toward a better understanding of the problem. A thorough scientific examination of the topic is beyond the scope of this section and text, but a brief description of the basic tenets of the approach should be useful in understanding the merits of an interdisciplinary view of the research problem. Chapter 7 will address this approach in greater detail in reference to *neuronal group selection theory, coordinative structures,* and *dynamic systems theory.*

Lockman and Thelen (1993) note that Bernstein (1967) introduced the term *biodynamics* in his writing on the genesis of motor coordination. The researcher's basic premise was that coordination and control emerged from continual and intimate interactions between the nervous system (brain) and the periphery (body). The central question Bernstein asked was, How can the brain control individually all the diverse elements (e.g., neurons, muscles, and joints) and multiple linkages associated with the production of movement? To address the problem, Bernstein introduced the notion of *synergies*—classes of movement patterns involving collections (groups) of muscle or joint variables that act as basic units in the regulation and control of movement. Bernstein also proposed that there must be an inseparable relation between the brain and associated movement components (e.g., hands, arms, and legs), and they must act and develop collectively. This basic premise set the agenda for the efforts of different disciplines to address the interface between perception and action.

This basic theme—interaction between perception and action—and variations have been addressed using, for example, mathematical techniques of nonlinear dynamics, principles of biomechanics, neural modeling, and, as previously mentioned, considerations of the context in which the development and behavior occurs. In addition to computer modeling and the use of robotics and animals, experimental observations have included humans (usually infants) performing a variety of upper limb (reaching, and grasping), locomotor (walking), and reflexive/spontaneous movements.

Dynamic systems research, an applied branch of developmental biodynamics, has stimulated considerable inquiry in recent years. Originating from Bernstein's problem with brain and body control, Kugler, Kelso, and Turvey (1980, 1982) introduced the dynamic systems approach, which focuses on the developmental perspective, that is, the emergence, or unfolding, of motor behavior. Most traditional views on how human movement evolves have been based on the descriptive-maturational perspective, that is, the orderly and sequential emergence of behaviors linked to development of the nervous system (e.g., spontaneous/reflexive behavior, crawling, and walking). Although this type of research has contributed to the understanding of when motor skills emerge and what they look like, one criticism has been that it falls short in explaining *how* (i.e., the processes of change) motor behavior emerges. The dynamic systems perspective suggests that coordination and control emerge as a result of the dynamic properties of the muscle collectives (i.e., *coordinative structures*). This view of development emphasizes the importance of the *dynamic* and *self-organizing properties* of the motor system to the individual's developing motor competencies. Along with biological considerations, this perspective (as a feature of biodynamics) suggests that change is stimulated by characteristics of the environment and demands of the specific task (contexts). Since its inception dynamic systems research has done much to provide a better understanding of how motor behavior emerges. Further elaboration on this important perspective will be given in chapters 7 and 8.

Obviously, no single theory described in the chapter entirely explains the complexity of lifelong motor behavior. As mentioned earlier, each in its own particular way casts some light on explaining what influences change. With this in mind, you are encouraged to use an **eclectic theoretical perspective** when viewing behavior broadly, an orientation that does not follow any one theory but incorporates what seem to be the best or most useful elements from various approaches. This method, of course, depends on the perspective desired and goal of observation. Is the goal to explain multiple influences on behavior, or is it to delineate change due to a specific factor? With today's advanced scientific technology for observing motor behavior, new theories are emerging which, in most cases, require developmentalists to rethink their original perspective.

THINK ABOUT IT

Why is there no single theory that can explain all aspects of human development?

■ *Careers in Motor Development*

As a course of study and as a research field, motor development has experienced considerable growth in recent years. With this growth, developmentalists have found work in a wide variety of settings as *teachers, researchers,* and *consultants.* In addition to the common higher-education setting, developmentalists may now find excellent opportunities, for example, in hospitals, business/industry, government agencies, professional education associations, private research facilities, and in a variety of schools where they can address a wide range of ages.

It is becoming more common for developmentalists to work for business/industry as consultants and researchers on projects such as play environments for children, toy development, educational publications (publishing companies), and media programming (e.g., TV, internet). Developmentalists can also be found working for state education divisions and with federal agencies such as the National Science Foundation, National Institutes of Health, Centers for Disease Control and Prevention, and the Department of Education. A considerable part of our federal government's current social policy related to education and research is devoted to early childhood and the older adult, suggesting that the future is bright for individuals who wish to focus on this field as a career. A program of study in motor development also provides an excellent background for those who wish to pursue professional schools such as physical and occupational therapy and medicine.

Summary

Motor development is a field of specialized study that examines patterns of growth, development, and motor performance (behavior) across the life span. With the development of a lifelong perspective on motor development has emerged the multidisciplinary approach to studying associated behavioral change. This approach has added significantly to our understanding of total human development and behavior. The major objective of the developmentalist is to identify and explain the characteristics associated with change across the life span. To understand the factors that influence change, the developmental systems perspective is appropriate. This view recognizes the changing relationship (interaction) between the developing person and changing multilevel environmental context. In general, development is a dynamic and self-organizing process.

In the study of human development, several fundamental observations (assumptions) have relevance to motor development. In brief, development appears stagelike, but its bases are underlined by processes that are likely continual and cumulative; the study of human development is a holistic process; environmental context plays a major role in development; there are critical and sensitive periods in development; development is aided by positive stimulation; there is much plasticity in development; motor skill development is a dynamic process; with advanced aging, regression of most skills is inevitable; and, primary to this text is the observation that biological and environmental systems are interactive factors in development.

From a descriptive view, complementing the age-related periods of life-span development are the seven phases of motor behavior: reflexive, rudimentary, fundamental movement, sport skill, growth and refinement, peak performance, and regression. This developmental continuum provides an outline for the study of lifelong growth, development, and motor performance.

Motor development is a scientific and applied discipline. Through motor development research we learn to better understand the capabilities of individuals in order to guide their development and improve their health and performance. The scientific method of studying human development and performance may employ a variety of research designs. The most popular method for collecting information and the basic tool of any science is systematic observation. This can be conducted in either a natural or structured setting.

Much of our present understanding of human development is derived from various traditional and contemporary theoretical models. Whereas earlier approaches to explaining development were more descriptive, using a systematic cataloging of norms and age-related behaviors, more contemporary approaches attempt to explain the mechanisms and processes accounting for change. Included in the comprehensive study of lifelong development are considerations of the biological systems and environmental context in which development occurs.

For those individuals who wish to pursue motor development as a career, there are promising opportunities as teachers, researchers, and consultants.

Think about It

1. Why is it important to have a general understanding of human development in order to gain insight into lifelong motor behavior?
2. In addressing the limitation of correlation research, how many different explanations are there for the observation that children who watch more TV have more body fat?
3. Think of a few major role models in your life and describe how they have affected your development, in general and with regard to motor development.
4. How have your environmental surroundings influenced the person you are today, in general and with regard to physical being and motor skills?
5. Why is there no single theory that can explain all aspects of human development?

Suggested Readings

Bronfenbrenner, U. (2000). Ecological theory. In A Kazdin (Ed.), *Encyclopedia of Psychology.* New York: American Psychological Association and Oxford University Press.

Lerner, R. (2002). *Concepts and theories of human development.* 3rd ed. Mahwah, NJ: Lawrence Erlbaum.

Lewis, M. (2000). The promise of dynamic system approaches for an integrated account of human development. *Child Development* 71(1):36–43.

Lockman, J. J., & Thelen, E. (1993). Developmental biodynamics: Brain, body, behavioral connections (Special section introduction). *Child Development* 64:953–959.

Plomin, R., & McClearn, G. E. (Eds.). (1993). *Nature-nurture and psychology.* Hyattsville, MD: American Psychological Association.

Santrock, J. W. (2002). *Life-span development.* 8th ed. Dubuque, IA: McGraw-Hill.

Shaffer, D. R. (2002). *Developmental psychology* (6th ed.). Belmont, CA: Wadsworth.

Thelen, E. (2000). Motor development as foundation and future of developmental psychology. *International Journal of Behavioral Development*, 24(4), 385–397.

WebLinks

Esther Thelen's Infant Motor Development Laboratory at Indiana University
http://php.indiana.edu/~gormleyf

The Jean Piaget Archives (Highlights of Jean Piaget and his theory of cognitive development)
www.unige.ch/piaget

The Jean Piaget Society: www.piaget.org

International Society on Infant Studies: www.isisweb.org

National Association for Sport & Physical Education
www.aahperd.org/naspe

North American Society for the Psychology of Sport and Physical Activity
www.naspspa.org

Society for Research in Child Development: www.srcd.org

Major Organizations

American Academy of Kinesiology and Physical Education: www.aakpe.org

American Academy of Pediatrics: www.aap.org

American Alliance for Health, Physical Education, Recreation, and Dance
www.aahperd.org

American College of Sports Medicine: www.acsm.org

Centers for Disease Control and Prevention: www.cdc.gov

National Association for the Education of Young Children: www.naeyc.org

National Institute on Aging: www.nih.gov/nia

National Institute of Child Health & Human Development: www.nichd.nih.gov

American Physical Therapy Association: www.apta.org

Biological Growth and Development

PART TWO provides information related to the structural and functional elements of human development and motor behavior. Although each chapter in this section addresses the process of physical growth, the specific topics have been placed in a broader context to provide a more explicit interpretation of developmental activity. Keep in mind that these topics are strongly interrelated. Chapters 2 and 3 focus on the hereditary, neurological, and physical aspects of human development typically manifested as structural growth. Chapter 4 builds upon that information in discussing change related to functional processes. Finally, chapter 5 describes the variety of other factors that may influence growth and development, such as prenatal care, nutrition, environmental agents, hormones, and physical activity.

chapters

2 Heredity and Neurological Changes

3 Physical Growth Changes

4 Physiological Changes

5 Factors Affecting Growth and Development

2 *Heredity and Neurological Changes*

OBJECTIVES

Upon completion of this chapter, you should be able to

2.1 Define the term *heredity* and describe its primary characteristics.

2.2 Identify the three primary functions of the nervous system.

2.3 Outline the basic structure of the central and peripheral nervous systems and briefly describe their functions.

2.4 Explain the basic structure and function of a neuron and identify the various types of neurons.

2.5 Identify the terms *motor unit* and *motor pathways*.

2.6 Describe how nerve impulses are conducted.

2.7 Outline and describe the sequence of early developmental changes in the central nervous system.

2.8 Identify the primary developmental changes that occur in the brain.

2.9 Explain brain lateralization in terms of both brain structure and its effect on motor behavior.

2.10 Outline and briefly describe the primary neurological changes that occur with aging.

KEY TERMS

heredity

genotype

phenotype

central nervous system (CNS)

peripheral nervous system (PNS)

motor unit

nerve conduction velocity

integration

differentiation

synaptogenesis

myelination

myogenic behavior

neurogenic behavior

critical periods

brain lateralization

Heredity

Objective 2.1

➤ **Heredity** is the total set of characteristics biologically transmitted from parent to offspring. From the moment of conception, two primary factors interact to determine the developmental patterns of the individual: genetic makeup and the environment. The environment, even during prenatal development, modifies and interacts with heredity to shape the individual and to control the extent to which maximal potential will be realized. The *nature-nurture* relationship suggests the significant influence of these two factors. Today behavioral scientists know that nature (heredity) and nurture (the environment) both contribute continually and inseparably to an individual's development. There is no organism in which one part is influenced *only* by genes and another segment *only* by the environment. The capacity of a living thing to respond to experiences in the environment is as genetically determined as the maturation of its neurological system. However, a gene is only a probability for a given trait, not a guarantee.

A *gene* is the basic unit of heredity found within a chromosome. Each human cell contains 46 *chromosomes* (in 23 pairs) in its nucleus. Each chromosome consists of more than 1,000 genes strung together in a chainlike formation. Genes are made up of molecules of *DNA* (deoxyribonucleic acid) packed tightly into the cell nucleus. During normal cell division, or *mitosis*, the DNA unzips, breaking its rungs and forming two separate strands. In this fashion, all 46 chromosomes of the single cell reproduce themselves.

The DNA molecule contains the genetic code that determines what hereditary information is to be transmitted from one generation to the next. The code contains instructions for creating an individual with a sex type and basic human characteristics like head, limbs, and hair (rather than fins or feathers). Only one of the 46 pairs of chromosomes determines whether the new human being is male or female. The female has two X chromosomes; the male has one X and one Y chromosome. Females always contribute an X chromosome to the offspring, so it is the male who determines the sex of the next generation. The code also provides the directions for creating a new individual with his or her own unique combination of characteristics such as intelligence, height, blood type, and eye color. To get from blueprint to creation, information in the DNA molecules is transcribed into molecules of *RNA* (ribonucleic acid). These molecules take the code from the DNA into the cytoplasm of the cell, which contains the raw material for making protein. It is out of the proteins, made according to instructions from the RNA, that the functioning parts and capabilities of each human being are developed. The human body contains about 100,000 genes, of which approximately half are involved in brain function.

TABLE 2.1

Estimated Genetic Contribution

Component	Genetic Contribution
Body Weight	40%
Stature	60%
Body Fat	25%
Regional Fat Distribution	30%
VO$_2$max (aerobic performance)	30%
Maximum Heart Rate	50%
Anaerobic Performance	50%
Physical Working Capacity	70%

Modified from Bouchard & Perusse (1994) and McArdle, et al. (2001)

The **genotype** is all of an individual's genetic inheritance. The actual expression of the genotype as the person's visible characteristics and behavior is referred to as the **phenotype.** The phenotype depends not only on the individual's genetic makeup but also on all the environmental elements that affect the person from the moment of conception. The observable characteristics of a phenotype include physical traits such as height, eye color, skin pigmentation, and psychological characteristics such as intelligence, creativity, and personality. Heredity also influences aging, puberty, time of tooth eruption, muscle fiber type ratio, body fat, and the development of skeletal age. Although body weight and aging are primarily the product of heredity, both can be significantly affected by environmental factors such as diet and exercise.

Much of our information about the genetic component of behavior has come about through the comparison of identical and nonidentical twins. Because identical twins have the same genetic material, variability in their behavior is due, in theory, primarily to environmental factors such as learning. Although the answers are far from complete, data such as these suggest that selected motor performance activities are significantly influenced by genetic factors.

A review of these studies by McArdle, et al. (2001) notes a significant effect of inherited factors on individual aerobic capacity and endurance performance. Table 2.1 shows the estimated genetic contribution of selected biological components.

THINK ABOUT IT

List some of the phenotype characteristics you have and from which parent you inherited them. Can you think of ways that the environment affects phenotype over time?

■ *Neurological Changes*

Objective 2.2   ➤ Of all of the systems of the human body the nervous system is one of the most important. Everything that takes place consciously or unconsciously, voluntarily or as a reflex, has its primary initiation within the nervous system. Growth, development, and motor behavior all depend on the efficient functioning of this system. The effectiveness of a motor response is significantly influenced by the quality and capability of the nervous system and the brain. According to Guyton (1991), the nervous system has three primary functions: (a) a sensory function, (b) an integrative function, which includes the memory and thought processes, and (c) a motor function.

Basic Structure and Function

Objective 2.3   ➤ A basic review of the anatomy of the nervous system is important to the further discussion of the neurological changes that occur across the life span. The nervous system has two major parts: the **central nervous system (CNS),** which consists of the spinal cord and brain, and the **peripheral nervous system (PNS),** which is made up of all the nerve fibers that enter or leave the brain stem and spinal cord to supply the sensory receptors, muscles, and glands. Essentially, the PNS represents the lines of communication, whereas the CNS is the center of coordination and the mechanism that determines the most appropriate response to incoming impulses.

Central Nervous System   The structures of the CNS basically function to transmit information about the environment and the body to the brain where it is recorded, stored in memory, and compared with other information (figure 2.1 on page 40). The CNS also carries information from the brain to muscles and glands, thus producing motor responses and the body's adaptations to environmental demands. The following discussion provides a brief description of selected parts of the CNS deemed most relevant to the study of motor development.

SPINAL CORD. The spinal cord has an essential role in the input and response phases of information processing and motor behavior. Its primary function is to act as a transmission pathway; it carries to the brain all sensory information from the body and all motor commands sent down from the brain to muscles (and glands). The spinal cord also has an important function in reflex behavior.

THE BRAIN. The brain is the principal integrative area of the nervous system. It is the location where memories are stored, thoughts are

■ *Figure 2.1*

■ *Figure 2.1*

Anatomy of the
central nervous
system

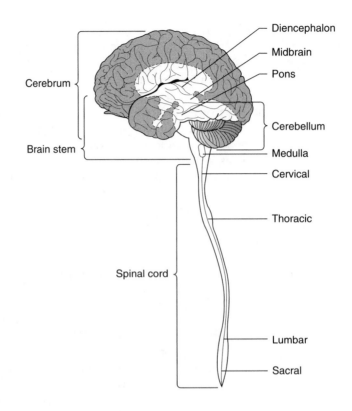

developed, emotions are generated, and complex control of motor
behaviors is performed.

The *brain stem* is that part of the brain primarily responsible for several involuntary (reflexes) and metabolic functions. The brain stem also
sets the rhythm of breathing and controls the rate and force of breathing movements and heartbeat.

Several important fiber tracts pass both upward and downward
through the brain stem, transmitting sensory signals from the spinal cord
mainly to the thalamus and motor signals from the cerebral cortex back
to the spinal cord. The major structures of the brain stem are the pons,
midbrain, medulla, diencephalon, and reticular formation. The *medulla*
contains a number of sensory tracts for carrying information to the brain
and motor tracts for carrying information to the muscles and glands.
The medulla serves primarily to regulate vital internal processes such as
respiration, blood pressure, and heart rate. The ventral and dorsal parts
of the *pons* contain several nerve tracts that allow for coordination and
involuntary influences on automatic movement and posture. The *midbrain* is involved with reflex movements caused by visual and auditory
stimulation. The *diencephalon* consists of two areas: the thalamus
and hypothalamus. The *thalamus* is an important integration center
through which most sensory information passes. The *hypothalamus* is the

structure where neural and hormonal functions work to create a constant internal environment (body temperature). The *reticular formation* plays an important role in attention and activation of the individual for cognitive and motor activity.

The *cerebral cortex* is the outermost layer of the cerebrum and is composed of an estimated 75% of the total neurons in the CNS. It is the functional head of the nervous system in its responsibility for higher-order critical thinking and information processing. Basically the cortex mediates (a) the reception and interpretation of sensory information, (b) the organization of complex motor behaviors, and (c) the storage and use of learned experiences. The principal functional area of the cortex controlling motor activities is called the *motor area*. The motor area occupies the posterior half of the frontal lobe and consists of the motor cortex, premotor cortex, and Broca's area. The *motor cortex* controls the specific fine motor muscles throughout the body (e.g., of the fingers, feet, toes, and lips). The *premotor cortex* elicits the coordinated movements that involve either sequences of individual muscle movements or the combined movements of a number of different muscles simultaneously. In this area much of the individual's knowledge of learned skilled movements is stored. *Broca's area* has the primary function of controlling the coordinated movements of the larynx and mouth to produce speech.

The *basal ganglia* area of the brain is made up of a group of nuclei located in the inner layers of the cerebrum. The basal ganglia integrates the sensory motor centers and is involved with unconscious behavior, such as the maintenance of muscle tone required in upright posture. A major function of the basal ganglia is to control very fundamental gross body movements, whereas the cerebral cortex plays prominently in the performance of more precise movements of the arms, hands, fingers, and feet.

The *cerebellum* is an important part of the motor control system. Even though it is located far away from both the motor cortex and the basal ganglia, it interconnects with both of these through special nerve pathways. It also interconnects with motor areas in both the reticular formation and spinal cord. Its primary function is to determine the coordinated sequence of muscle contraction during complex movements. Its functions are also associated with vestibular awareness (balance), postural adjustments, and reflex activity.

Peripheral Nervous System The peripheral nervous system (PNS) is a branching network of nerves. It is so extensive that hardly a single cubic millimeter of tissue anywhere in the body is without nerve fibers. The PNS is divided into two systems: the somatic and the autonomic. The *somatic system* controls all the skeletal muscles (contracted through voluntary initiation); the *autonomic system* is primarily responsible for regulating the automatic functioning of the smooth muscles of the internal organs such as the heart, liver, lungs, and endocrine glands. The activities of the autonomic system are seldom subject to voluntary control.

PNS nerve fibers are of two functional types: *afferent fibers* for transmitting sensory information into the spinal cord and brain, and *efferent fibers* for transmitting motor impulses back from the CNS to the peripheral areas, especially to the skeletal muscles. The peripheral nerves that arise directly from the brain itself and supply mainly the head region are called *cranial nerves*. The remainder of the peripheral nerves are *spinal nerves*.

Objective 2.4

➤ NEURON. A *neuron* (nerve cell) is the basic structural unit of the nervous system. There are billions of neurons in the nervous system; the average neuron is a complex structure with thousands of physical connections with other cells. Nerve impulses travel along neurons to relay information from one cell to another (and through the nervous system). The junction between two cells across which the information must pass is called a *synapse*. The three basic parts of the neuron are the cell body (soma), dendrites, and the axon (figure 2.2).

The *cell body (soma)* is the metabolic center of the cell. It contains the nucleus, which is responsible for regulating the various processes of the cell. Neuron cell bodies are located mostly within the central nervous system. Clusters of cell bodies are called nuclei. A *dendrite* is a nerve fiber that extends from the cell body. Each neuron can have from one to thousands of dendrites. Dendrites are the receiving part of the neuron, serving the important function of collecting information and orienting it toward the cell body. Although many dendrites branch from the cell body of a neuron, there is only one axon. The *axon* is the nerve cell structure that carries information away from the cell body to other cells. As previously noted, nerve impulses travel along neurons to transmit information. An impulse is an electrochemical process that travels in a chainlike sequence from the dendrite or cell body of one neuron to its axon, to the dendrite or cell body of another neuron, and so on, through the length of the nerve tract. The functional connection between the axon and another neuron is the *synapse*.

Neurons are generally classified according to their function. *Afferent neurons*, also referred to as sensory neurons, carry nerve impulses from the sensory receptors into the spinal cord or brain of the central nervous system. *Efferent neurons* transmit impulses from the central nervous system to the muscles and glands. Efferent neurons passing impulses to muscles are commonly called *motoneurons*. Over 95% of all neurons are classified as *interneurons*. This type of neuron originates and terminates solely within the CNS.

Along with the neuron, the other basic types of nervous system tissues are supporting and insulating cells. These cells have the important function of holding neurons in place and preventing signals from spreading between the neurons. In the CNS these cells are collectively called

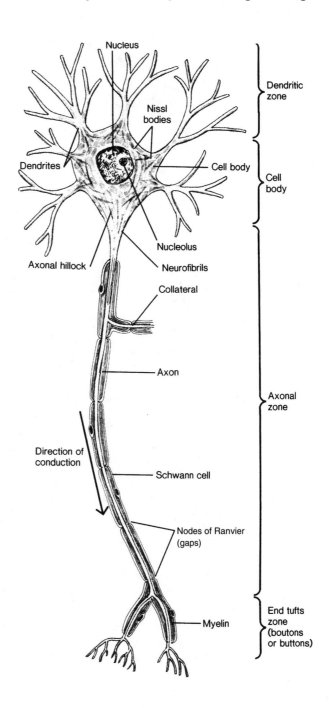

■ *Figure 2.2*

The basic parts of
a neuron

neuroglia and referred to specifically as *glial cells.* In the PNS they are
referred to as Schwann cells. *Schwann cells* wrap myelin sheaths around
the large nerve fibers, thus insulating the pathway for an electrochemical nerve impulse.

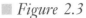
Figure 2.3

A motor unit

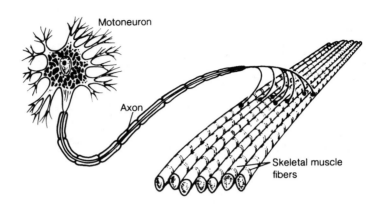

Objective 2.5

➤ THE NEUROMUSCULAR (MOTOR) UNIT. Each motoneuron axon branches into several synaptic terminals, and each of these terminals provides the nerve supply to a muscle fiber. A neuron and all the muscle fibers innervated by it are referred to as a **motor unit** because all the muscle fibers contract as a unit when stimulated by the motoneuron (figure 2.3). Each of the muscle fibers making up the small delicate muscles of the eye may be supplied by a motoneuron, but larger postural muscles may only have one motoneuron to supply as many as 150 muscle fibers.

MOTOR PATHWAYS. Nerve impulses travel through two major motor pathways on their way to producing muscular contraction or relaxation. The *pyramidal system* is made up of those neurons that originate in the cerebral cortex (premotor area), the axons of which descend through a direct channel to the spinal cord (figure 2.4). The neurons of the cortex that send their axons down the pyramidal tract provide a direct channel from the cortex to the spinal neurons, which, in turn, cause either muscle contraction or relaxation. Functions of the pyramidal system are primarily associated with specific movement patterns.

The *extrapyramidal system* includes all of the motoneuron axons not included in the pyramidal system. These neurons originate in the motor area of the cortex as well as in other cortical areas. Instead of traveling a direct pathway to the spinal neurons as happens in the pyramidal tract, several axons on the extrapyramidal tract are interrupted synaptically to terminate in various subcortical structures, especially in the basal ganglia, cerebellum, and thalamus. The extrapyramidal system is primarily associated with general rather than specific movement patterns.

Objective 2.6

➤ IMPULSE CONDUCTION. Neurons send information through their axons in the form of brief impulses, or waves, of electricity in the form of single electrical clicks called *action potentials*. **Nerve conduction velocity** is the speed at which information travels; this rate is greatly

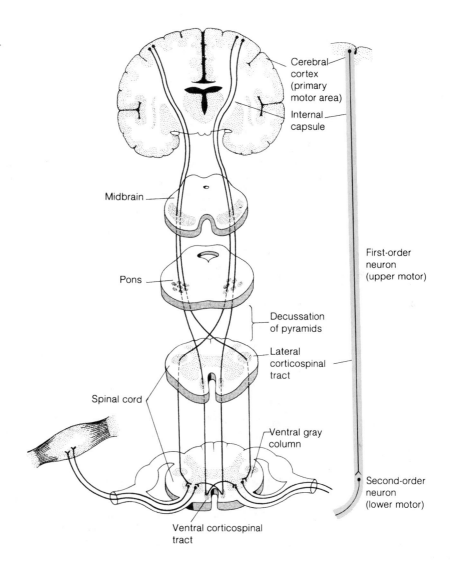

■ *Figure 2.4*

The pyramidal
motor pathways

Cerebral
cortex
(primary
motor area)

Internal
capsule

Midbrain

Pons

First-order
neuron
(upper motor)

Decussation
of pyramids

Lateral
corticospinal
tract

Spinal cord

Ventral gray
column

Second-order
neuron
(lower motor)

Ventral corticospinal
tract

affected by the presence or absence of a material called *myelin* around
the axon. *Myelin* is a fatty material that forms a sheath around many
axons both within and outside the CNS. The myelin sheath is formed
from a type of insulating cell called a *Schwann cell.* These cells wrap
around the axon and form a jelly-roll-type structure that serves as an
effective insulator of electrical currents. The myelin sheath is interrupted
every millimeter or so by gaps called *nodes of Ranvier* (see figure 2.2).
The neuron membrane is active only at the nodes, so the impulse is conducted when the action potential jumps from one of these nodes to
another. This type of impulse conduction is known as *saltatory conduction* and is significantly faster than conduction in nonmyelinated axons.

Saltatory conduction also requires less metabolic energy, enabling myelinated axons to fire nerve impulses at higher frequencies for longer periods of time. Research has also indicated that there is higher conduction velocity, lower threshold, shorter latency, and higher amplitude coincident with the time of appearance and the degree of myelination. Another factor in conduction velocity is the size of the axon. Basically, the larger the cross-sectional diameter, the faster the speed of conduction. Apparently axon conduction velocity is related to the urgency of the information it is called upon to transmit. Axons with greater speed potential are concerned with the control of movement, especially in the mediation of rapid reflexes; axons that transmit visceral information are small, generally unmyelinated, and slow.

Early Developmental Changes

Objective 2.7 ➤ A mature brain contains more than 100 billion neurons intricately connected with one another in ways that make possible the amazing functions that underlie our behavior. Perhaps most remarkable is the precision of neural circuitry (wiring) that develops between connections that occur; each neuron links up with thousands of others to form trillions of connections. The total length of wiring between neurons is estimated at 62,000 miles (Coveney & Highfield, 1995)! It was once believed that the wiring diagram for each person was predetermined by one's genetic blueprints. However, the contemporary perspective is that although the main circuits may be prewired for responses such as breathing, control of heartbeat, and reflexes, stimulation from the environment can shape the trillions of finer connections that complete the architecture of the brain. This critical effect, which has profound implications for our nature-nurture theme and motor development in general, will be discussed in the latter part of this section.

Normal CNS development appears to follow a dynamic sequence of integrated biological events; these include the processes of *cell proliferation, migration, integration* and *differentiation, myelination,* and *cell death.* Basically the developmental process begins with immature neurons (cell proliferation). These cells become specified regarding their function and location within the system. When their location has been determined, the different cell types migrate to various sites and integrate with other cells. At the site of integration, neurons begin to elaborate axons and dendrites in preparation for establishing the functional connection (synapse) between cells (differentiation). In their final stage of morphological development, most nervous system pathways become coated with myelin to allow them to transmit impulses more effectively. Many neurons are eliminated during early development of the nervous system (cell death), which is believed to be a normal part of the development process.

It should be reemphasized that while the developmental sequence is rather exact, it is also a complex and intricate process. The sequence described only represents highlights in the process. The following discussion elaborates in greater detail significant events that occur within the sequence of early neurological development.

Cell Proliferation and Changes Neurons first appear in the brain during the second prenatal month and virtually all of the *cell proliferation* process (growth in number) is completed by birth. At this time, a baby's brain contains about 100 billion neurons and a trillion glial cells, which form a honeycomb that protects and nourishes the neurons. Not only do neurons multiply very rapidly during early development, but they also grow in size as well. The period of dramatic increase in neuron size seems to occur from the sixth prenatal month through the first year of life.

Beginning around the third trimester of gestation and continuing into at least the fourth year is a period of rapid brain growth and development called the *brain growth spurt.* The general period also includes development in terms of cell proliferation, myelination, dendritic and synaptic growth, and refinement of certain enzyme systems. A considerable body of evidence suggests that the brain has a critical period for laying down its foundation (wiring of circuits) for optimal development. After this critical period, there are limits to the brain's ability to reorganize (plasticity). It is also important to note that the timing of the growth spurt cannot be altered; the time line for development is predetermined genetically. However, as will be discussed later, the extent of development is *activity-dependent,* that is, it is significantly affected by experience and stimulation. This fact points to the importance of prenatal care and a stimulating postnatal environment, especially during the early years.

The genetic structure of the cell nucleus plays a primary role in controlling cell proliferation and differentiation. As noted earlier, about half of the body's total genes (50,000) are involved in forming and maintaining the CNS. Although their role during growth is vital to the wiring of basic functional circuits, there are simply not enough of them to specify the trillions of finer connections made after birth.

Along with the process of cell proliferation several developmental changes occur in the axon and dendrite structures. Once the neurons have *migrated* to their final location in the CNS, they begin to elaborate their axon and dendritic structures in readiness to accept impulses through synaptic interconnections. Again, neurons may be categorized as sensory (afferent, sending signals to the CNS), motor (efferent, sending signals from the CNS to the muscles), and central or interneurons (originating and terminating in the brain or spinal cord). This specification is likely biochemically set. The axons of sensory neurons must often travel relatively long distances to reach their synaptic conjunction.

Terminal targets of motor neurons do not appear to be as specific as those for sensory neurons, but complex specificity is still evident in the growth process. The growth of the axon of a motor neuron is guided somewhat by the chronological order in which it matures and differentiates as well as by its biochemical properties. When a motor neuron innervates a muscle, the axon makes contact and induces biochemical specificity into the muscle, thus allowing the two structures to match up biochemically. Once specificity of the neuromuscular junction is established, sensory and central neurons form their synaptic connections.

One of the major events in cortical neuronal differentiation is the elaboration of dendritic structures. Dendrites are important because they are the main receptors for the neuron. At the synaptic junctions the dendrites of each neuron can receive signals from literally thousands of other neurons. It has been estimated that dendrites of cortical neurons provide more than 95% of the targets for transmitting information through the system. Not until approximately the eighth fetal month do the first signs of thick dendrites with conspicuous spines start to appear on cells

| At birth | 1 month | 3 months | 15 months | 24 months |

■ *Figure 2.6*

Representation of dendritic development

in the visual cortex. Even though the motor cortex is noted as being more advanced in dendritic development than the visual cortex at that time, the appearance of dendritic spine development is not as evident. At around 30 weeks of gestation, the dendritic spines show obvious immaturity; they are few in number and irregular in shape. But by 8 months (postnatal) the number of well-formed, lollipop-shaped, stubby spines has multiplied. Figure 2.6 represents the various stages of dendritic development in large pyramidal neurons (Lund, 1978).

Integration and Differentiation As cells begin to multiply, migrate to their final location, and elaborate, they also undergo the concurrent processes of integration and differentiation (i.e., wiring of the brain). **Integration** refers to the intricate interweaving of neural mechanisms toward their target destination. **Differentiation,** on the other hand, is the process by means of which structure, function, or forms of behavior become more specialized. This term also refers to the progression of motor control from gross, poorly controlled movements to precise, complex motor behavior. Differentiation cannot occur until **synaptogenesis** has taken place (i.e., the synapses [connection] between neurons have formed).

Estimates for the average number of neuronal connections range from 1,500 to 15,000, depending on the type and function of the neuron, producing trillions of connections. The formation of synapses occurs at different times and in different parts of the brain, with the sequence tied with the emergence of various functions and skills

(Chugani, 1997, 1998). Neuronal connections begin to form during embryonic development when each differentiating neuron sends out an axon (the transmission lines of the nervous system) tipped at its leading point by a *growth cone*. The cone migrates through the dense environment to its synaptic targets. Current theory suggests that the growth cone navigates itself (at times, relatively long distances) to the target using guidance mechanisms (cues) involving various chemical attractor and repulsion processes (Tessier-Lavigne & Goodman, 1996). By the time of birth, the infant's brain has already formed trillions of neuronal connections (synapses). Areas already wired prior to birth include functions for breathing, circulation, heartbeat, reflexes, and basic (spontaneous) movement. In the first months of postnatal life, the number of connections will increase 20-fold. Synaptogenesis begins in the motor cortex at about 2 months of age—a time when basic reflexes (e.g., startle and rooting) begin to phase away and purposeful movement emerges (e.g., reaching). Tied closely to this event is synaptic formation in the visual cortex at about 3 months, allowing the infant's eyes to focus on an object. Shortly after, the brain, in a phase of biological exuberance, begins to produce trillions more connections than it can possibly use. Around the age of 10 years, the brain selectively eliminates (also referred to as *pruning*) connections that are infrequently or never used.

Some interesting data reported by Chugani (1998) provide what has been referred to as a glimpse of the period of exuberant connectivity and a testament to the general *critical period* for wiring of the brain (figure 2.7). These data show the human brain's consumption of glucose (metabolic rate of glucose utilization) from birth to adulthood. As shown, the rates at birth through about 10 years are more than twice that of adults. The suggestion is that these high levels of consumption are devoted to extraordinary activity in neurogenesis, more specifically, an increase in the number of dendrites per neuron and synaptogenesis. Supportive data comparing the brains of children that died early show similar age-related developmental change (Huttenlocher, 1994; Huttenlocher & Dabholkar, 1997). For example, in one layer of the visual cortex, the number of synapses rise from around 2,500 per neuron at birth to as many as 18,000 about six months later. While different areas of the brain develop at different rates, in general, there is a rise in the rates of glucose utilization from birth until about age 4, at which time the child's brain uses over twice as much glucose as that of an adult. From 4 to about 9 to 10 years these levels are maintained, after which there is a gradual decline. Once again, comparative data with animals and cadavers show that after this period of exuberance begins a pruning phase, with surviving neurons showing a decline in synaptic density. Hypothetically, neurons stimulated adequately during the critical period show less elimination and support the idea of activity-dependent stabilization. Correlations between regional glucose consumption and behavior provide much of the basis

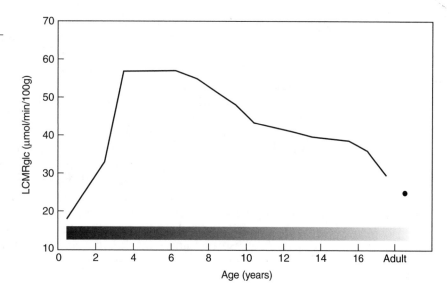

■ *Figure 2.7*

Average glucose
utilization levels
in four areas
of cortex

Source: Adapted from
Chugani (1998)

for what has become known as the optimal windows of opportunity for
wiring and efficient learning.

THE EFFECTS OF EXPERIENCE As alluded to in chapter 1 and in
this section, scientists now believe that to achieve the precision of the
mature brain, neural function and stimulation during infancy and early
childhood are necessary. That is, optimal development is activity-
dependent (e.g., Nelson, 2000). Dr. Bruce Perry, a noted researcher in
this field, sums up the findings on this topic by stating that "Experience
is the chief architect of the brain" (*Time*, February, 1997; refer to the
set of articles in the Suggested Readings regarding early brain development for further reference).

   The general notion is that while genetics play a major role in determining the main neural circuits of the brain, positive stimulation significantly influences the trillions of finer connections made after birth.
Experience appears to exert its effects by strengthening synapses. That
is, stimulation from the environment produces a signal that forms various connections. Connections that are not made, or are weak, are pruned
away. If the neurons are used, they become integrated into the circuitry
of the brain. Thus, due to differences in experience, not even identical
twins are wired the same.

   How do scientists know this? They invasively examine (invade tissue) the brains of animals after experimental manipulation and nonin-
vasively study infant brain structure and activity using sophisticated
neuroimaging techniques. Most research on this topic has been conducted with regard to development of the visual system in mammalian

species (cat, rat, and ferret). Although the measurement techniques are more sophisticated, several modern studies have followed the general experimental manipulation popularized by Hubel and Wiesel in the 1970s. That is, either one or both eyes of the animal are deprived of stimulation prenatally or postnatally for as long as several weeks. Scientists then make comparisons of anatomical and physiological changes to control animals, or between visual cortex areas within the animal. Common observations include (for example) number of synapses, neuron and axon size, and biochemical characteristics. The general conclusion from these experiments suggests that optimal functional and structural organization of the brain (wiring of the visual system) requires a level of stimulating experience. In addition, several interesting experiments have compared rats raised in various environmentally enriched settings (e.g., toys, treadmills, and obstacle courses) to rats kept in deprived environments (e.g., isolated and confined movement). These studies also confirm that stimulation (of this general type) is a significant factor in brain development (Cotman & Engesser-Cesar, 2002; Jones & Greenough, 1996; Kempermann & Gage, 1999).

Studies with humans provide a provocative parallel. For example, researchers have measured the size of cortical and subcortical areas of a child's brain, as related to stimulation or environmental deprivation. These studies, in general, found that the human brain grows in size, develops complexity, makes synaptic connections, and modifies as a function of the quality and quantity of sensory experience. It is speculated that during early childhood, exercise and play provide vital sensory and physiological stimulation resulting in increased nerve connections. This general effect (of stimulation) has also been used to explain results of studies conducted in more naturalistic settings. For example, Craig Ramey has found that intensive early education using blocks, beads, and a variety of games has long-term positive effects on IQ and academic achievement. This conclusion is the result of three separate studies conducted on children aged 4 months to 8 years who live in disadvantaged environments (Ramey & Ramey, 1994). Perhaps most noted is the finding that the earlier the children enrolled in the program, the more enduring the long-term result; those enrolled after age 5 derived little comparative benefit, suggesting a *critical period* effect.

There is no question that this line of research has added a great deal to our understanding of brain development, and the future looks quite promising. However, at this point, it is still quite unclear as to the specific types of experience and how much is optimal to stimulate the formation of particular neural connections.

DOES THE BRAIN DEVELOP NEW NEURONS AFTER BIRTH (IN ADULTHOOD)? Recall from our discussion of neuron proliferation that virtually all neurons are present at the time of birth. A long-standing belief was that neurons were produced only during the fetal period and for only a short time after birth, if then. However, due in large part to new techniques for observing brain processes, that belief has changed dramatically. Researchers now know the brain does indeed generate new neurons on a rather regular basis throughout much of the lifespan (Eriksson et al., 1998). The number of neurons is relatively small, and the location appears to be limited to the hippocampus, which is involved in memory and learning processes. Most interesting, however, is compelling evidence that environmental manipulations affect adult neurogenesis (Kempermann & Gage, 1999; Van Praag et al., 1999). This has been shown in animal studies as evidenced by exercising mice (running on a treadmill) that produce 2.5 times the growth of new neurons compared to animals housed in more sedentary conditions. This line of research supports the theory discussed earlier that environmental manipulations may affect neurogenesis in a positive manner.

Myelination   The developmental process of **myelination** has been one of the most extensively examined indicators of neurological growth. Much of the early growth in brain size and weight can be attributed to myelination. Evidence has already been presented to show that neurons have slower transmission rates before myelination, are more prone to fatigue, and are more limited in their rate of repetitive firing. The relative rates of myelination in different areas of the brain give a rough estimate of when these areas reach adult levels of functioning (e.g., Bronson, 1982). The degree of myelination is also closely related to maturation (and readiness) in acquisition of motor skills during early childhood. The ages at which myelination begins and ends seem to vary from one brain structure to another, as does the time required for the myelination process itself.

The formation of myelin begins in the spinal cord about halfway through fetal development, continues through adolescence and adulthood and, in some areas of the brain, perhaps into old age. Figure 2.8 on page 54, provides an approximate time line of the myelination process in selected structures and pathways within the CNS. Both sensory and motor roots begin myelination four to five months before birth. The motor roots are the first parts to develop myelin; the sensory structures exhibit a rapid increase about one month later. Motor mechanisms of the spinal cord appear to be fully myelinated and functional by the end of the first month after birth. Once again, the sensory mechanisms lag behind somewhat and do not show myelin growth in the cord until approximately six months after birth.

The primary sensory tracts to the cortex appear to mature at slightly different times during the life span. The myelination of auditory pathways begins as early as the fifth prenatal month, and the visual pathways begin around the time of birth. However, once the developmental process of the visual pathways begins, it proceeds very rapidly and is completed sometime during the first five months of postnatal life.

*Width and length of bars indicate increasing density of myelination; blacked-in areas at end of bars indicate approximate age range of completion of myelination process.

■ *Figure 2.8*

An estimated time line of the myelination process

Auditory myelination, on the other hand, is not completed until approximately 4 years of age. The higher somesthetic pathways related to touch show myelin growth about the eighth prenatal month, and by birth these pathways are myelinated through to the cortex. Evidence of this level of development is exhibited by newborns who are normally quite sensitive to touch stimuli. Significant growth continues in the somesthetic pathways until the child is between 1 and 2 years of age.

The pyramidal tract, the major efferent pathway from the motor cortex, begins myelination a month before birth. Although the pathway does not achieve full maturity for about two years, it is probably functional by 4 to 5 months, when intentional (voluntary) motor behavior can be observed in the infant (Bushnell, 1982; McDonnell, 1979). The part of the brain that integrates information (cerebral commissures) exhibits a rapid increase in myelin about the third month after birth and this process continues until approximately age 10. The reticular formation associated with the attention processes begins a period of rapid myelination at birth and continues to mature in an individual until sometime after the second decade. This observation has led to the belief that a person's capability to selectively attend to a task is still being modified until early adulthood. Last to undergo myelination are the areas of the brain associated with memory. These structures, called association areas, begin to show significant myelin growth that starts around the third month after birth and continues into and beyond the third decade of life.

The development of myelin and the characteristics of early motor behavior present an interesting developmental parallel. Prior to the initiation of voluntary motor control, movement is exhibited in the form of *myogenic, neurogenic,* and *reflex* behaviors. **Myogenic behavior** is movement that is the result of direct muscle stimulation rather than stimulation that arrives at the muscle through some intervening neural structure. Myogenic movement can sometimes be elicited in the fetus prior to the appearance of myelin.

After the appearance of myelin in the spinal cord at about the fourth fetal month, movement can be elicited through the motor neuron's connection with the muscle. This type of behavior, which is affected by neural structures, is called **neurogenic behavior.** At approximately 6 months (prenatal), myelination is more complete in the spinal cord and *reflex arcs* appear, meaning that the fetus can receive sensory input and reflexively translate the information into a behavior or motor response. Touch stimulation can elicit such movement behaviors as the primitive grasp reflex of the hands and the Babinski reflex of the feet. By the eighth fetal month the cord is close to fully myelinated, and the direction of growth proceeds upward toward the higher brain regions such as the medulla, midbrain, and thalamus. At this point several important developmental motor responses can be observed: respiratory movements, primitive sucking, the Moro reflex, tonic neck reflexes, and other righting reflexes.

At birth and during the neonate period, and as the motor pathways from the cortex are myelinated, voluntary motor behavior becomes possible. Since the somatosensory pathways are the most advanced of the sensory tracts, the infant responds readily to tactile stimulation on almost any part of its body. Although myelination of the optic tracts trails somewhat behind at this point, the neonate is capable of visual fixation and simple tracking movements as well as some form and depth perception awareness. As previously noted, myelination of the auditory pathways develops at a slower rate than the other sensory tracts; therefore, in comparison, the infant's responses are less mature (e.g., exhibiting primarily gross reactions to a sharp, loud sound) during the first month of life.

Cell Death   Although we may never be able to get an honest count of neuronal loss, researchers do believe that there is considerable *cell death,* or natural elimination of neurons, during early development and as we age. During early development some structures may lose 40% to 75% of neurons initially generated. Cell death of neurons in this instance is believed to be a normal part of the developmental process of

TABLE 2.2

Summary of Developmental Events Associated with the General Sequence of Early Brain Neurogenesis

1. With *proliferation*, the brain produces many more neurons than it needs, then eliminates the excess.

2. These neurons *migrate* to their final location.

3. Once cells have reached their target destination (*integration*), they spin out axons that connect to other neurons via dendrites (*synaptogenesis*). Spontaneous bursts of electrical activity strengthen some of these connections, while others die.

4. During this process, *myelination* (insulation of the neural pathway) and *differentiation* (greater specialization of function) occurs.

5. After birth, the brain experiences a second growth spurt (in neuronal size) reflected by an explosion in the number of dendrites, that is, new connection sites. Additional sensory stimulation fine-tunes the brain's circuitry by making and strengthening new connections.

6. Connections not made or stimulated adequately are *pruned* away.

7. *Cell death* is a natural, lifelong process.

establishing synaptic connections (i.e., differentiation), first, in a phase of synapse overproduction, followed by selective elimination (i.e., pruning) or preservation to yield a more specific neural connection. It has been hypothesized that proliferating cells compete with each other for a limited number of synaptic sites or for some function that is vital to their existence. Table 2.2 provides a summary of the sequence of early neurological development.

Critical Periods (Windows of Opportunity) One of the strongest implications of the research described is the observation that during the developmental period of exuberant connectivity, there is a relatively high degree of brain plasticity. That is, there are **critical periods** in neuronal development in which experience may be most effective in forging connections (wiring the brain). From another perspective, these critical periods have more recently been referred to as *windows of opportunity*, the theory that nature opens certain windows for the experience effect starting before birth and then closes each opportunity, one by one. In theory, there are a series of windows for developing motor control, vision, language, feelings, etc. With increasing age, the brain's plasticity declines. The child who misses an opportunity may not develop the brain's circuitry to its full potential for a specific function. For an applied example, recall the Ramey research noted in the previous section; the critical period for early intervention was before age 5 (not

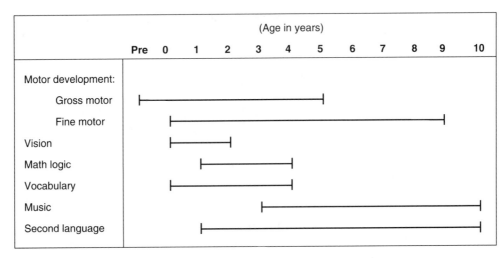

■ *Figure 2.9*

Windows of Opportunity

Source: Data compiled from *Newsweek* (1997) and *Time* (1997) articles noted in Suggested Readings

THINK ABOUT IT

From this discussion, describe the role of nature/nurture in early brain development. If you were designing a motor development (physical activity) program for 3- and 4-year-olds, what would it look like based on this information?

in the 5- to 8-year-olds). Figure 2.9 shows estimates of the critical periods (windows of opportunity) for different functions in which neuronal development is most receptive to experience. Keep in mind that these projections are estimates of general functions.

Most relevant to our discussion is the general window of opportunity estimated for motor development. For basic motor skills, it appears to be from the prenatal period to around the age of 5 years. Keep in mind once again that this is a period in which experience is vital to forging the foundation of brain circuits dedicated to motor control. Other factors such as myelination are also important. The main circuits for reflex (involuntary) behavior are wired prenatally. The window for the primary circuits that control posture and general movement, housed in the cerebellum, is open for about the first two years. It is during this time that children begin to gain considerable experience in the world as they move about in the environment. Once again, this suggests that physical activity may be a strong determinant in early development of the brain, not just motor control (as suggested earlier in reference to Greenough's work). In regard to finer muscle control and timing (which follows gross-motor development), it seems reasonable that the general window would be open from shortly after birth to about age 9. Also evident in figure 2.9 is general closure of the window of opportunity around the age of 10, especially for second language development. This is the period when the balance between synaptic connectivity and pruning abruptly shifts.

Objective 2.8

➤ **Changes in Major Brain Structures**   Throughout brain growth from early periods, the appearance of function approximates maturation in structure. Keep in mind that structure is influenced by experience, therefore making age predictions gross estimates. However, general trends have been documented. The adult brain weighs about 3½ pounds, and although it makes up only about 2.5% of the total body weight, it requires 15% of the body's blood supply and about 25% of all the oxygen consumed. From two to eight weeks following conception the nervous system begins to develop as a long, hollow tube on the back of the embryo. As the system develops, brain size increases into a mass of neurons, losing its primitive tubular appearance. At birth, the infant's brain weighs about one-fourth of its adult weight. After birth, nerve cell size increases, other supporting cells called neuroglia are formed, and the myelin develops, causing the brain to double in volume. By age 3 the brain has reached nearly 90% of its adult size, and by age 6 it has basically achieved its full size. In contrast, total body weight at birth is just 5% of young adult size and by age 10 it is only 50% of the weight that will eventually be attained. The part of the brain most fully developed at birth is the midbrain. As previously mentioned, the midbrain is the part of the CNS that controls much of the early reflex behavior. The midbrain, pons, and medulla occupy approximately 8% of the total brain volume at 3 fetal months of age, but by birth this proportion has fallen to around 1.5%. During the first decade of life, these percentages increase slightly due to fiber tract growth. After the midbrain (in developmental progression) comes the cerebrum, and considerably later, the cerebellum.

Growth and differentiation of the cortical regions of the brain are landmark features in the functional maturity of the CNS. As previously noted, the cortex is composed of an estimated 75% of the total neurons found in the brain; this is an estimated 75 billion, interconnected by about 50 miles of axons and dendrites. Yet in actual size, it accounts for only a very small portion in forming the outermost layer of the cerebrum—about one-fourth inch in thickness. While thickness of the cortex normally reaches adult levels by approximately 2½ years of age, functional maturity of the cortical areas in general is usually not achieved until later early childhood.

According to Tanner (1990), two clear gradients of development occur during the first two years after birth. First, is the order in which general functional areas develop, and second, the order in which bodily localizations advance within the areas.

The rate of development among the cerebral lobes is quite varied. Each lobe has its own rate of development, each area in each lobe has its own developmental rate, and each layer of those areas has different rates of development. In order of increasing maturity, the occipital lobe (visual functions) matures first, the parietal lobe (somatosensory functions) next, and the temporal (auditory and memory functions) and frontal (memory and motor functions) lobes are the slowest to reach full maturity. The most advanced part of the cortex is the primary motor

■ *Figure 2.10*

The concept of lateral dominance of limb control

area, which initiates most basic movement. Next is the primary sensory area, then the primary visual area in the occipital lobe, then the primary auditory area in the temporal lobe. The association areas lag behind the corresponding primary areas.

Following the basic principle of cephalocaudal development within the motor area, control of the legs generally evolves later than the capabilities for upper body movements. The same is generally true in the sensory area. By about 2 years, the motor and sensory areas are similar in maturity and the association areas add considerably to function. The cerebellum, the area of the brain primarily responsible for controlling coordinated motor responses, lags behind the midbrain, areas of the spinal cord, and cerebral cortex in development. Closely linked to its functional maturity is myelination of the tracts between it and the cortex, which reaches potential about age 4.

Objective 2.9   ➤ **Brain Lateralization and the Corpus Callosum**   Although the two hemispheres of the brain appear symmetrical, in functional terms they are quite different. Each hemisphere has its own specialized functions (i.e., functional asymmetries), a characteristic known as **brain** (hemispheric) **lateralization.** In most humans, the left hemisphere is associated with the governance of language, logic, and sequential processing, whereas the right hemisphere is specialized for nonverbal, visuospatial functions (e.g., music awareness, map reading, and figure drawing). Of more direct relevance to motor behavior is that the cortex of the right hemisphere controls muscular activity in, and receives sensory input from, the left half of the body (figure 2.10); whereas the left hemisphere has a complementary role in conscious movement on the right side of the body.

Dividing and connecting the two hemispheres of the brain is a tough band of myelinated tissue called the *corpus callosum.* One of its primary functions is to provide the link for shared information between the two hemispheres, in essence allowing the right hand to know what the left hand is doing. Thus, the corpus callosum is important for the functional integration of the two cerebral hemispheres and possibly for the manifestation of functional asymmetries. Evidence to date suggests that the corpus callosum plays a significant role in high-level attentional and cognitive functions (Hoptman & Davidson, 1994). The callosum undergoes marked growth in overall size and myelination during postnatal development and by 4 to 5 years, its development is fairly advanced (Witelson & Kigar, 1988). With regard to sex differences in cerebral lateralization of function, some research has indicated that neither the male brain nor the female brain is more asymmetrically organized. This includes actual callosum area and its growth curve during development (Peters, 1988a). Further discussion of this topic will be provided in chapters 8 and 9 in relation to theoretical and applied considerations of functional (motor) asymmetries (i.e., the development of handedness, footedness, and eye preference).

Neurological Changes with Aging

Objective 2.10 ➤ There are considerable individual differences in aging of the brain. In addition, the many components of the brain itself vary in degree of age-related change. The loss of neurons in various regions is accepted as a significant part of the aging process. It is estimated that this loss is about 5% to 30% by old age. The brain loses about 7% of its weight from the time when we are younger adults. This amount could be substantially more if some form of organic brain disease or other secondary aging element (e.g., drugs, diet, alcohol, or health of the cardiovascular system) is present. It is generally believed that the brain has such remarkable recovery capabilities (plasticity) that, even though significant neuron loss may occur, the brain may only lose a small portion of its ability to function. In fact, it has been reported that to compensate for losses, older brains literally rewire themselves for a given task (Rapaport, 1994).

In addition to a significant loss of neurons, other important changes appear to be occurring within the neurons themselves. One of the most critical of these changes involves the gradual shrinking and withering away of the dendrites (density) and axons (i.e., interconnectivity among neurons) while other mutations may include the cell body. Process deficits normally associated with advanced aging include a decrease in neuron connectivity, delay in new axon growth and myelination, decrease in neuron excitability, and an estimated two-fold increase in synaptic delay (Scheibel, 1996). Several of the characteristics listed have been associated with the older adult phenomenon known as *psychomotor slowing* (to be discussed in greater detail in chapters 7 and 11).

In general, aging may be constituted by a proliferation of abnormal material and functions referred to as vacuoles, plaques, and tangles. *Vacuoles* are thick granules surrounded by fluid; and although they are most common in diseased brains, they show up in three-fourths of the brains checked from people over 80 years of age (Adams, 1980). *Senile plaques*, collections of debris consisting of cells, silicone, and macrophagic elements, are frequently found in the frontal and occipital lobes of the brain. *Neurofibrillary tangles*, tangled clumps of double-helical strands of protein, appear in older brains, but no one clearly understands their effect. Tangles tend to be particularly prominent in the cerebral cortex as a whole and in the thalamus, basal ganglia, and spinal cord. Eckert (1987) notes that plaques and tangles appear to some degree in the brains of 99% of all individuals older than 80 years of age. Senile plaques and neurofibrillary tangles have been found in brains of people who had primary degenerative dementia (i.e., Alzheimer's disease). Studies have also noted that as neurons and dendrites deteriorate, neuroglia (the connective tissue that fills the spaces between neurons) increase in number. Bodies of *astrocytes*, star-shaped neuroglia, get larger in the aging brain and may prevent neurotransmitters from building up between nerve cells.

One of the most dramatic decreases in basic neurological function related to motor behavior is the deterioration of vestibular awareness (balance). Neurons in one layer of the cerebellum die off fairly rapidly after the age of 60. With this decrease is an estimated 40% loss of vestibular hair and nerve cells by 70 years. As previously noted, the cerebellum functions to coordinate voluntary motor behavior and vestibular awareness. Balance as measured by speed-of-return-to-equilibrium and body sway deteriorates significantly during old age. (e.g., Shumway-Cook & Woollacott, 2001). The topic of balance in older persons will be discussed in chapter 11.

Another basic neural process crucial to motor behavior is nerve conduction velocity. This function also declines with increasing age. The loss appears to be more prominent in the distal segments of the body and in the lumbosacral regions. The results of such a loss have been evidenced by several studies showing how reaction and movement time slow with increased age. In general, the decline of both functions tends to occur most rapidly in the lower parts of the body and in areas of most frequent use, such as the fingers. The general rate of decline appears to be affected by the complexity of the task.

Table 2.3 on the following page presents a summary list of selected neurological functions that normally show signs of deterioration with aging.

THINK ABOUT IT

Name some reasons why there are large individual differences in brain function of the elderly.

TABLE 2.3

Selected Basic Neurological Changes with Aging

Neurological Structure	Function
Brain weight	Decreases
Number of neurons	Decreases
Dendritic density	Decreases
Nerve conduction velocity	Decreases
Connectivity	Decreases

Summary

The blueprint for our heredity is contained in the genes found within the 23 pairs of chromosomes of a human cell nucleus. Along with such traits as sex and eye color, heredity influences numerous developmental factors such as aging, puberty, general body type, height, muscle fiber type, and skeletal age. These factors can also be affected by the environment as evidenced by the documented effects of diet and exercise on body weight and aging.

The nervous system serves three primary functions: (a) sensory, (b) integrative, which includes the memory and thought processes, and (c) motor. The basic function of the CNS is to transmit information about the environment and the body to the brain, and to carry information from the brain to muscles and glands, thus producing motor responses and bodily adaptations to environmental demands. The PNS is a branching network of nerves consisting of two distinct systems: the somatic and autonomic. The somatic system controls all the skeletal muscles, whereas the autonomic system is concerned with the automatic regulation of the smooth muscles.

The basic parts of a neuron (or nerve cell) are the cell body, dendrites, and axon. Dendrites are the receiving part of the neuron, whereas the function of the axon is to carry information away from the cell body to other cells. The functional connection between the axon and another neuron is called a synapse. The pyramidal and extrapyramidal motor pathway systems provide the channels through which nerve impulses travel on their way to producing muscular contraction or relaxation. Messages are sent through the nervous system in the form of chemical impulses (waves of electricity). How fast the information travels depends to some degree on the presence of myelin, which forms an insulating sheath around many axons.

Development of the CNS can be described in a sequence of six integrated biological events: cell proliferation, migration, integration, differentiation, myelination, and cell death. The process of proliferation is virtually completed by birth. As proliferation occurs, cells migrate to their final location and elaborate, which is evidenced by the developmental changes that take place in the axon and dendrite structures. Neurons are also involved in an intricate interweaving process to target cells (integration) and, in turn, become more specialized (differentiation). A significant influence in the wiring process is stimulation provided by the environment. During this general process, the critical formation and development of myelin (myelination) also transpires. A normal part of the developmental process is cell death.

The human body's central computer, the brain, undergoes several rapid quantitative and developmental (level of functioning) changes during the first few years. During the course of brain development, each hemisphere establishes its own specialized functions; this is referred to as lateralization. Related to this concept is the notion that hand and foot motor control on one side of the body are controlled by areas of the brain in the opposite-side hemisphere.

Several neurological changes occur during the latter stages of aging. Along with the loss of neurons and brain weight, important functional (process) changes are also evident. Advanced aging may produce abnormal material such as vacuoles, plaques, and tangles. Other materials (e.g., astrocytes) may also develop and fill spaces between neurons, thus inhibiting neural transmission. There are several motor behavior functions that normally show signs of deterioration with aging. Among the most affected by age are vestibular awareness (balance) and nerve conduction velocity (a slowing of movement).

Think about It

1. List some of the phenotype characteristics you have and from which parent you inherited them. Can you think of ways that the environment affects phenotype over time?
2. From this discussion, describe the role of nature/nurture in early brain development. If you were designing a motor development (physical activity) program for 3- and 4-year-olds, what would it look like based on this information?
3. Name some reasons why there are large individual differences in brain function of the elderly.

Suggested Readings

Early brain development (magazine reports):
  The brain. *Newsweek* (special issue), Spring/Summer, 1997.
  Fertile minds. *Time* (special report), February 3, 1997.
Malina, R., & Bouchard, C. (1991). *Growth, maturation, and physical activity.* Champaign, IL: Human Kinetics.
Sanes, D., Reh, T., & Harris, W. (2000). *Development of the nervous system.* New York: Academic Press.
Scheibel, A. B. (1996). Structural and functional changes in the aging brain. In J. Birren and K. Schaie (Eds.), *Handbook of the psychology of aging.* 4th ed. New York: Academic Press.

WebLinks

The Visible Embryo (Resource on prenatal development)
  www.visembryo.com

Society for Neuroscience
  www.sfn.org

3 *Physical Growth Changes*

OBJECTIVES

Upon completion of this chapter, you should be able to

3.1 Provide a brief summary of the major changes in physical growth that take place over the course of the life span.

3.2 Define the terms *physical anthropology, anthropometry,* and *growth curve.*

3.3 Outline and briefly describe the significant growth and development events that occur during the prenatal period.

3.4 Discuss the major characteristics and changes associated with the pubescent (adolescent) growth spurt.

3.5 List and briefly describe the major changes in body proportions and physique that take place during normal growth and development.

3.6 Discuss how height and skeletal growth measurements typically change during development.

3.7 Identify the major changes in body mass that accompany lifelong development and the methods used to assess those changes.

3.8 List and briefly describe the various ways of estimating physical maturity.

3.9 Discuss maturity variations among developing individuals.

3.10 Explain secular trend.

3.11 Discuss the implications for motor performance of change in physical growth characteristics.

KEY TERMS

physical anthropology

anthropometry

growth curve

pubescent growth spurt

menarche

growth hormone (GH)

somatotype

ossification

body mass

biological age

secular trend

IN THE PREVIOUS CHAPTER you learned about the growth and development characteristics of the basic neurological structures. This chapter will focus on changes in the physical growth over the life span. Specific discussions will cover a general overview of physical growth, prenatal development, the adolescent growth spurt, body proportions and physique, height and skeletal growth, and body mass. Methods of estimating maturity level and maturity variations will also be examined.

An Overview of Physical Growth and Development

Objective 3.1

➤ The new perspective on lifelong human development stresses the fact that the developmental process evolves along a continuum from conception to physical death. This perspective is supported through the observation of physical growth changes. Although the first two decades of life are a period of significant growth increases, marked changes also occur during later stages of the aging process.

Growth and maturation begin in a cephalocaudal and proximodistal pattern. With the cephalocaudal pattern, growth (especially during the prenatal stage) first occurs in the head and gradually proceeds its way downward to the neck, shoulders, and trunk. At the same time, proximodistal growth proceeds from the center of the body and moves toward the extremities (e.g., the hands and fingers). Individuals grow at a faster rate during gestation and the first year after birth than they will at any other time in their lives. During the early childhood years, physical growth progresses at a relatively uniform and steady rate. In middle and late childhood, growth is a relatively slow, consistent process that may be characterized as the calm before the dramatic biological change that occurs during early adolescence and the onset of puberty. The pubescent growth spurt represents a landmark in physical growth with regard to sex differences and motor performance. Later in early adulthood, physical development usually begins to slow down. And as people age they generally get shorter, lose muscle mass, experience a change in body proportions, and get heavier. Interestingly, in old age there is a tendency for individuals to become lighter than they were during middle adulthood.

Objective 3.2

➤ We have learned that motor development is tied closely to developmental psychology; the field of **physical anthropology** also provides information and scientific procedures related to the study of biological growth and development. Physical anthropology is basically concerned with the meaningful understanding of the nature, distribution, and significance of biological variation in humans. The branch of science concerned with biological growth and body measurement is referred to as **anthropometry,** which is one of the basic tools used in growth studies.

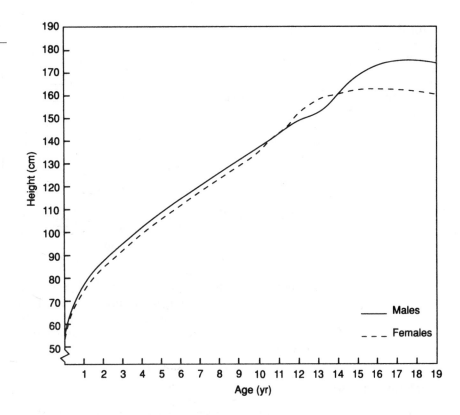

■ *Figure 3.1*

Typical distance curves for change in height

Each physical growth topic discussed in this chapter will include a description of anthropometric measurement techniques. For a detailed description of anthropometric techniques, refer to the excellent training module provided by the Centers for Disease Control and Prevention (CDC) (2000), which complements the selected growth charts shown in this chapter (see Suggested Readings which includes the CDC Web site address).

Anthropometric data used to assess growth take the form of mean value comparisons, percentile rankings, and growth curves. Perhaps a less-known but frequently used procedure in growth studies is to plot the pattern of physical change in individuals or groups on a **growth curve.** One type of curve is called a *distance curve*, which is used to plot growth from one year to the next. The distance curves for males and females exhibit a gradual height increase before a leveling off occurs, as shown in figure 3.1. It depicts typical individual height curves based on data from many individuals. If the values of only one individual were plotted, the graph would be unlikely to show such a smooth curve.

Another technique is to measure the rate of growth using what is known as *velocity curve*. This type of measurement better reflects the individual's growth state at any particular moment than it does the

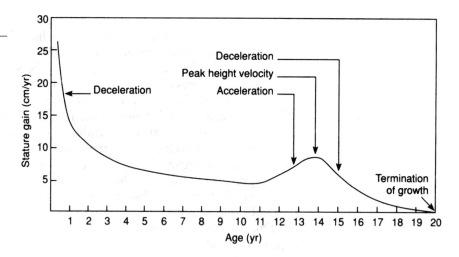

■ *Figure 3.2*

An example of a velocity curve for height indicating the different phases of growth

distance or change in growth achieved in preceding years. The velocity of growth refers to increments in growth value from year to year and is represented by points of deceleration or acceleration. Figure 3.2 illustrates a hypothetical velocity curve with different phases of growth rate for height.

Prenatal Development

Objective 3.3 ➤ The prenatal period (conception to birth) plays a significant role in human development. Events that take place during this period forge the foundation for future development across the life span. In comparison to the other developmental stages of life, the prenatal period presents the greatest variation in human growth and development.

Conception Life begins at *conception* when a single male sperm cell unites with the ovum (egg) in the female's fallopian tube. Fertilization occurs within several days after the egg begins its journey from the ovaries through the fallopian tubes to the uterus.

Germinal Period The *germinal period* lasts for approximately 14 days after conception. Almost immediately, the 23 chromosomes from the sperm cell nucleus combine with the 23 chromosomes from the ovum to produce 46 chromosomes. The chromosomes then split, yielding 46 pairs, which serve as the template in the development of the individual. Two major developmental events occur during the next 10 to 14 days. One is continued cell differentiation, and the other is the firm attachment of the ovum to the wall of the uterus. During this time the divided cells gradually form a spherical mass, which separates into inner and outer segments. The outer segment eventually forms part of the mother–fetus barrier, and the inner mass becomes the fetus.

Embryonic Period By two weeks after conception, the embryonic disk has folded and formed the distinct layers of cells called an embryo. The *embryonic period* lasts from about two to eight weeks after conception. During this period human form begins to take shape. Although the embryo after eight weeks is only about 1 inch (2.5 cm) and weighs only half an ounce (14 g), the basic parts of the body—the head, trunk, arms, and legs—can be identified. Some of the finer features such as the eyes, ears, fingers, and toes are also discernible. The central nervous system (CNS) is relatively developed and the internal organs (e.g., the heart, lungs, reproductive organs, liver, and kidneys) are beginning to function to some degree. All of these developments take place according to a master blueprint that dictates that development starts at the head, then moves to the trunk, and then to the lower extremities, in cephalocaudal order. This developmental blueprint also calls for development to proceed proximodistally from the midline of the body (centering around the spine and heart) outward to the extremities (the shoulders, arms, and hands).

Fetal Period The *fetal period* of development begins about the eighth week, when the embryo becomes a recognizable human being, and lasts until the time of birth.

By the third month, the fetus is about 3 inches (7.5 cm) long and weighs approximately 1 ounce (28 g). The sex organs are developed to the point where sex can be determined and a number of physical and anatomical features are better defined. The forehead is more prominent, and the eyelids, nose, and chin are clearly distinguishable. Although the process may have begun during the embryonic period, it can now be seen that flexible cartilage is being replaced by bone in a process called *ossification*. The fetal period also marks the time at which the first muscle movements in the mouth and jaw probably occur. By the ninth week the muscles of the arms and legs are capable of responding to tactile stimulation.

The fourth month (16 weeks) of fetal development is a period of significant growth. The fetus will increase its length to about 6 inches (15 cm) and weight to approximately 4 ounces (110 g). Whereas a considerable amount of growth has already occurred in the upper body, there is now a growth spurt of the lower parts of the body in the cephalocaudal direction. The toes and fingers have separated, and fingerprint and footprint patterns begin to emerge.

By the end of the fifth month (20 weeks), the fetus is approximately 12 inches (30 cm) in length and weighs about 1 pound (450 g). Features of the skin have become more differentiated, and distinctive fingernails and toenails are present.

During the sixth month (24 weeks) the eyes and eyelids are completely formed, the eyelids open for the first time, and a fine layer of hair has begun to form on the head. At this point, the fetus weighs approximately 2 pounds (900 g) and is about 14 inches (36 cm) long.

The seventh month (28 weeks) is sometimes called the age of viability—meaning that the fetus has matured enough to have a 50% chance of surviving outside of the womb if birth comes prematurely. The internal organs are functioning, and the brain now can regulate breathing, body temperature, and swallowing. The fetus is about 16 inches (40 cm) long and weighs close to 3 pounds (1,350 g).

The eighth and ninth months are a period of rapid weight gain. The fetus gains about half a pound per week for a total of 5 pounds (2,250 g) for the two-month period, on the average. Just a few weeks prior to birth (and at delivery), the average fetus is 20 inches (50 cm) long and weighs about 7 pounds (3.2 g). During these months fatty layers are developing that will help to nourish the fetus after birth.

Table 3.1 summarizes the major physical growth changes that occur during the prenatal period. Figure 3.3 shows the general body form changes of a developing fetus.

The Pubescent (Adolescent) Growth Spurt

Objective 3.4 ➤ Next to the period of prenatal growth, the pubescent growth spurt, which occurs during early adolescence, represents the life span's most dramatic period of biological change. This period also has landmark significance for the evolution of motor performance and gender differences. These will be discussed in detail in subsequent chapters. At the beginning of adolescence a number of rapid changes occur in physical maturation and growth. This period of biological development is known as *puberty;* hence the term **pubescent growth spurt.** These changes are controlled primarily by genetic factors and hormones. Along with rapid changes in body size and proportions, sexual maturation is one of the most prominent aspects of the pubertal process. In this context, puberty is referred to as the stage of maturation in which the individual becomes physiologically capable of sexual reproduction.

The pubescent growth spurt generally begins at about 10 to 13 years of age in females and 12 to 15 years of age in males, and it lasts for two to three years. Females also go through the pubertal period in a somewhat shorter time than males and thus are typically about two years ahead of males in maturity (see figure 3.16 with regard to height). Add to this the wide range of ages at which individuals enter puberty, and the general picture of the possible variation in individual differences becomes quite evident.

In females, the growth spurt usually designates the beginning of sexual maturity, when breasts and pubic hair also first appear. This period of development is highlighted by a universal maturity landmark known as **menarche,** or the time of the female's first menstrual flow. The average age at menarche is about 12.5 years; for many girls the

TABLE 3.1

Major Physical Growth Changes from Conception to Birth

Period	Age (weeks)	Height (cm)	Weight (g)	Notable Characteristics
Germinal	(0–2)			Cell differentiation begins
				Inner and outer mass formed
Embryonic	(2–8)	2.5	14	Human form takes shape (ears, eyes, arms, legs)
				Internal organs begin to develop (heart, lungs, reproductive, liver, kidneys)
Fetal	12	7.5	28	Sex can be distinguished
				Movement
				Bone replacing cartilage
				Head growth, facial features
	16	15	110	Growth spurt in lower part of body
				Fingerprints and footprints emerge
	20	30	450	Skin structures form
				Fingernails and toenails present
	24	36	900	Eyes, eyelids formed
				Head hair forming
	28	37.5–40	1,110–1,350	Internal organs functioning
				Age of viability
	32–36	40–50	1,800–3,600	Rapid weight gain
				Layer of fat forming beneath skin
				Bones of head are soft

Source: From John W. Santrock, *Life-Span Development,* 2nd edition. Copyright © 1986 Wm. C. Brown Publishers, Dubuque, Iowa. All Rights Reserved. Reprinted by permission.

Weeks of prenatal development

■ *Figure 3.3*

General body form changes of a developing fetus

event may occur as early as the age of 10 or as late as 15.5 years. Maturity indicators for males include the appearance of pubic and facial hair, a change in voice, and an increase in the size of the reproductive organs. Sexual maturity, including menarche, will be discussed in greater detail in subsequent sections of the text.

Hormonal Influence   Hormonal change is another prominent feature of the adolescent growth spurt. Primary agents of this change are the hypothalamus (a part of the brain) and the pituitary (master) gland, which regulates the endocrine system. The other primary glands include the gonads (sex glands), thyroid gland, and the adrenal glands (which plays a supportive role). See chapter 5 (figure 5.2 on page 160) for an illustration of the general location of these structures. In addition to regulating the endocrine system, the pituitary produces **growth hormone (GH),** one of the primary agents that stimulates the adolescent growth spurt.

How does this complex system work (figure 3.4)? Basically, puberty begins as increased levels of hormones (via the endocrine system) enter the bloodstream in response to signals from the hypothalamus. These signals instruct the pituitary to release GH and stimulate production of thyroxine (from the thyroid) and sex hormones (from the gonads). Together GH and thyroxine contribute strongly to the tremendous gain in body size and completion of skeletal maturation during puberty. In addition to stimulating growth in most tissues, GH also is one of the major regulators of metabolism.

Perhaps as significant is the interaction between GH and androgens produced by the gonads. Throughout childhood, the male and female bodies produce approximate levels of estrogens and androgens. After a signal from the hypothalamus, the pituitary sends a signal via *gonadotropins* to stimulate the production of estrogen in the ovaries (female) and androgens (mostly testosterone) in the testes (male). When secretions of these hormones reach critical levels, the pituitary produces more GH; the result is the growth spurt in both sexes.

Androgens play a significant role in hastening the fusion of epiphyseal growth plates in the bones and stimulating the protein synthesis required for the development of muscle tissue. Nottelman and Associates (1987) found that testosterone levels increased 18-fold in boys but only 2-fold in girls during puberty; in contrast, estrogen levels increased 8-fold in girls but only 2-fold in boys. Note that both hormones are present in both sexes, but that testosterone dominates in the male. Thus, it appears that adolescent boys experience larger growth spurts than girls primarily because of significantly greater testosterone levels. Estrogen, although important to the growth spurt and bone development in females, promotes the accumulation of body fat. Although females may continue to develop muscle tissue (due to the presence of GH and

■ *Figure 3.4*

Hormonal influence on the body at puberty

THINK ABOUT IT

Consider some ways
the phenomenon of
puberty can influence
participation in
sports.

androgens), the effects of estrogen may account for the greater amount
of fatty tissue in comparison to males. In addition, estrogens cause a
quicker closure of the epiphyseal (bone) plate than does testosterone; as
a result females usually do not reach the same height. With regard to
androgens produced by the adrenal glands (above kidneys), recent
thoughts are that they play a secondary (supportive) role to other hormones in promoting the development of muscle and bone (Tanner,
1990).

Table 3.2 on page 74 provides a list of selected anatomical gender
differences that emerge during the adolescent growth spurt due to
genetic and hormonal influence. This information will be useful in coming chapters that describe motor performance changes as age increases.

TABLE 3.2

Selected Anatomical Gender Differences

Height and weight: males taller and heavier

Shoulder width: males wider, more rotation torque

Forearm length: males longer, more lever torque

Hip shape: insertion of femur more oblique in females

Elbow and knee joints: males parallel; females shaped

Leg length: relatively longer in males

Chest girth: males greater thoracic cavity

Center of gravity: males higher, females lower

Fat-free weight: males more muscle, bigger bones

Changes in Body Proportions and Physique

Objective 3.5   ➤ Although the development of the human body follows a relatively consistent cephalocaudal/proximodistal pattern of development, specific body parts show varying rates of growth. During the course of development from birth to adulthood, the head size will double, trunk length will triple, the length of the upper limbs will quadruple, and the length of the lower limbs will quintuple. Along with these differential growth rates, observable changes in body proportions and general body build (physique) can be noted.

Body Proportions

Body Proportion Changes Relative to the Head Figure 3.5 shows general postnatal body proportion changes with age. Most notable are the proportional changes of head size in relation to total body length. The head of the newborn accounts for approximately one-fourth of its total height and its legs make up only about three-eighths of its stature. In comparison, the adult head accounts for about one-eighth of total height and leg length for approximately half of stature. The principle of cephalocaudal development is clearly evident here. Also interesting to consider is that in the newborn, head width is very close to that of the shoulders and hips, whereas head width of adults is only about one-third of shoulder width. After birth, shoulder width is generally greater than hip width. During postnatal development, the legs grow at a faster rate than other body parts in moving toward the adult model of body proportions.

Head circumference is a common anthropometric measurement is used to estimate the rate of brain growth among infants and young

■ *Figure 3.5*

Postnatal body
proportion changes

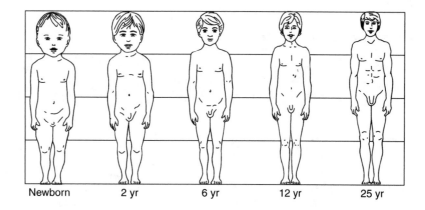

Newborn   2 yr   6 yr   12 yr   25 yr

children. The head circumference measurement is taken at the level of
the plane passing just above the bony ridge over the eyes and the most
posterior protrusion on the back of the head (figure 3.6). Normal head
circumference values fall within a relatively narrow range for any
given age group, with the variance remaining almost constant for the
entire growing period. Although there are slight sex differences, with
males having a greater circumference, the difference generally does not
exceed 1 centimeter at any age. Table 3.3 on page 76 provides information on average head circumferences for individuals from birth to
20 years of age.

During the early months of postnatal life, growth in head circumference is very rapid and then begins to decelerate. During the first four
months there is an increase of about 5 centimeters that doubles by
the end of the first year. From that point until age 18, head circumference only increases another 10 centimeters. Head circumference norms,
apart from being used as an estimate of brain growth, are also used to

■ *Figure 3.6*

Measuring head
circumference

TABLE 3.3

Average Head Circumference

	MEAN				MEAN	
Age	Inches	Centimeters	Age	Inches	Centimeters
Birth	13.8	35	5	20.0	50.8
1 mo	14.9	37.6	6	20.2	51.2
2	15.5	39.7	7	20.5	51.6
3	15.9	40.4	8	20.6	52.0
6	17.0	43.4	10	20.9	53.0
9	17.8	45.0	12	21.0	53.2
12	18.3	46.5	14	21.5	54.0
18	19.0	48.4	16	21.9	55.0
2 yrs	19.2	49.0	18	22.1	55.4
3	19.6	50.0	20	22.2	55.6
4	19.8	50.5			

Source: Data from Lowrey (1986)

identify significant abnormal trends such as hydrocephalus. Figures 3.7 and 3.8 (see page 78) provide incremental (velocity) growth charts for males and females up to 36 months. Charts such as these are frequently used in clinical settings to examine changes in the rate of growth over a specific period of time.

Head size in the very young may have biomechanical implications for motor skill performance. It would seem quite possible that even if the newborn were neurologically ready to attempt walking, a top-heavy body would present problems in maintaining balance. Another commonly seen example is that of a 4- to 5-year-old attempting to perform a backward roll. Due to the larger proportional head size of younger compared to older children, the task of completing a smooth roll over the back of the head often presents difficulty. Few, if any, research findings have shed real light on performance differences attributable to proportional diversity among children.

Changes in Ratio of Sitting Height to Stature   The ratio of sitting height to stature measures the contribution of the legs and trunk to total height. Sitting height is measured as the height from the seat of the chair in which a person is sitting (with spine erect) to the vertex, or top of the head (see figure 3.9 on page 79). Measures of the change in head and trunk height can then be compared with measures of total stature, which includes leg length.

■ *Figure 3.7*

Head circum-
ference for age
percentiles: Boys,
from birth to
36 months

Source: Developed by
the National Center
for Health Statistics
in collaboration with
the National Center
for Chronic Disease
Prevention and Health
Promotion (2000)

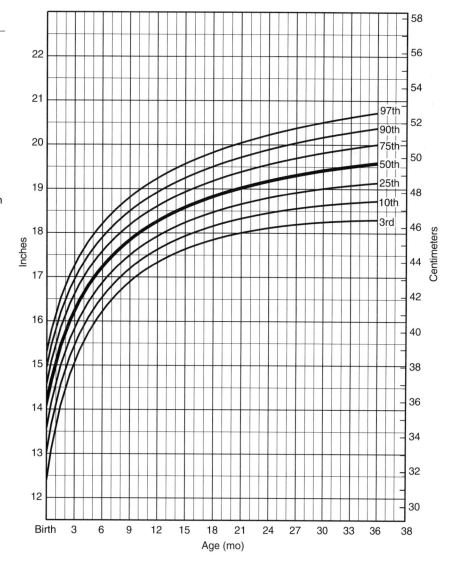

Sitting height is typically 60% to 70% of total body length in the early years and decreases to about 50% when mature height is reached. The most noticeable changes occur in the legs and trunk; the head actually contributes very little to height change after birth. Figure 3.10 on page 79 depicts the ratio of sitting height to stature for individuals up to 18 years. The rapid growth of the legs is evidenced by the decrease in the ratios over time. The ratio is highest in infancy and declines throughout childhood into adolescence. Females reach the lowest ratio point around 12 to 13 years, whereas males hit theirs about two years later (from age 13 to 15). Until approximately 12 years of age, 55% to

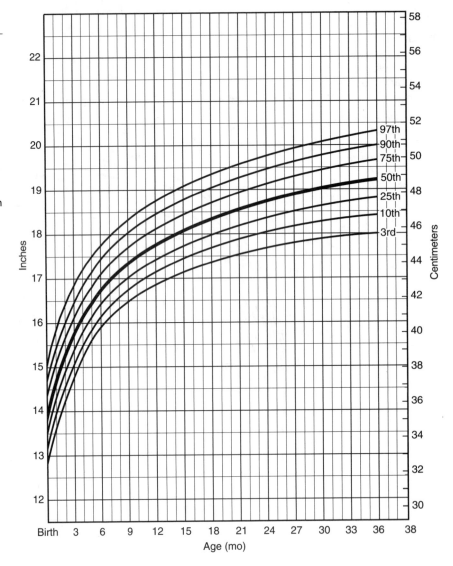

■ *Figure 3.8*

Head circum-
ference for age
percentiles: Girls,
from birth to
36 months

Source: Developed by
the National Center
for Health Statistics
in collaboration with
the National Center
for Chronic Disease
Prevention and Health
Promotion (2000)

60% of overall height gains for both sexes are attributed to leg growth
because males and females experience almost identical increases in sitting height (trunk length). Prior to adolescence males and females are
proportionately similar in terms of relative leg and trunk length. However, after that point in time, females exhibit, for an equal stature, relatively shorter legs than males.

Changes in Shoulder and Hip Width The shoulder/hip ratio serves
as a basic descriptor of proportional growth in the human body. It
also provides information with biomechanical implications for motor

■ *Figure 3.9*

Measuring sitting height

performance. The shoulder/hip ratio is determined from two measurements: (a) biacromial breadth (or shoulder width)—the distance between the right and left acromial processes (figure 3.11 on page 80); and (b) bicristal breadth (or hip width)—the distance between the right and left iliocristales.

Although hip and shoulder width appear almost equal in the newborn (refer to figure 3.5 on page 75), shoulder width is typically greater than hip width for all individuals. Figure 3.12 on the next page illustrates shoulder (biacromial) and hip (bicristal) width values for males and

■ *Figure 3.10*

Ratios of sitting height to stature

Source: Data from Hansman (1970) as reported by Malina (1984)

■ *Figure 3.11*

(a) Measuring biacromial (shoulder) width
(b) Measuring bicristal breadth (hip width)

a.

b.

THINK ABOUT IT

What is the relationship between specific body proportions and motor performance after pubertal change?

females from 6 to 17 years of age. Although there are differences between the sexes prior to adolescence, the variances are generally minimal. Beginning with the pubescent growth spurt, the obvious broadening of the shoulders relative to the hips is characteristic in males, whereas females experience greater hip breadth gains relative to the shoulders and waist. The biacromial/bicristal ratio remains relatively constant in males from ages 6 to 11 years, then exhibits a marked increase that continues up to around 6 years. This increase is due primarily to the fact

■ *Figure 3.12*

Shoulder and hip width values

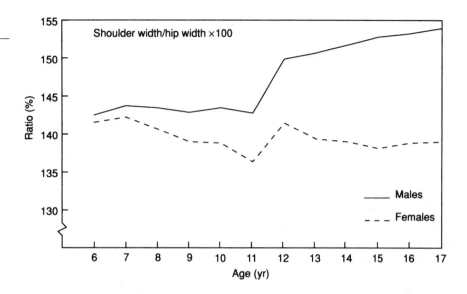

▨ *Figure 3.13*

Shoulder and hip
width ratios

that shoulder breadth is increasing at a more rapid rate than hip breadth. After peaking at approximately 12 years of age, the ratio for females steadily declines as a result of increased hip growth relative to shoulder breadth (figure 3.13).

Physique

Also referred to as body build, *physique* is a composite of body proportion relationships and body composition characteristics. An informal assessment of body build is made when an individual is identified using terms such as *stocky*, *lean*, *muscular*, or *soft-bodied*. Various ratios of body mass (weight) to height have been used to provide a simple and convenient estimate of physique; however, several limitations have been noted. Because body proportions change with growth, it is very difficult to develop a scheme of body typing for use over the life span. The best-known and most widely used method of classifying body builds was developed by Sheldon, Dupertuis, and McDermott (1954).

Sheldon's somatotype classifications are a complex rating of standardized photographs used in combination with a height/weight index score. The Sheldon method uses three general body build components to categorize an individual's **somatotype,** or body build: endomorphy, mesomorphy, and ectomorphy. *Endomorphy* describes a body type that is soft and round in contour, suggestive of a tendency toward fatness and obesity; *mesomorphy* describes a body with well-defined muscularity and balanced body proportions; *ectomorphy* describes the leanest of the body types, with characteristics typically associated with an extremely thin individual.

Each somatotype is viewed as a continuum for that particular body build rather than as a discrete and separate category. Individuals are rated from one to seven (seven is the highest) on each of these body types. For example, a somatotype rating of 2-6-2 (endomorph-mesomorph-ectomorph) describes a mesomorph with only slight endomorphy and ectomorphy characteristics. An important limitation of Sheldon's method is that the ratings were not developed to classify females and children. Furthermore, somatotyping is not a highly scientific method because it is primarily descriptive and subjective. Subsequent investigators have modified Sheldon's method to make the rating process more objective by incorporating data on body composition, by using anthropometric measures, and by including children and females (Carter & Heath, 1990; Peterson, 1967).

There appears to be a void in the literature related to changes in physique during the growing years. Some evidence suggests a strong genetic link based on the high percentage of children who acquire their parent's body build. Still, there is no strong evidence indicating consistency in physique from the early years to maturity. There have been reports that males, in general, are more mesomorphic from preschool through young adulthood and that females consistently exhibit more endomorphic characteristics. A rather consistent observation is that considerable variation exists within sex, racial, and geographic groups in children and adults. For an excellent discussion on this topic refer to Malina and Bouchard (1991).

THINK ABOUT IT

Describe how nature/nurture can affect physique.

Changes with Aging

As individuals reach middle age, mesomorphic characteristics tend to diminish due to loss of muscle mass; consequently, more endomorphic and ectomorphic traits are exhibited. As a result of bone tissue loss with a decrease in total height, changes in body proportions also tend to occur with aging.

Structural Development

Height

Objective 3.6

➤ The measurement of body length is one of the simplest and most common measures of structural growth. Height is determined by measuring the individual either while lying down or in a standing position. Until the infant can stand erect without assistance, total body length is measured in the supine position from the vertex (top of head) to the heel. A special slide ruler (figure 3.14) or anthropometer is used to measure the distance to the nearest ⅛ inch (0.1 cm). The preferred measurement of body length is standing height (stature), which is the distance between the vertex and the floor. To gain greatest accuracy, measurements are taken without shoes, using a sliding headboard (figure 3.15).

■ *Figure 3.14*

Measuring recumbent length in infants

We learned earlier that the embryo at about 8 weeks begins to take human form and has a body length of approximately 1 inch (2.5 cm). During the remainder of prenatal development, a phenomenal rate of growth produces an average length at birth of 20 inches (50 cm). The growth rates that occur during the nine months preceding birth and the first year of life are the fastest the body will experience. A typical child will increase its birth length by 50% at 1 year and reach

■ *Figure 3.15*

Measuring standing height (stature)

TABLE 3.4

Expected Increase in Height per Year

Age (yr)	Increase (in)		
Birth	[Average height = 20 in]		
0–1	9.8		
1–2	4.8		
2–3	3.1		
3–4	2.9		
4–5	2.7		
5–6	2.7		
6–7	2.4		
7–8	2.2		
8–9	2.2		
9–10	2.0		
10–11	1.9 Male	2.3 Female	
11–12	1.9	2.5	
12–13	2.2	2.6	
13–14	2.8	1.9	

Source: Modified from Lowrey (1986)

approximately ½ of adult height by 2 years of age (see table 3.4). After age 2, the growth rate slows somewhat to average about 2 inches per year until the onset of the pubescent growth spurt. It is not uncommon for children to experience a *midgrowth spurt* in height around the age of 7, although this change is usually less dramatic than the adolescent spurt. Growth accelerates before and during puberty, with peak rates of between 3 and 4 inches per year. Until puberty, males on the average are slightly taller than females; however, there is a large overlap, with some females taller than males. Females generally enter the height growth spurt two years earlier than males and typically complete the process in a shorter period of time (figure 3.16); however, the age of onset and completion can vary considerably.

Females, on the average, complete their peak growth period by 16½ years of age, whereas males continue to gain in stature for another two years or so. Males are 4 to 6 inches taller than females when they reach mature height. According to Tanner (1990), maximum growth of the long bones may not be reached until about age 25 and of the vertebral column until approximately 30 years, at which time an individual may add ⅛ to ¼ inch to his or her height. As illustrated in figure 3.17, height remains relatively stable until sometime after the third decade of life when total height begins to regress. Figure 3.18 (see page 86) and

■ *Figure 3.16*

Typical velocity
curves for males
and females
illustrating height
gain per year

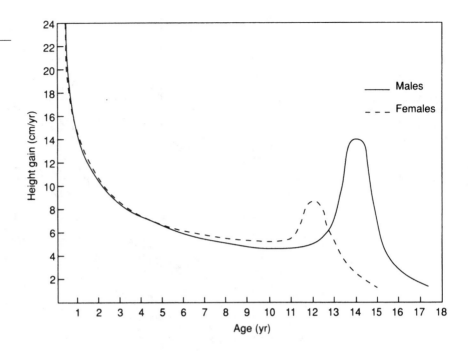

■ *Figure 3.16*

Typical velocity
curves for males
and females
illustrating height
gain per year

■ *Figure 3.17*

Distance curves
for stature

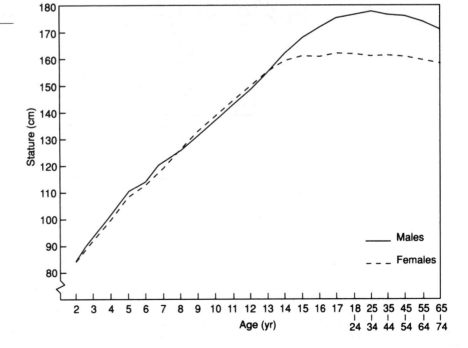

■ *Figure 3.17*

Distance curves
for stature

■ *Figure 3.18*

Stature-for-age percentiles: Boys, from 2 to 20 years

Source: Developed by the National Center for Health Statistics in collaboration with the National Center for Chronic Disease Prevention and Health Promotion (2000)

figure 3.19 provide percentile charts for comparing individual growth values (from 2 to 20 years).

Skeletal Growth

The process of bone growth and development that will lead to skeletal maturation begins with the formation of mesoderm cells in the embryo about 16 days after fertilization. Approximately five to six weeks after conception, the first ossification centers appear in the jawbones and collarbones. This is also the approximate time that the long bones of

■ *Figure 3.19*

Stature-for-age percentiles: Girls, from 2 to 20 years

Source: Developed by the National Center for Health Statistics in collaboration with the National Center for Chronic Disease Prevention and Health Promotion (2000)

the upper arm and leg appear in a cartilage form. Soon after the cartilage takes the shape of a long bone at about 2 months (fetal age), a ring of true bone begins to form. At the same time, primary ossification centers begin to appear in the midportion (*diaphysis*) of the long bones. In most bones, the primary ossification center appears by the third month of fetal life. The developmental status of a human fetus skeleton at 18 weeks is shown in figure 3.20 on page 88.

Ossification is the transformation of cartilage to true bone. It proceeds from the center of the shaft outward in both directions until the entire shaft is ossified. More than 800 ossification centers appear in the

■ *Figure 3.20*

A fetal skeleton at 18 weeks. Dark areas denote ossified portions and spaces between cartilage models.

body after birth. Shortly after birth, secondary ossification centers appear at the end of the shaft (*epiphyseal area*), forming the epiphyseal plate, or growth plate. Basically, cartilage cells are nourished by the blood in a reservoir next to the epiphysis. They begin to increase in size in the *proliferating zone* before moving on to the *hypertrophic zone* where the cells arrange themselves in vertical columns. At that point, the cartilage cells erode, and true bone begins to grow as collagen is secreted by *osteoblasts* (the bone cells engaged in producing true bone). *Osteocytes*, the principal cells of mature bone, become trapped in the tissue matrix and collect calcium and phosphorus. Essentially bone is a matrix composed primarily of collagen fibers and noncollagenous proteins. When full maturity is completed, the epiphysis fuses to the *metaphysis* (the area between diaphysis and epiphysis) and the growth plate is erased (figure 3.21).

■ *Figure 3.21*

(Left) Long bone with upper and lower epiphyses (Right) General process of bone formation

Source: Modified from Tanner (1990)

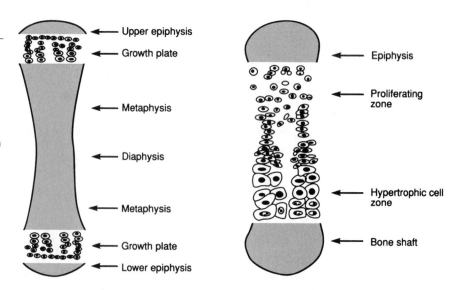

The mechanism controlling bone girth (appositional growth) is not as complex as the cartilage replacement processes responsible for growth in length. New rings of bone are added in circular layers on top of the old layers formed earlier. The bone has a compensating mechanism that controls thickness. As new rings are added old layers are removed from the inner circumference of the bone sleeve, permitting the shell to become thicker. This process continues until each of the long bones reaches full maturity in late childhood to early adulthood.

Another important mechanism of long bone growth is modeling resorption. At birth the bone shaft tends to flare out at its ends, hence creating a thinner middle. As the bone grows in length, the end becomes wider and the shaft heavier. The mechanism for maintaining the linear form of the bone is called *modeling resorption*. As the ends become increasingly thick, the excess bone tissue is removed by a process of resorption or breakdown, thus permitting the bone to maintain its linear shape while it is growing longer.

During the growth of short bones of the wrist and fingers, the core of the bone in the center of the cartilage steadily enlarges. At the same time, the original cartilage itself is growing appositionally as more cartilage is deposited on its surface. Growth of new bone tissue proceeds faster than growth of cartilage; thus more and more bone is added to the developing structure. This continues until the bone matures fully.

Epiphyseal plate closure, indicative of long bone maturity, generally starts somewhere between 13½ and 18 years of age, beginning at the distal humerus. Most of the long bones reach maturity from about 16 to 18 years of age in females and 18 to 21 in males. Cranial development follows a different postnatal growth curve. The majority of growth is completed by 3 years, with 50% attained by the ninth month. There are areas of the braincase, however, that do not reach maturity until well into adulthood.

Females, from birth, typically have a more developed skeleton than males. Females are approximately 20% more advanced in skeletal maturity than boys, which in practical terms is a difference of about two months at age 1 and two years at age 10. There are also indications that there is less variability in rate of ossification for females. Greater size in the male after puberty is due to the longer growing period (approximately two years) and the increased production of adrenal androgens and testosterone. As will be noted later in the discussion of maturity estimates, skeletal age may precede or lag behind chronological age by as much as a year.

Changes with Aging

Normal aging causes the bones to lose mass and the total height to decrease. Women begin to lose bone mineral at about age 30 and men at approximately 50 years of age. Stature decreases with age because of

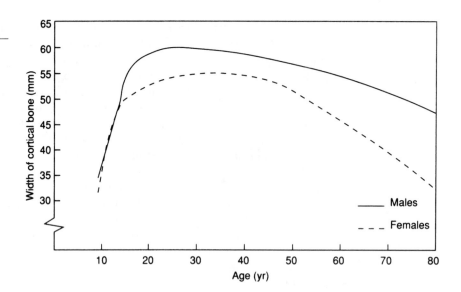

Figure 3.22

Age changes in width of cortical bone (second metacarpal)

an increase in postural kyphosis (rounding of the back), compression of intravertebral disks, and deterioration of vertebrae. Estimates of height decreases from 35 to 75 years of age are about 1 inch for males and 2 inches for females.

The loss of bone mass presents a more complex problem, especially in women. Bone loss in women begins slowly during the third decade (0.75% to 1% per year) and can increase to a higher rate (2% to 3% per year) shortly before and after menopause. The total bone mineral mass loss by age 70 is approximately 25% to 30%. Bone loss estimates for men at age 70 are about half what women experience (12% to 15% by age 70). The amount of bone loss is specific to the individual and varies considerably in different types of bone. Age- and sex-related changes in the width of cortical bone are illustrated in figure 3.22; figure 3.23 depicts loss of spine and femur bone density in females with advanced aging.

Figure 3.23

Loss of bone density in females

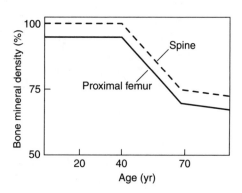

Osteoporosis has become a familiar term to the general public; it refers to the loss of total bone mass to such an extent that the skeleton is unable to maintain its mechanical integrity. The development of this condition is a complex process influenced by a variety of nutritional (related primarily to calcium), physical, hormonal (primarily estrogen), and genetic factors. In the scientific community there is some debate concerning the dividing line between normal aging of bones and the more pronounced brittleness of bones generally associated with osteoporosis. As a result of osteoporosis bones tend to break more easily, which increases the risk of fracture. Almost one–half of all women over the age of 60 are affected by osteoporosis.

■ *Body Mass*

Objective 3.7

➤ Body weight and body composition are terms frequently used to describe an individual's **body mass.** Body weight is a general descriptor of total body mass that is a composite of all tissue components. Body composition, in contrast, is a description of the various independent tissue components—namely, lean body mass (fat–free weight), and body fat. Thus, body weight equals lean body mass plus fat. The following discussion of body composition will focus on skeletal muscle tissue (lean body mass) and body fat. It should be noted, however, that lean body mass (for body weight measures) encompasses all of the body's nonfat tissues including skeleton, muscle, water, connective tissue, organ tissues, and teeth. The growth and development of cardiac (heart) muscle tissue will be discussed in chapter 4.

Body Weight

The assessment of body weight is the most common anthropometric measure used to estimate body mass. Instrumentation is relatively simple in that the individual stands on clinical scales (preferably beam-type) without shoes and dressed in as little clothing as possible (preferably briefs or bathing suit). Infant scales and bed scales are typically used for the disabled, elderly, or other individuals not capable of standing without aid. Weight is measured to the nearest tenth of a kilogram (or quarter of a pound).

The embryo at 8 weeks weighs about half an ounce (14 g); by the end of the fifth month the fetus weighs about 1 pound (450 g). The last two months of prenatal life is a period of rapid weight gain. The fetus gains about half a pound (225 g) a week for a total of 5 pounds (2,250 g) on the average. Just a few weeks before birth (and at delivery), the average fetus weighs about 7 pounds (3.2 g). Females, on the average, are about half a pound smaller than males at birth.

■ *Figure 3.24*

Distance curves for
body weight

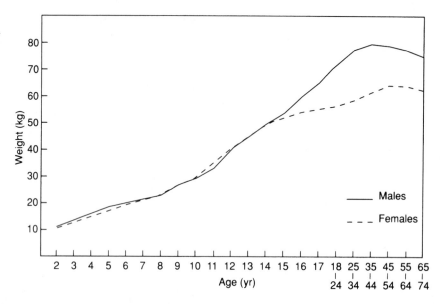

Total body mass generally decreases during the first few days after birth due to transition factors such as maternal milk supply and level of physiological stress. However, birth weight is usually regained within two weeks. Body weight doubles after three to four months, triples at one year, quadruples by the second year, and by age 7 increases seven times the birth weight (Lowrey, 1986). Most children will reach one-half of their mature body mass by age 10. Figure 3.24 illustrates a distance curve for body weight among individuals 2 to 74 years of age.

The pubescent growth spurt for body weight is similar to the height curve except that it generally continues for a longer time. Female growth patterns reveal a particularly rapid weight gain between the ages of 12 and 13. As in the growth pattern for height, males begin the growth spurt later than females and add more body size. Males increase their body mass by about 45 pounds (20 kg) and females by approximately 35 pounds (16 kg) by early adulthood. Mature body weight is about 20 times that of birth weight. Total body mass begins to decline with aging as a reflection of bone and muscle tissue losses. Figures 3.25 and 3.26 (see page 94) compare individual growth values using percentile charts (from ages 2 to 20 years).

Body Composition

Body weight is a general measure of body mass and therefore does not break down the contribution of different tissues making up this collective measurement. A measure of body composition, however, independently assesses two types of tissue: muscle tissue (lean body mass) and body fat. A variety of measurement techniques are available to estimate

▪ *Figure 3.25*

Weight-for-age
percentiles: Boys,
from 2 to 20 years

Source: Developed by
the National Center
for Health Statistics
in collaboration with
the National Center
for Chronic Disease
Prevention and Health
Promotion (2000)

total body fatness, lean body mass, or both. All of the measurement
descriptions that follow are only *estimates* because they are indirectly
determined. The only direct way of taking the measurements is by making a biochemical analysis of cadavers.

Some of the more common techniques for measuring body
composition are underwater weighing, radiographs (X rays), anthropometric dimensions (skinfolds), and body mass index. Although
potassium–40 (a naturally occurring isotope) is also used to measure and
predict body composition (i.e., lean body mass), this method is almost
completely restricted to research because the necessary equipment is so
expensive.

■ *Figure 3.26*

Weight-for-age percentiles: Girls, from 2 to 20 years

Source: Developed by the National Center for Health Statistics in collaboration with the National Center for Chronic Disease Prevention and Health Promotion (2000)

Underwater (hydrostatic) weighing is considered the most accurate indirect means of measurement and serves as a standard for other methods such as skinfold measurement. In underwater weighing, the percentage of body fat is computed by finding the ratio of body weight to body volume, called body density. Body volume is equal to the loss of weight in water with the appropriate temperature correction for the density of water. Using other equations, total body fat and lean body weight can also be measured. The equations used to predict body density with underwater weighing were formulated from the chemical analyses of human adult cadavers. The use of the same equations for younger populations has been known to give problems in developmental interpretation.

In the past, the body fat content of children was estimated from an adult model on the assumption that the child's body composition was chemically equivalent to that of a mature individual. Evidence suggests, however, that pre- and postadolescent children are not chemically mature and may have a fat-free body density lower than that of an adult. Body density, in this context, refers to water content and bone mineral content of the fat–free body. Water content of the fat-free body typically falls from about 81% at birth to around 72% in adulthood. The adult level appears to be reached around 15 years of age. Bone mineral content also varies between the adult and child models. In general, bone density increases with age from the early fetal period to adulthood; male bones are heavier than female bones. In addition, there is some evidence that the bones of blacks are heavier than those of whites.

In summary, children and youth are likely to have higher body water content and lower bone mineral than adults, which result in a lower fat-free body density. Therefore, body composition estimates for children from adult equations may over–estimate values. Updated equations based on better estimates of children's fat-free body composition are available (see Lohman, 1989, 1992). These estimates may provide more accurate information about children's body composition in particular, and about patterns of growth and development in general.

Radiographs (X rays) are used to assess regional changes in fat, muscle, and bone during growth. When proper laboratory facilities are not available, subcutaneous skinfolds can also provide accurate regional information about growth changes. In nonlaboratory field situations, skinfold measurements and body mass index are popular. The rationale for using skinfold measurements is based on the fact that a relationship exists between the amount of fat located directly beneath the surface of the skin and body composition (internal body fat). Skinfold equations are derived using statistical techniques of multiple regression that predict the results of the underwater weighing procedure. It is essential for individuals to be measured using an equation derived from a compatible population; this has implications for measuring children and adults. The triceps skinfold and the more recently introduced medial calf skinfold correlate more closely with body density data derived from underwater weighing procedures. Limitations of this method include its use for measuring very thin or obese individuals, skinfold caliper accuracy, and tester reliability.

Body mass index (BMI) is a calculation of body fat based on height and body weight:

$$BMI = body\ weight\ [kg]/height^2\ [m]$$

This method has been used more in recent years as an alternative to skinfolds because it can be easily administered. The predictive accuracy

■ *Figure 3.27*

Body mass index-for-age percentiles: Boys, from 2 to 20 years

Source: Developed by the National Center for Health Statistics in collaboration with the National Center for Chronic Disease Prevention and Health Promotion (2000)

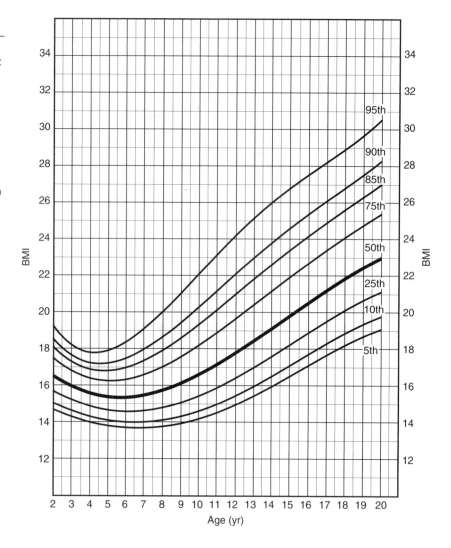

of this as an estimate of body fat has not been extensively studied. The existing data indicate that it warrants only a fair rating and is less accurate than the triceps skinfold method. The basic limitation of BMI is that it ignores the possibility that muscle tissue rather than fat may contribute to excessive body weight relative to height. Figures 3.27 and 3.28 show BMI valves from 2 to 20 years of age.

On the average, males at all ages have greater body densities and greater lean body mass than females (Malina & Bouchard, 1991). While the differences are closer during the childhood years, females have greater amounts of body fat across the life span. This difference is magnified as adolescence approaches and continues on through development.

■ *Figure 3.28*

Body mass index-for-age percentiles: Girls, from 2 to 20 years

Source: Developed by the National Center for Health Statistics in collaboration with the National Center for Chronic Disease Prevention and Health Promotion (2000)

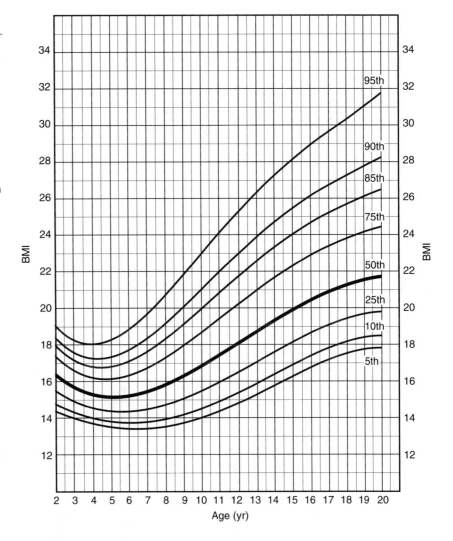

Figure 3.29 on page 98 shows selected body composition values for ages 7 to 70. During the pubescent growth spurt, males experience a rapid increase in lean body mass and a decrease in percentage of fat. Females also experience an increase in lean mass, although less than males, and an increase in body fat. Figure 3.30 on page 99 depicts estimated changes in fat-free mass, fat mass, and relative percent fat during the first 20 years.

Body Fat Growth Body fat layers appear in the fetus between the seventh and eighth prenatal months. Between birth and 6 to 9 months, body fat mass will increase 10% to 20% before tapering off to a plateau that may last from five to seven years. On the average, percentage of body

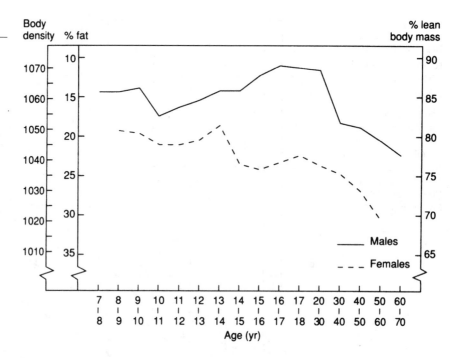

■ *Figure 3.29*

Body composition change as a function of age

fat increases from about 16% at birth to between 24% and 30% at 1 year. By age 6 body fat decreases to approximately 14% of body weight. Some individuals will experience an increase during the mid-growth spurt of 5½ to 7 years, which generally ceases after that period in males but continues in females through the adolescent years. As noted earlier, females have more body fat (absolute and relative) than males at all ages, with differences being more apparent during and after puberty.

Fat and muscle cells grow both in number (*hyperplasia*) and in size (*hypertrophy*). The adult of average body size has between 25 to 50 billion fat cells. Obese individuals may have 75 billion or more (McArdle, et al., 2001). The size of fat cells in children up to 1 year is about ¼ that of adult fat cells. Fat cell size triples during the first 6 years, then remains relatively stable until the onset of puberty. At this time, very little information is available on fat cell development during adolescence. What exists suggests that cell size increases during the growth spurt because the cells of adults are significantly larger than cells at age 13 or in late adolescence.

By the end of the first year of life, the number of fat cells is about three times what it was at birth. It is believed that most of the fat cell production takes place during the last trimester before birth. After the first year, the number of cells increases gradually until the onset of the pubescent growth spurt, at which time the number increases significantly

■ *Figure 3.30*

■ *Figure 3.30*

Body composition
across age for
boys and girls

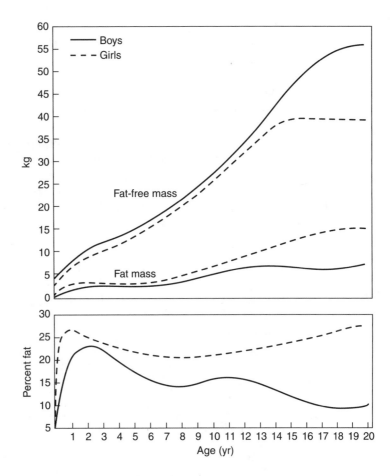

(Dietz, 1997). Although the evidence is not decisive, there is speculation that fat cells are particularly prone to overmultiplying if overfeeding occurs during the early stages of life (Hager, et al., 1977; Oscai et al., 1972). Relationships have been drawn between overfeeding, excessive fat cell multiplication, and the weight control problems that individuals may experience in later life. There are also indications that reduced fetal fat deposition in late pregnancy (i.e., less intake by the mother) may lead to subsequent greater leanness in the infant (Dietz, 1997).

Although there is some disagreement, it is generally believed that by adulthood (or perhaps before) the number of cells becomes fixed and increases in size only, except in cases of extreme obesity. When individuals gain fat tissue as a result of overeating, their fat cells enlarge but no new cells are created. Complementing this line of information, Dietz describes three critical periods for the development of obesity: the prenatal period, between 4 and 6 years of age, and adolescence (especially in females). As noted in chapter 2, about 25% of the variation among people in percent body fat is genetically determined; thus there is considerable environmental effect.

Skeletal Muscle Tissue Growth   Muscle fibers develop in the premuscular mesodermic tissue. After the 16th week of fetal development, the first muscle fibers can be identified. Growth of voluntary muscle during the prenatal period is both hyperplastic and hypertrophic. The hyperplastic phase continues until shortly after birth, after which cell growth is predominantly achieved by increasing cell size hypertrophy. The increase in mass of a skeletal muscle of up to 50 times during postnatal development is due almost exclusively to a massive increase in the size of individual fibers (Lang & Luff, 1990). Thickness of the muscle fibers at birth is approximately one-fifth that in an adult. Protein, the essential element in muscle composition, increases gradually during the fetal period and, by birth, reaches a level very near that found in adults. Approximately 15% of total body mass of the fetus halfway through its development consists of skeletal muscle tissue. This percentage increases progressively to about 25% of birth weight for both sexes. Approximately 40% to 50% of body mass in the adult male is skeletal muscle. Females generally do not show a significant increase in lean body mass during puberty; and at maturity they have only about 60% of the muscle mass and force characteristics of males.

The differentiation of fiber types and sizes is frequently used to describe muscle growth and development. Basically, in the adult, *type I fibers* (described as slow twitch) are relatively fatigue resistant, and are associated with the performance of aerobic endurance activities (e.g., long-distance running and cycling). *Type II fibers*, in contrast, are *fast twitch* and have the capacity to contract more rapidly and forcefully, but they also fatigue rapidly. Fast-twitch fibers are associated with the performance of short-duration (anaerobic) activities (e.g., sprinting, jumping, and weight lifting). At birth and through childhood, type I fibers constitute approximately 50% to 60% of all muscle fibers. During this same period, only about 25% of type II fibers are found. The amount of undifferentiated fibers ranges from 15% to 20%. In adults there are very few, if any, undifferentiated fibers (Baldwin & Haddard, 2001; Jesper et al., 2000).

Studies that have investigated muscle fiber changes during adolescence have noted the possible significant effects of pubertal hormones on growth and differentiation. Researchers have found a relatively high percentage (7% to 13%) of transitional fibers in adolescents. In *transitional fibers* the functional features of the enzyme system may develop as either aerobic (type I) or anaerobic (type II), depending on the physical training to which the fibers are treated. These fibers supposedly develop after infancy due to the influence of pubertal hormones. Such factors may have implications for motor programming and training with adolescents.

With regard to muscle fiber size, the typical adult has a fiber diameter of 50 to 60 micrometers. At about the 14th or 15th week of fetal development the fiber is approximately 6 micrometers; by birth the diameter has doubled. By the end of the first year the fiber size will be about 30% of adult size; at 5 years it will reach approximately 50%. It should be noted, however, that size (and type) of muscle fiber can vary considerably in fetuses of the same age. There does not appear to be any major differences between upper and lower extremities or proximal and distal muscles, or any significant variance between the sexes. Although several hypotheses have been proposed concerning how muscle growth and differentiation take place in both the prenatal and neonatal period, the strongest is that the pattern is inherited and genetically coded in the nucleus of the muscle cell.

Changes with Aging

THINK ABOUT IT

Using a distance curve format, illustrate the major physical growth milestones across the life span. Then, briefly summarize each event.

Significant changes in body fat and lean muscle mass take place with aging. Whereas height decreases with age, weight increases steadily beginning in the third decade and continues until 55 to 60 years of age, when it declines (Frisancho, 1990). An increase in body weight is usually accompanied by gains in body fat and a decrease in lean body mass. After age 60 or so, total body weight decreases despite the increase in body fat, due in part to loss of muscle and bone mass. At 17 years of age, the average male is 15% fat and by 60 years increases to about 28%. Females change from about 25% body fat at 17 years to approximately 39% at 60 years. These values can vary to quite an extent depending on lifestyle and tend to be less in individuals who are physically active. Refer to figure 3.29 for selected estimated body composition values for age.

As individuals age, the distribution of body fat also tends to change. With advanced aging there is an increased general tendency for a large proportion of the total body fat to be located internally rather than subcutaneously (Schwartz et al., 1990). As females age they tend to accumulate fat in the hip, thigh, and breast region, while in males, the abdomen is the specified site (Bemben et al., 1995). To some extent, these patterns of distribution are inherited.

Lean body (fat-free) mass tends to decrease with age. This overall effect is due primarily to the loss of bone mass (15% to 30%) and the reduction of muscle mass. Most individuals experience a marked deterioration in muscle mass with aging. For people over 60 years of age, the loss of muscle mass can be as high as 30% to 50% of that in young adults. Overall lean body mass loss approximates losses in muscle and bone. Table 3.5 summarizes physical growth changes with advancing age.

TABLE 3.5

Summary of Physical Growth Changes with Aging

Physical Growth Characteristic	
Stature	Decreases
Bone mass	Decreases
Body weight	Increases/Decreases (after 60)
Percent body fat	Increases
Lean body (muscle) mass	Decreases
Distribution of fat	More internal

Maturity Estimates

Objective 3.8

➤ Because maturation is a qualitative process, it can be a challenge to determine in quantitative terms how far an individual has progressed along his or her road to full maturity. Level of maturity is generally estimated from chronological age and biological (developmental) age characteristics.

Chronological age refers to the age of an individual in relationship to standard calendar days. To estimate level of maturity using this method alone is of limited value because of the wide variance in growth and development that is possible at any single age. An accurate calculation of chronological age does provide the basic factor with which measures of growth and development are compared when estimating level of maturity. The measurement of **biological age** generally provides a better method for estimating maturity by providing information that may be compared with the individual's age. Characteristics commonly used in a measurement of biological age include estimates of morphological age, dental age, sexual age, and skeletal age.

Morphological Age

The term *morphology* refers to the form or structure of an individual. Morphological age is usually estimated from height. A measure of height is easy to attain, and there are several height percentile charts that indicate where an individual ranks for a given age and sex. A frequently used general assessment of a person's maturity might indicate that he or she is above or below average for age and sex. A measure of height alone, however, is not a good estimate of maturity because individuals differ in mature height. To be assessed as above average in height at a specific time in a child's life may signify either a rapid pace of growth or an average rate of growth for a child who will be above average in height as an adult.

Dental Age

The age at which teeth erupt may also provide information on approximate level of maturity. Eruption of both deciduous (temporary) and permanent teeth in most individuals occurs fairly predictably. The deciduous dentition erupts from 6 months to 2 years; permanent teeth generally appear from about 6 to 13 years of age. One limitation of using dental age to gain a complete perspective of full maturity is the lack of available information on dentition growth between the ages of 2 to 6 years and after age 13. Recent research has focused on dental calcification seen in X rays as a promising indicator of dental age.

Sexual Age

This biological estimate of sexual age refers to the assessed maturity of primary and secondary sexual qualities. Subjective maturity rating scales are often used to evaluate the status of sexual development in the reproduction organs, pubic hair, and breast development and menarche in females. Of the sexual characteristics of females, the age of menarche (first menstrual flow) is the most common standard of maturity.

In most cases, menarche occurs relatively late in the adolescent growth period, after growth in height has peaked. Approximately 96% of females experience menarche between the ages of 11 and 15. It can also be estimated from this data that most females will have their first menstrual flow between 12 and 13 years of age. Although menarche indicates maturity in uterine development, it does not always denote full maturity of the female reproductive system. Initially menstrual cycles may be very irregular, and it may be several years after periods begin that a female becomes fertile. Figures 3.31 and 3.32 on page 104 illustrate the normal range of the development of selected sexual characteristics in males and females.

Skeletal Age

Perhaps the best method of maturity estimate is derived from evaluating the successive stages of skeletal growth as seen in X rays. Also referred to as bone age, skeletal age provides a good estimate of maturity because its development spans virtually the entire period of active growth and maturation. All normally developing people, regardless of whether they are early, average, or late maturing, will eventually reach a stage of complete skeletal maturity. Skeletal maturity is usually

■ *Figure 3.31*

Average age and range of sexual development in males

Source: Tanner (1990)

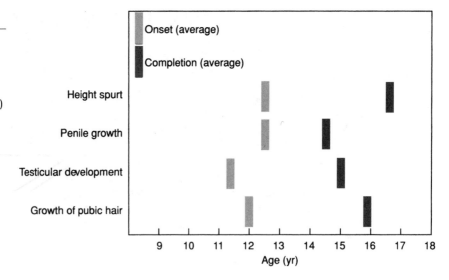

measured by x-raying the bones of the left wrist and hand complex, which consists of some 29 separate ossification centers. The hand and wrist, however, only provide useful information for those about 18 months of age and older. Other parts, such as the leg, knee, and foot, have also been recommended for measuring the skeletal age of younger and older populations. The progressive enlargement and change in shape of ossification centers can be detected on X ray and compared

■ *Figure 3.32*

Average age and range of sexual development in females

Source: Tanner (1990)

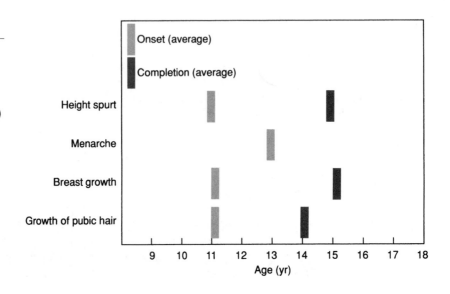

■ *Figure 3.33*

X ray of the hand showing the skeletal maturity of a male at 48 months or a female at 37 months

with other X rays standardized to represent skeletal ages at six-month and one-year intervals (figures 3.33 and 3.34).

Along with the differences in skeletal growth, these X rays can differentiate the male and female maturity rates. Females, in general, are more biologically mature than males. Areas that appear as spaces between the wrist and fingers (black or grayish in appearance) are cartilaginous bone not yet calcified. As the bone matures, or ossifies, it becomes more dense and thus is more visible in the X ray. Females are approximately 20% more advanced in skeletal maturity than males. In practical terms, the difference is about 2 months at age 1, and 2 years at age 10. Popular atlases of skeletal maturity include those developed by Greulich and Pyle (1959) and Tanner and Associates (1983).

■ *Figure 3.34*

X ray of the hand showing the skeletal maturity of a male at 156 months or a female at 128 months

Maturity Variations

Objective 3.9

➤ Although diet and other health factors may influence the rate of maturity, the biological clock within the individual sets the pace of maturation. Individuals are generally grouped into categories of early, average, and late maturers, according to where they fit on various maturational scales. We are often concerned with the development of individuals who appear to be late maturers or early maturers. As noted earlier, it can be difficult to quantify a rather qualitative aspect of growth and development. However, the extremes can be established with more accuracy than levels in the midrange of maturity.

Early maturers are those in whom the maturity characteristics are in advance of their chronological age, whereas late-maturing individuals are behind in relation to the standard. For example, an individual with a chronological age of 10 and a skeletal age of 13 is categorized as ahead (early maturing) of the normal maturation pace. A female who experiences menarche at 10 years (when the average is 12.5 years) is also an early maturer. In contrast, a female who does not experience menarche until her 15th birthday is considered late maturing, as is the female who is 8 years old with a skeletal age of 6 years.

What is early or late? Keogh and Sugden (1985) suggest that when comparing chronological age with skeletal age, a 20% difference from mean skeletal age should be considered early or late, respectively. For example, if a 10-year-old is average maturing, he or she has a skeletal age of 10 years; a skeletal age of 8 years is considered late maturing, and a skeletal age of 12 years, early maturing. These, however, are arbitrary cutoffs, and clinical practice often uses up to one to three years on either side of chronological age. Early maturers, on the average, take four to five fewer years to achieve full skeletal maturity and tend to complete the pubertal growth period faster than late maturers.

THINK ABOUT IT

Can you think of any advantages of being a late-maturing person?

Although differences in maturity levels are apparent prior to the pubescent growth spurt, they appear to be most pronounced during adolescence. Early maturers are generally taller and heavier for their age than late-maturing peers. Late maturers, however, catch up to early maturers in stature during late adolescence or early adulthood. Various maturational rates also may affect body build. Early-maturing males are generally more mesomorphic, and early-maturing females more endomorphic. Later-maturing males and females tend to have less weight for stature, whereas early maturers of both sexes generally have more body fat during adolescence.

In terms of interaction with peers, early maturation appears to be advantageous. Early maturers are more likely to be elected to class offices, rated as popular, and excel in athletics. The superior size and advanced physiological characteristics (e.g., strength, and speed) associated with early maturing are in accord with male sex-role expectations.

■ *Figure 3.35*

Secular trend for menarche

For an excellent discussion of maturity-associated variation refer to Malina and Bouchard (1991) in the Suggested Readings.

Objective 3.10

➤ These maturational differences are *individual* differences. As a group, today's population is taller and heavier and matures earlier than the population of generations past. These observations are referred to as **secular trend.** Today the average female reaches adult height two years earlier than did females at the turn of the century. Figure 3.35 illustrates the secular trend for menarche. Note that menarche occurred around age 17 for Norwegian girls in 1840, compared with just over 13 years of age in 1969. For American girls, the mean age of menarche has been declining an average of about four months per decade. Thus, due primarily to improved health conditions and nutrition, females are maturing earlier (sexually).

Most males today reach adult stature by age 18 or 19, whereas about 75 years ago most males did not reach maximal height until age 25 or 26. Since 1900 children from average households have increased in height between the ages of 5 and 7 years by approximately 1 to 2 centimeters each decade. Secular differences in stature appear to be most evident during the adolescent growth period due to the faster rate of maturation in more recent generations. The difference between a 15-year-old male of 1880 and 1960 was approximately 5½ inches (14 cm). The difference in maximal adult height during that same period was of a lesser magnitude—about 3 inches (8 cm) (Eveleth & Tanner, 1990).

It has been suggested that secular trend in size and maturation in individuals from developed countries has leveled off in recent years.

THINK ABOUT IT

Considering the secular trend, speculate on the difference between the 15-year-old of today and the 15-year-old of the year 2050. What type of research design would you use to study this?

Speculation is that the factors associated with secular trend, in general, such as improvement in nutrition, reduction in the incidence of disease, better health practices, and greater genetic hybridization, have been maximized. A negative secular trend noted in recent years is that children carry more body fat than their counterparts of the 1960s (Centers for Disease Control, 2000). In addition, there is evidence that teenagers are less physically active than they were a decade ago and considerable speculation that the same general trend (due to such factors as watching more TV, etc.) applies to children. This topic is discussed in greater detail in chapter 5.

Implications for Motor Performance

Objective 3.11 ➤ All of the physical growth characteristics described in this chapter are related in some manner to motor performance. Although research has produced few conclusive findings, especially with young populations, some generalizations can be offered.

One of the original lines of study followed up in recent years is the relationship between body length and weight at birth to the onset of independent walking. A common finding of all investigations has been that infants who are longer for their weight tend to walk at an earlier age in comparison to shorter and fatter babies. However, follow-up studies have revealed that delayed groups usually catch up quickly and that initial walking patterns of the early group are quite immature. Similar inconclusive findings concerning young populations have also been reported concerning the relationships between body size, body mass, body fat, selected anthropometric measures, and strength-related tasks (e.g., Gabbard, 1982, 1985).

With school-age and older populations, research has demonstrated rather clearly an inverse relationship between excess body fat and performance on tasks that require the body to be propelled (e.g., running, and jumping), and particularly in endurance activities (Boileau, 1996; Claessens et al., 1999). In tasks requiring that an object be propelled or force be applied, increasing body size (fat-free mass) usually has a positive effect on performance. It should be noted, however, that the overall contribution of age, stature, and body mass to variation in motor performance is generally low to moderate at best.

Similar relationship levels have also been found in regard to strength performance and somatotype. In general, mesomorphy and endomorphy are related positively to strength, whereas ectomorphic characteristics are not. Relationships between body build and motor performance (especially with activities involving body propulsion and agility) are generally low between endomorphy and task performance. The inconsistency here is that correlations between individuals having mesomorphic qualities and motor performance are generally positive but low.

As noted earlier, the proportion of the infant's head in relationship to the remainder of the body may influence motor performance. Because infants are relatively top heavy, their ability to balance and perform such tasks as body rolling may be hindered. As body proportions change during childhood an individual's center of gravity may also vary considerably. Although the center of gravity remains relatively constant in proportion to total height with age, the center of gravity is higher in children because they carry a greater proportion of weight in the upper body. In general, females have a lower center of gravity than males, which contributes to the better performance of females in tasks requiring balance. From the age of 6 fetal months to 70 years the center of gravity descends gradually from the level of the seventh thoracic vertebra to the level of the first sacral (pelvis) segment (Swearingen et al., 1969).

The structural and anatomical changes that occur during adolescence also may contribute to motor performance differences between the sexes. As a result of the pubescent growth spurt, males generally become taller and heavier, develop wider shoulders and longer legs and forearms, and gain in lean body weight. Females during this period will develop a lower center of gravity.

The implications of these characteristics for performing motor tasks are not decisive but warrant consideration from a biomechanical perspective. The female's lower center of gravity and shorter legs give her better balance. Shorter leg length and wider hips, however, are disadvantageous in running (especially sprinting) and jumping events, when compared to the performance of males whose legs are proportionately longer and their hips narrower. The male's longer arms and wider shoulders also may provide a mechanical advantage for motor tasks involving throwing and striking. Research findings have estimated that body size and structure may account for 10% to 25% of the variance in motor performance scores (Haubenstricker & Sapp, 1985).

Summary

Characteristic of the changes in lifelong physical growth are the cephalocaudal and proximodistal patterns of development. The study of these changes can be measured using a variety of instruments and techniques.

Individuals grow faster during gestation and the first year after birth than at any other time in the life span. After conception, three major periods of physical growth are associated with the rapid changes that occur before birth: the germinal period, the embryonic period, and the fetal period.

Next to the rapid changes in growth that appear during the prenatal stage, the growth spurt that takes place with puberty represents the life span's most dramatic period of biological alteration. In males puberty is characterized by significant sexual, anatomical, and physiological changes. For females the changes are less dramatic, but a major milestone reached during this period is menarche—the first menstrual flow and the universal indicator of sexual maturity.

Along with the rapid changes in physical maturation and growth are the emergence of several landmarks in motor performance. One of the primary mechanisms at work in the changes associated with puberty is the endocrine system and the increased levels of hormones it releases. The hormones that have the greatest impact at this time are androgens, estrogens, and the growth hormone. Of those hormones, the greater quantities of androgens produced in males account, to a large extent, for the oftentimes significant differences found between the sexes.

Specific body parts undergo dramatic changes during the course of physical growth and development. Along with a doubling of head size, there are also comparable changes in limb length (especially the legs), trunk length, and shoulder and hip width. Prior to puberty, males and females appear to have similar body builds; however, noticeable differences occur thereafter, as evidenced by higher mesomorphic rating in males. With advancing age, mesomorphic characteristics tend to diminish and more endomorphic and ectomorphic traits appear. Changes may also occur in body proportions due primarily to a loss of bone tissue.

A typical child will increase birth length by 50% at 1 year of age and reach approximately one-half of mature height at 2 years of age. Most females complete their peak growth period by age 16½, while males continue to gain in stature for at least another two years.

The elaborate process of bone ossification begins shortly after conception and continues until maturity when epiphyseal plates and fusion areas are closed. Although growth of the long bones is generally complete by the early twenties, portions of the braincase do not reach maturity (or become fused) until well into adulthood.

With normal aging, stature decreases slightly, and the body has a tendency to develop kyphosis. More dramatic, however, is the loss of bone mass that occurs, especially in females. By the age of 70, some females may lose as much as 30% of total bone mineral mass. Related to bone loss is the condition of osteoporosis, which causes bones to break more easily and fractures to occur in old age. Bone loss estimates for males are about one-half the estimates for females.

Body mass characteristics (body weight and body composition) also undergo numerous changes over the life span. The growth spurt for body weight is similar to the height curve, except that it generally continues for a longer time. Males usually begin the spurt later and add more body size. Due primarily to the normal loss of bone and muscle tissue with advancing age, total body mass declines in later years.

Males at all ages have greater body densities and greater lean body mass than females. During the pubescent growth spurt, males experience rapid gains in lean body mass and decreases in the percentage of body fat. Most females, on the other hand, characteristically have greater amounts of body fat than males throughout the life span, with the difference more evident after puberty. With advancing age, body weight usually increases as body fat increases and lean body mass decreases. The loss of muscle mass in individuals over the age of 60 may be as high as 30% to 50%.

Estimating the level of physical maturity is best accomplished using measures of biological age rather than chronological age. Of these methods skeletal age, which is derived from comparisons of radiographs, is perhaps the most accurate estimate of physical maturity.

Individuals are often categorized as early, average, or late maturers, according to where they fit on various maturational scales. In general, early maturers are taller and heavier for their age than their late-maturing peers. However, late maturers often catch up to others during late adolescence or early adulthood.

Observations of secular trend indicate that today's population is maturing earlier and is taller than that of about 75 years ago. The explanation for this trend is complex but includes the factors of improved nutrition, reduced incidence of disease, and better health practices.

Though few conclusive findings have been reported, several generalizations can be made about the implications of change in physical growth for motor performance. One of the most evident is the relationship between the specific structural and anatomical changes that occur during adolescence and selected motor performance differences between the sexes.

Think about It

1. Consider some ways the phenomenon of puberty can influence participation in sports.
2. What is the relationship between specific body proportions and motor performance after pubertal change?
3. Describe how nature/nurture can affect physique.
4. Using a distance curve format, illustrate the major physical growth milestones across the life span. Then, briefly summarize each event.
5. Can you think of any advantages of being a late-maturing person?
6. Considering the secular trend, speculate on the difference between the 15-year-old of today and the 15-year-old of the year 2050. What type of research design would you use to study this?

Suggested Readings

CDC (2000). *CDC growth charts*, United States. National Center for Health Statistics, U.S. Department of Health and Human Services. Web site includes charts and measurement training module (http://www.cdc.gov/growthcharts/)

Malina, R. M., & Bouchard, C. (1991). *Growth, maturation, and physical activity.* Champaign, IL: Human Kinetics.

Spirduso, W. W. (1995). *Physical dimensions of aging.* Champaign, IL: Human Kinetics.

Tanner, J. M. (1990). *Fetus into man.* 2nd ed. Cambridge, MA: Harvard University Press.

WebLinks

Health Status Internet Assessments (Body mass index calculator)
http://healthstatus.com/bmi.htm

National Center for Health Statistics (CDC growth charts)
www.cdc.gov/growthcharts

American Academy of Pediatrics (Information on puberty)
www.aap.org/family/puberty.htm

March of Dimes
www.modimes.org

The Visible Embryo (Information on prenatal development)
www.visembryo.com

World Health Organization Global Database on Child Growth and Malnutrition
www.who.int/nutgrowthdb

4 *Physiological Changes*

OBJECTIVES

Upon completion of this chapter, you should be able to

4.1   Outline and briefly describe the basic structure and functions of the cardiorespiratory system.

4.2   Identify significant growth and development changes that occur during the part of the life span prior to puberty.

4.3   Distinguish between the terms *aerobic power* and *anaerobic power* and describe the lifelong developmental changes that take place in these characteristics.

4.4   List the major changes that occur over time in heart rate, cardiac output and stroke volume, and vital capacity and pulmonary ventilation.

4.5   Describe the ways in which the body's blood characteristics change as individuals age.

4.6   Define *basal metabolic rate* and briefly note how it changes over the life span.

4.7   Distinguish between the various types of muscular strength and describe how their characteristics may vary through the lifelong developmental process.

4.8   Discuss what determines flexibility and its developmental characteristics.

4.9   Describe the effects of advanced aging on each of the basic physiological functions in both general and specific terms.

KEY TERMS

maximal oxygen uptake (VO$_2$max)

aerobic power

anaerobic power

cardiac output

vital capacity

basal metabolic rate (BMR)

muscular strength

flexibility

IMPORTANT TO ANY COMPREHENSIVE DISCUSSION of lifelong motor development is an understanding of the basic physiological changes associated with exercise and motor skill performance. In the context of this aspect of developmental exercise physiology and motor development, this chapter will focus on the cardiovascular and respiratory systems, basal metabolic rate, muscular strength, and flexibility. Along with the functions of the central nervous system, these components provide the basis for motor skill performance and lifelong physical fitness. In recent years, the term *health-related fitness* has been used to describe those aspects of physical fitness related to functional health and preventive medicine (aerobic fitness, muscular strength and endurance, flexibility, and optimal body composition), rather than motor performance (speed, power, agility, and coordination).

The next chapter will discuss the particular effects of physical activity and exercise on the basic physiological components of change outlined in the following pages. For a more detailed discussion of physiological change as a result of various intensities of exercise, refer to the Suggested Readings.

Cardiorespiratory Development

The term *cardiorespiratory* in this discussion refers to selected aspects and functions of the cardiovascular and respiratory (pulmonary) systems. Early system growth and development, as well as the developmental aspects of selected functions and capabilities of these systems, will be covered.

Basic Structure and Function

Objective 4.1 ➤ The *cardiorespiratory system* consists of the heart, its cardiovascular network of arteries, capillaries, and veins, and the respiratory (pulmonary) system. The heart is a four-chambered muscular organ that weighs less than 1 pound yet has the power to beat approximately 40 million times per year. The heart may be viewed as two separate pumping units. The chambers that compose the right side of the heart receive blood returning from all parts of the body and then pump blood to the lungs. The left side of the heart receives oxygenated blood from the lungs and pumps it into the aorta for distribution throughout the body by way of the circulatory system (figure 4.1).

The heart is composed of three layers: the pericardium, the outer layer composed of fibrous and adipose tissues; the myocardium, the middle layer composed of cardiac muscle tissue; and the endocardium, or inner layer. Cardiac muscle tissue differs from skeletal muscle tissue in that cardiac muscle is involuntary. The individual fibers of cardiac tissue

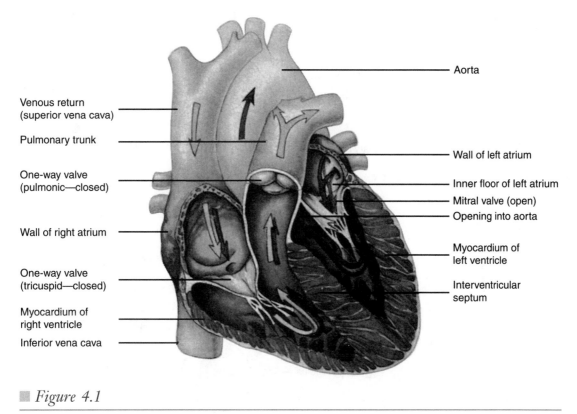

Venous return (superior vena cava)

Pulmonary trunk

One-way valve (pulmonic—closed)

Wall of right atrium

One-way valve (tricuspid—closed)

Myocardium of right ventricle

Inferior vena cava

Aorta

Wall of left atrium

Inner floor of left atrium

Mitral valve (open)

Opening into aorta

Myocardium of left ventricle

Interventricular septum

■ *Figure 4.1*

The heart and direction of blood flow

are multinucleated cells interconnected in a close network. Consequently, when an individual cell is stimulated, the action potential, or impulse, speeds through the entire heart and causes it to function as a unit.

The process by which air is brought into and exchanged with the air in the lungs is referred to as pulmonary (respiratory) ventilation. Air enters through the nose and mouth and flows into the ventilation system where it is adjusted to accommodate body temperature. The air then is filtered and humidified as it passes through the trachea. The inspired air then passes into two bronchi, the large tubes serving as primary conduits in each of the lungs. The bronchi further subdivide into numerous bronchioles that conduct the air to be mixed with existing air in the alveoli, or terminal branches of the respiratory tract (figure 4.2 on page 116).

Early Growth and Development

Objective 4.2 ➤ **Heart Growth** The heart begins its development as a single tube. Its first pulsations may occur as early as the third week of conception, even though there is no blood for it to circulate because the fetus is getting oxygen through the umbilical cord. By 12 weeks the circulatory system is

■ *Figure 4.2*

■ *Figure 4.2*

Basic structure of
the respiratory
(ventilatory) system

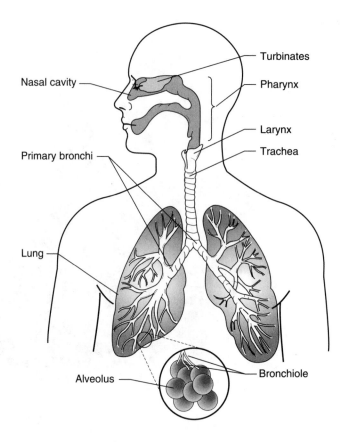

operating. By sometime between the fourth and fifth fetal months, the heartbeat is regular and strong enough to be heard using a stethoscope. The greatest increases in heart weight occur after the first month of postnatal life. The weight doubles during the first year, quadruples by age 5, and has increased six times by age 9. From 9 to 16 years of age the heart undergoes a second phase of rapid growth that parallels the general growth rate during that period. All of the functional mechanisms found in the adult electrocardiogram (ECG) are also evident in the fetus after about five weeks.

In the fetus, the vessels that develop from the main trunk of the heart grow in direct proportion to the parts of the body supplied. This indicates that a relationship exists between caliber of growth and the volumes or weights of the regions supplied. At birth the right ventricular muscle outweighs the left by about 13%, but by the fifth month they become equal in weight. By 7 years of age the left wall is 2 to 3 times thicker than the right, as it is in the adult.

The thickness of the walls of the major veins doubles between the time of birth and puberty, and cavity size increases approximately 2½ times by early maturity. In newborns, the total blood volume of the heart, one indicator of size, is approximately 200 milliliters. By the end of the first year, this value doubles, and at the time of maturity, blood volume for males is 5,500 milliliters and 4,200 milliliters for females. There is little difference between the sexes until puberty; after that, the male heart is about 15% larger, even with adjustment for body weight. As a general rule, heart size is related to body size, so children have smaller hearts than adults do. This accounts for much of the endurance performance differences observed.

Respiratory Component Growth   By the sixth fetal week, the trachea, bronchi, and lung buds are evident, and migration toward the thoracic region begins. By the third fetal month the journey is almost complete, and thereafter the lungs gradually begin to descend into their destined location. At birth the larynx is approximately one-third of its adult size, but it is about the same size in relation to the rest of the body as it is in the adult. From about the third year on, the larynx is longer and wider in males than in females. At the time of delivery the trachea is roughly one-third (about 4 cm) of its adult length; by puberty it will increase both its anteroposterior and lateral diameters nearly 300%.

Anatomical growth of the lungs follows individual patterns for each of the major ventilatory components. Development of the lungs begins as a lung bud protrusion that appears between the third and fourth fetal week. Growth proceeds when this protrusion branches, and by about the 16th fetal week the bronchial tree is completely formed. The airways canalize around 20 weeks and, a little later, alveoli develop from the distal branches of the airway. Bronchial cartilage begins to form at 10 weeks; by 25 weeks its distribution resembles the adult model. At about 13 weeks, mucous glands appear; they are functional by 24 weeks. Cilia make their appearance around the 13th fetal week and extend to the peripheral bronchi. By 15 weeks bronchi sensory and motor nerves can be detected along the pathways to the most distal passages. Capillaries appear about the 20th week and multiply rapidly near the developing airways when the alveoli begin to grow. Development of the alveolar-capillary interface for the exchange of oxygen and carbon dioxide is essential for independent existence after birth; this process is seldom complete before the 26th fetal week.

The weight and capacity of the lungs double in the first six months, triple by age 1, and increase approximately 20-fold by maturity. There also will be an increase of two to three times in the diameter of the airway. The diameter of the bronchi doubles by age 6 and that of the bronchioles and trachea by approximately age 15. About 20 million primitive alveoli are present at the time of birth. During the first three years after birth, the increase in lung size primarily is due to increases in the number of alveoli. By age 8 there are about 300 million alveoli—about the same number found in the adult. After age 8 the alveoli begin to increase in size until the chest wall ceases growing.

Aerobic Power

Objective 4.3 ➤ Sometimes referred to as maximal oxygen consumption and maximal aerobic power, **maximal oxygen uptake (VO$_2$max)** is the maximum amount of oxygen an individual can use per unit of time. This amount usually is expressed in liters or milliliters of oxygen per minute. Maximal oxygen uptake is considered the best measure of cardiorespiratory fitness, as indicated by graded maximal working capacity tests using either a cycle ergometer or a treadmill.

The association between VO$_2$max and aerobic power lies with the energy sources of the body. For the body to do mechanical work, it depends on the splitting of adenosine triphosphate (ATP) to release energy for muscle contraction. This can be supplied from (a) limited stores of phosphagens, (b) glycolysis, which produces lactic acid, or (c) the conversion of substrates to carbon dioxide and water in a phase of carbohydrate breakdown called the Kreb's cycle, which is coupled with the electron transport system. The first two sources are considered anaerobic processes because additional oxygen is not required. Muscle contractions that result from anaerobic sources generally cannot be sustained longer than 40 or 50 seconds. Motor performance activities considered more anaerobic are sprints, jumping, weight lifting, and other movements where the required power intensity is high and the duration relatively short. In contrast, the third conversion method requires oxygen, meaning that it uses **aerobic power.** Muscle contractions using oxygen as an energy source can last several minutes and, in trained individuals, several hours. Activities primarily, though not exclusively, associated with aerobic power include long-distance running, cycling, cross-country skiing, and swimming. These activities also involve anaerobic processes to a degree.

Figure 4.3 illustrates the relationship between maximal oxygen uptake and age. As a general trend, maximal oxygen uptake increases with growth through childhood; both sexes have similar values until approximately 12 years of age. Maximal oxygen uptake in males continues to increase until about age 18, while females show little improvement beyond age 14. The increase in VO$_2$max for males in puberty appears to correspond with the peak increase in height and with the time when androgen secretion increases dramatically. After about age 25, capacity declines steadily. Both children and adults have shown improvements in aerobic capacity through training; average increases range from 5% to 20%.

Maximal oxygen uptake is strongly related to lean body mass, which accounts to a great extent for the difference between the sexes after puberty. As noted earlier, lean body mass that follows puberty tends to level off in females as additional mass, primarily in the form of body fat, is added. Males, in contrast, continue to gain lean body mass. Approximately 70% of the individual differences in VO$_2$max can be explained simply by differences in body mass (McArdle et al., 2001). Values for

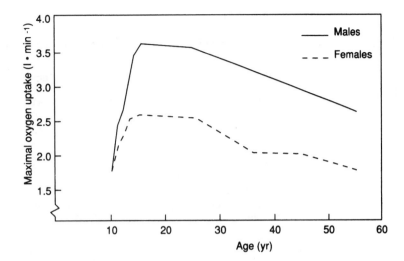

■ *Figure 4.3*

Figure 4.3

Maximal oxygen
uptake as a
function of age

young adult females are typically 15% to 30% lower than males. Among
trained athletes, the difference ranges from 12% to 20%. Although aerobic capacity has been shown to increase with growth through childhood, when expressed relative to body mass, aerobic capacity remains
the same or decreases with age.

Along with training and physical characteristics, maximal oxygen
uptake also is influenced by heredity. Based on the findings that genetic
factors appear to influence the growth of body size and mass as well as
muscle fiber type, the heritability estimate for maximal oxygen uptake
(which itself accounts for about 30%) is believed to be over 90%.

Body weight is the major physical determinant in maximal oxygen
uptake capacity; however, several other factors also are related. These
factors include cardiac output, vital capacity, heart rate, stroke volume,
and the oxygen-carrying properties of the blood, including blood volume and hemoglobin. Differences between the sexes primarily are
related to differences in the values associated with these factors and differences in heart size. Table 4.1 on page 120 indicates adult gender
differences in maximal oxygen uptake.

Anaerobic Power

In contrast to the characteristics of aerobic power, **anaerobic power** is
the maximum rate at which metabolic processes can occur without additional oxygen. Sustained aerobic activity depends on a continuous transport of oxygen to the working tissues, as measured by VO_2max. However,
when exercise continues longer than a few seconds, more energy for
ATP resynthesis must be generated through the anaerobic reactions of
glycolysis. More intense, all-out activity requires levels of energy that far
exceed what the respiratory processes alone can generate. Consequently,

TABLE 4.1

Gender Differences in Maximal Oxygen Consumption (50th Percentile)

Age (yr)	Males	Females
20–29	40.0	31.1
30–39	37.5	30.3
40–49	36.0	28.0
50–59	33.6	25.7
Over 60	30.0	22.9

Source: Data from Pollock, M. L., J. H. Wilmore, & S. M. Fox, *Health and Fitness through Physical Activity.* Copyright © 1978 John Wiley & Sons, Inc., New York, NY.

the anaerobic reactions of glycolysis predominate, and large amounts of lactic acid accumulate within active muscle and in the bloodstream. The level of lactic acid in the blood is the most common indicator of anaerobic activity. As the intensity of exercise increases and VO_2max is reached, the amount of lactic acid in the blood increases quickly. Under these conditions, work can be maintained only for a few minutes. Anaerobic power generally is measured in tests requiring that a supramaximal exercise be performed for a minute or less. Popular tests include sprinting up a flight of stairs (Margaria Power Test), arm or leg cranking on a cycle ergometer (Wingate Anaerobic Test), jumping-power tests, and short sprints.

Anaerobic power increases with age up to early adulthood no matter whether the values are expressed absolutely or relative to body weight (Inbar, 1996; Rowland, 1996). In anaerobic tests that last one minute or less, children exhibit significantly lower scores than adolescents and adults do. Whereas maximal aerobic power generally does not change and may even decrease relative to body weight, anaerobic power increases progressively with growth. Figure 4.4 provides an example of the increase across ages 8 to 14 years relative to body weight. The differences in anaerobic power cannot be accounted for by muscle tissue mass. The markedly lower capacity of young children reflects, to a great extent, a qualitative deficiency in the muscle. The major age-related difference appears to be in glycolytic capacity—the resting concentration of glycogen and the rate at which lactate is produced with its utilization. Although exercise lactate levels rise progressively during childhood, they are lower than in older populations. The level of acidosis at which the muscle still can contract also is used as an indicator of anaerobic capacity. Following a pattern similar to glycolytic capacity, children do not reach the levels of acidosis of which adolescents and young adults are capable. Irrespective of measured values, maximal acidosis also increases with age.

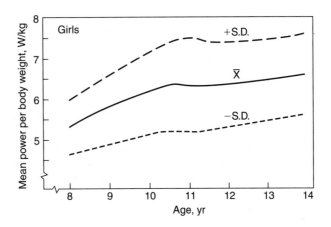

■ *Figure 4.4*

Relative mean
power (watt/kg)
from the Wingate
Anaerobic Test
across age for
boys and girls

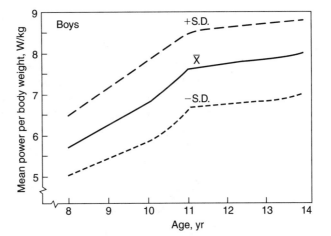

THINK ABOUT IT

What factors con-
tribute to making a
great sprinter and
long-distance runner
(nature/nurture)?

Females, in general, do not have the anaerobic power of males, especially after puberty. Inbar (1996) notes that gender-related differences cannot be explained merely by differences in body size. Although unclear at this time, the explanation likely is based in part on qualitative factors such as hormonal variation, muscle characteristics, or the nature of motor unit activation. As noted previously, individual differences can be explained in large part by genetic influence (about 50% contribution).

Heart Rate

Objective 4.4   ➤ Due to the relative ease of monitoring, *heart rate* has been one of the most commonly used measures of cardiovascular response to exercise and of energy expenditure. Because heart rate is the major determinant in cardiac output (the amount of blood pumped per unit of time), it is also an important factor in maximal oxygen consumption. Heart rate measures can be taken at rest, at a given rate of exercise (submaximal), and at maximal level of exercise (for maximal heart rate). A rough estimate of maximal heart rate can be obtained by subtracting a person's age from 220. A more direct and accurate measure is obtained by measuring the highest heart rate during a treadmill test that pushes the individual to maximal oxygen uptake.

Resting heart rate levels decrease with age; females average 5 beats per minute (bpm) higher than males do (table 4.2). A similar pattern exists for heart rate at a submaximal exercise level—namely, that submaximal heart rate also declines with age and that females exhibit higher rates. Under these exercise conditions, it is not unusual for a preadolescent child to have a heart rate 30 to 40 beats per minute higher than a young adult performing the same task. The difference is due in part to the greater relative exercise intensity performed by the younger individual and the physiological compensation for a lower stroke volume.

The reported reasons for the higher rates for females are not conclusive. A possible reason, at least among adults, is the lower blood hemoglobin levels of women. However, the hemoglobin levels of preadolescents are similar, and females still exhibit greater heart rates. Another explanation has been related to stroke volume differences between the sexes. Increased heart rate may compensate for the lower stroke volume and cardiac output of females.

TABLE 4.2

Average Heart Rate at Rest

Age	Average Rate*
Birth	140
1 mo	130
1–6	130
6–12	115
1–2 yr	110
2–4	105
6–10	95
10–14	85
14–18	82
20–29	66
30–39	65
Over 40	64

Source: Data recalculated from Lowrey (1986) and Pollock et al. (1978)
*Female values are an average 5 bpm higher than males.

Londeree and Moeschberger (1982) conducted a comprehensive review of existing information on maximal exercise heart rate among sampled individuals from 5 to 81 years of age. The review showed that maximal exercise heart rate declines with age, and that as age increases the decline accelerates slightly. It also was reported that no significant differences between the sexes or categories of race for maximal exercise heart rate are apparent. Although this general trend is evident in updated reports, there are indications that rates are more stable throughout the childhood and early teen years, and decrease across the life span (Rowland, 1996).

Cardiac Output and Stroke Volume

Cardiac output is the major indicator of the functional capacity of the circulatory system. Output refers to the rate blood is pumped by the heart (heart rate) and the quantity of blood ejected with each stroke (stroke volume). As previously noted, cardiac output is the primary determinant of maximal oxygen uptake.

In general, as heart volume increases with growth and age, maximal cardiac output gradually increases, much like the pattern of development in maximal oxygen uptake (see figure 4.3). Children have a significantly lower stroke volume than adults do at all exercise levels and thus a lower cardiac output. This is compensated for by higher heart rates. Males have a higher stroke volume than females at all levels of exercise (although the difference is not dramatic) partly due to the biological advantage of a larger heart that has greater volume and pump capabilities, especially after puberty.

Vital Capacity and Pulmonary Ventilation

Vital capacity refers to the total volume of air that can be expired voluntarily following maximal inspiration. Vital capacity consists of the tidal volume, the air moved during inspiration or expiration, plus the available reserve volumes. The movement of air in and out of the pulmonary system is called ventilation (breathing).

The growth pattern of vital capacity indicates that as males and females age and grow larger in body size, their vital capacity increases (figure 4.5 on page 124). Vital capacity is strongly linked to body size. Males and females experience similar increases until the onset of puberty, when the larger body size of the male allows for greater absolute values. At 20 years of age, males have approximately 20% greater vital capacity than females. Because females enter puberty earlier than males (from 10 to 12 years of age), body sizes are relatively equal at that time and their vital capacities are much closer to equal.

As with vital capacity, the absolute volume for pulmonary ventilation increases with age and body size until young adulthood (Fahey,

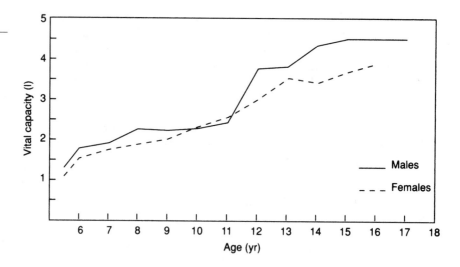

1990). An average 6-year-old may have a maximal ventilation of 30 to
40 liters per minute, whereas a young adult can reach 100 liters per
minute easily. However, children's maximal ventilation values are not
significantly different from adolescent and adult values when
expressed relative to body weight. Once again, due to body size differences, maximal ventilation is normally higher in males. Interestingly, however, due to the smaller lung capacity in children, their
respiratory rates are markedly higher than that of adults when performing a submaximal exercise task. Ventilation at any given oxygen
uptake is higher in children, and the ventilatory breaking point, which
signifies the onset of blood lactate, appears earlier than in adolescents
and adults. During a submaximal test, a child of 6 years can have a
ventilation value 50% higher than that of an individual of 17 years.
In fact, children breathe more rapidly than adults, with a decline in
maximal rate observed during childhood. Though not conclusive,
research related to ventilatory equivalent, a numerical expression of
ventilatory efficiency, suggests that it decreases with age. This indicates that children are less efficient at ventilating (Rowland, 1996).

■ *Blood Characteristics*

Blood Volume

Objective 4.5 ➤ The increase in total blood volume maintains a relatively constant
relationship to growth in body weight. The average newborn infant has
a blood volume of 85 milliliters per kilogram relative to body weight.
This increases to about 105 milliliters shortly after birth, then decreases
during the first few months. Thereafter, the average blood volume is

75 to 77 milliliters per kilogram, which is maintained through adolescence and adulthood. Males' larger body mass, especially after puberty, results in a greater total and relative blood volume than that of females. The relative difference is approximately 10 milliliters per kilogram.

Red Blood Cells Content

The red blood cell is one of the most specialized cells in the body. Its major compound, hemoglobin, accounts for more than 95% of the total protein and for about 90% of the dry weight of the cell. The function of hemoglobin is to combine reversibly with oxygen, which allows red blood cells to collect oxygen from the lungs and deliver it to the tissues.

By the second week of gestation the developing embryo begins to produce red blood cells. The production of these structures outside of the skeletal system peaks at about the fifth fetal month. Thereafter, production takes place in the bone marrow. The red blood cell count increases from approximately 1.5 million per cubic millimeter at 12 weeks of gestation to about 4.7 million at birth (Rudolph, 1982). A marked decrease in the rate of red blood cell production continues for six to eight weeks after birth. This period marks the peak of red cell destruction and decreased hemoglobin values. The life span of a red cell lasts about 90 days shortly after birth, compared to 120 days in adults. After this period, cell production increases gradually throughout childhood and adolescence.

The number of red blood cells and, consequently, the amount of hemoglobin (except for the two-month period in which both decrease) are closely related to growth in body mass and blood volume (figure 4.6 on page 126). Values in males and females first begin to diverge during adolescence. In the female, the gradual increase starts in preadolescence, continues into early puberty, and then levels off. In contrast, increases in the male appear to be related to sexual and physical maturity. The higher values of androgens in males after puberty have been associated with higher concentrations of hemoglobin. During adolescence in males, blood levels vary with sexual maturity. Higher hemoglobin levels in males help to explain higher anaerobic capacity.

Blood Pressure

Blood pressure is the product of cardiac output and peripheral vascular resistance; an increase in either cardiac output or peripheral resistance will raise blood pressure. Systolic pressure refers to how hard the heart is working and the strain against the arterial walls during ventricular contraction. Diastolic pressure is an indication of peripheral resistance, or the ease with which blood flows from the arterioles into the capillaries. Due to the higher contractile forces of the heart during exercise, there

■ *Figure 4.6*

Mean red blood
cell values in
relation to age

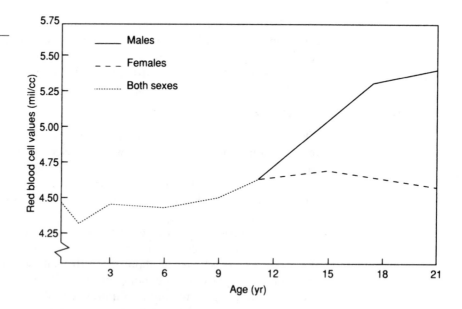

is a marked increase in systolic pressure compared to diastolic pressure. Diastolic blood pressure changes only slightly with physical exertion.

Systolic blood pressure rises steadily during childhood and increases at a much faster rate during adolescence until approximate adult levels are reached. The average systolic and diastolic blood pressure for young adults at rest is about 120/80 (mmHg), although this varies related to age and size. Comparatively, the typical pressure for a newborn is 70/55, and at 10 years the average is 100/62. During submaximal exercise, children respond with lower systolic and diastolic pressures than do individuals of adolescent age. Bar-Or (1983) notes this is associated with the child's lower cardiac output and stroke volume; it also may reflect a lower peripheral vascular resistance due to shorter blood vessels. Typically, males have a higher systolic pressure than females do after the age of 12. As with measures of other blood characteristics, this change first appears at about age 12 in females and rises markedly during puberty in males. Again, this difference between the sexes has been attributed primarily to the greater heart size and increased blood volume in males. Diastolic pressure changes very little during adolescence, with no apparent difference between the sexes.

Basal Metabolic Rate

Objective 4.6 ➤ **Basal metabolic rate (BMR)** refers to the amount of heat produced by the body during resting conditions. This physiological process reflects the minimum level of energy required to sustain the body's vital functions in the waking state. BMR usually is determined indirectly by measuring submaximal oxygen consumption and is recorded in terms of the heat produced per square meter of body surface. Individuals are measured after they have fasted for at least 12 hours so there is no increase in metabolism due to the energy required to digest food. The BMR frequently is used to establish an energy baseline for constructing programs of weight control.

Basically, BMR declines continuously from birth to old age (figure 4.7). The BMR per kg of weight in an infant is more than twice that of an adult. Males have slightly higher values at all ages; the values for adult females are 5% to 10% lower than those for adult males. This difference is largely because females generally have more fat tissue, and fat is metabolically less active than lean body tissue. This difference between sexes almost is eliminated when BMR is expressed relative to fat-free or lean body mass. The hormonal effects of increased androgens in males also has been mentioned as a possible contributing factor in sex differences. Overall, the decline can be explained by a decrease in the relative size of the major organs contributing to resting energy metabolic expenditure (Rowland, 1996).

■ *Muscular Strength*

Objective 4.7 ➤ Previous discussions regarding muscles have focused on their neurological structure and tissue development. This section will provide information concerning the force characteristics of a muscle and their relationship to motor performance. **Muscular strength** refers to the

■ *Figure 4.7*

Basal metabolic rate as a function of age and sex

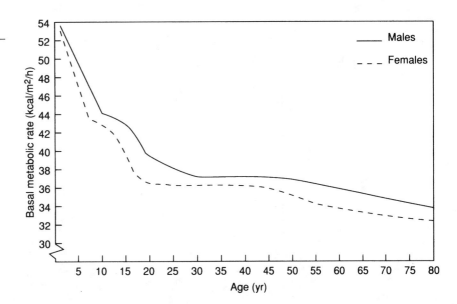

maximum force or tension generated by a muscle or muscle groups. Tension of the muscle in partial or complete contraction without any appreciable change in length is identified as *isometric* contraction. This type of muscular force is referred to as *static strength* and is generally measured using a dynamometer and tensiometer. If the muscle varies its length when activated to produce force, the contraction is *isotonic*. Isotonic force also is known as *dynamic strength*. It is usually determined by a one-repetition maximum, which refers to the maximum amount of weight lifted one time. Some exercise physiologists also refer to *isokinetic* contraction. This is a muscular contraction in which the muscle shortens at a constant velocity. For training purposes, isokinetic machines can be set to move at various specified velocity rates and resistance levels.

Most past descriptive studies of children have documented the development of static strength using either a hand-grip dynamometer or, for other parts of the body, a cable tensiometer. With more recent advances in scientific instrumentation and the emergence of microprocessor technology, it is now possible to update this body of information (especially with younger populations) by quantifying more accurately the muscular forces generated during a variety of movements.

Figures 4.8 and 4.9 show means of strength characteristics (absolute and relative to body weight) for individuals from 10 to 59 years of age. Basically, muscular strength increases with age in both sexes and reaches a peak between 25 and 29 years of age. There is, however, considerable variability within and between the sexes. The development of strength

■ *Figure 4.8*

Strength index (means) of right and left grip of arm

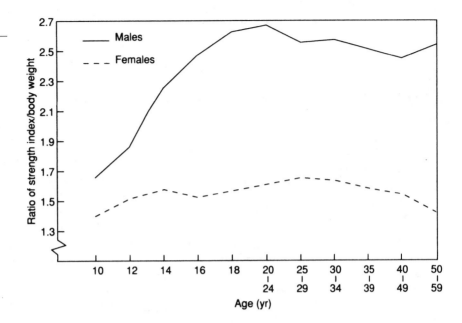

■ *Figure 4.9*

Ratio of strength index to body weight

is basically symmetrical on both sides of the body, although the dominant side is slightly stronger. The legs contribute approximately 60% to total body strength.

Reports of the development of strength during childhood show that both sexes demonstrate strength increase with age, with the values for boys slightly greater. This slight difference during childhood is apparent as early as 3 years of age (Rowland, 1996). However, at the onset of puberty, the picture changes. The significant physiological and structural changes associated with the adolescent growth spurt are reflected in both capacity and differences between the sexes (figures 4.8 and 4.9). Much of the difference is attributed to greater muscle mass (see figure 3.29 on page 98) and androgen production in males.

When evaluating the differences between the sexes, three approaches may be taken: (a) relative to muscle cross-sectional area, (b) on an absolute basis as total force, and (c) relative to body weight or lean body mass. Regardless of sex, human skeletal muscle, based on cross-sectional analysis, generates approximately 3 to 4 kilograms of force per square centimeter (McArdle et al., 2001). Here the difference is related to the size of the muscle cross section; for the same-size muscle section, there is little difference.

When strength is compared on an absolute basis, males usually are considerably stronger than females (figure 4.8). Males are typically 30% to 50% stronger than females in most muscle groups. The difference is generally less when comparing the strength of the trunk and legs, as opposed to the shoulders and arms. As noted earlier, much of this difference, especially after puberty, is related to higher androgen levels and larger lean body mass in males. Researchers also have noted that the greater levels of androgens are an advantage in muscle hypertrophy, an increase in muscle size in response to training. Adult males have about 10 times the amount of androgens as prepubescent children and women do.

When strength values are expressed relative to body weight, males are generally still stronger (figure 4.9). This difference is due in part to the fact that the measure of body weight reflects total body fat and lean body mass. Since females have more body fat and less lean body mass than males, their strength per unit of body weight is lower. When strength is calculated relative to lean body weight, the large absolute differences are reduced considerably. This information has led to the conclusion that sex differences are a function of differences in lean body weight and distribution of muscle and fat in the body segments.

The decline in muscular force production after it peaks (from 25 to 29 years of age) is closely related to the loss of muscle mass. A decrease in mass of approximately 25% to 30% takes place with aging.

Closely associated with strength and the ability of the muscle to produce force is *muscular endurance*. In the purest form, muscular strength refers to maximum force or tension generated by a muscle or muscle group in a single maximum contraction. Muscular endurance, on the other hand, is the ability of a muscle or muscle group to perform repeated contractions. That is, endurance is the ability to sustain strength performance. Commonly used tests of muscular endurance include push-ups, sit-ups, and pull-ups. According to two nationwide physical fitness surveys, children gain steadily in sit-up and pull-up performance from 6 to 9 years of age; males generally continue to increase through adolescence and females show indications of leveling off around the time of puberty (NCYFSI, 1985; NCYFSII, 1987). Figure 4.10 illustrates this pattern with bent-knee sit-ups. Other gross motor activities such as running, swimming, bicycling, and gymnastics require varying levels of muscular endurance. The primary component in the initiation of any muscular endurance task, however, is muscular strength.

THINK ABOUT IT

Recently, there has been controversy regarding weight training of prepubescent children. What do you suppose is the issue?

■ *Flexibility*

Objective 4.8

➤ **Flexibility** is the degree of ability to move body parts through a range of motion without undue strain. This is an essential component of health-related fitness for optimal performance of motor skills and for preventing muscle injury. Research on the basic tenets of flexibility has produced the following conclusions: (a) flexibility is specific to each joint, (b) flexibility is not related to the length of limbs, (c) strength development need not hinder range of motion, (d) activity levels are a better indicator of flexibility than age, and (e) females tend to be more flexible than males.

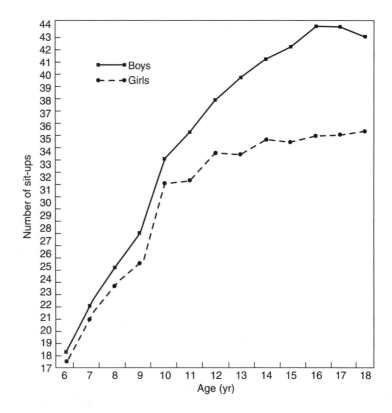

■ *Figure 4.10*

Average scores on bent-knee sit-ups (60 sec) for ages 6–18

Source: As reported by Ross & Gilbert (1985) and Ross & Pate (1987)

Most flexibility tests are classified as relative or absolute measures. Relative tests measure flexibility relative to the length or width of a specific body part; thus, the movement and influencing body parts are measured. Tests that measure only the movement are referred to as absolute. The most commonly used instruments for testing flexibility are various types of flexometers and goniometers (linear or rotary measuring devices) and the sit-and-reach box. In recent years the sit-and-reach test, which is an absolute measure of hamstring, lower back, and hip flexibility, has been used extensively in field studies.

In a comprehensive review of the literature, Clarke (1975) concluded that general range of motion increases steadily through childhood, with males starting to decline around age 10 and females beginning to decrease at about age 12. This conclusion is not decisive, however since several other reports have indicated both earlier or later initial declines. This is not surprising considering that flexibility is joint specific, rather than a general attribute, and these studies have not measured the flexibility of the same body parts. It also has been speculated that activity levels are a better indicator of flexibility than age.

When considering the best single test, the sit-and-reach task, it appears that flexibility begins to decline in the late teens (figure 4.11), with the trend continuing through adulthood. A rather consistent

■ *Figure 4.11*

Average sit-and-reach scores for ages 6–18

The zero point was located at 12 inches.

Source: As reported by Ross & Gilbert (1985) and Ross & Pate (1987).

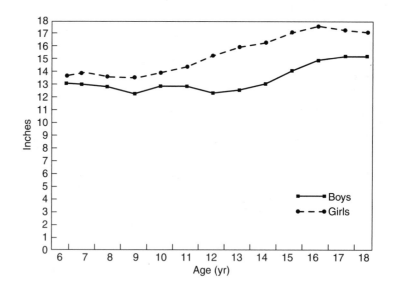

THINK ABOUT IT

Take a position that males are as flexible as females. Can you provide proof?

finding complementing this trend is that, in general, females are more flexible than males from age 5 to adulthood (e.g., Haubenstricker et al., 1997). Explanations for the difference only have been speculative but include relative differences in physical activity patterns, limb length, body size, and specific body composition and hormone levels. Another suggestion is that as body surface area increases, flexibility decreases; thus, during adolescence males would be at a disadvantage. This seems plausible, providing that the males do not participate in exercises that stimulate range of motion.

Before we begin the discussion of changes with advanced aging, which will be given more attention in chapter 11, table 4.3 summarizes

TABLE 4.3

Summary of Key Physiological Differences between Children and Adults

- Heart size is related directly to body size, so children have smaller hearts and thus lower stroke volume and cardiac output.
- Absolute aerobic capacity is lower in children. However, when expressed to reflect body size, there is little or no difference.
- Children are less economical runners because they require about 25% more oxygen per unit of body mass to run at a particular speed.
- Anaerobic capacity is lower in children, due in large part to a lower glycolytic capacity.
- Children are more susceptible to heart stress.
- Prepubescent children can increase muscle strength with resistance training, primarily through neural recruitment. However, significant increases are difficult due to relatively low androgen levels.

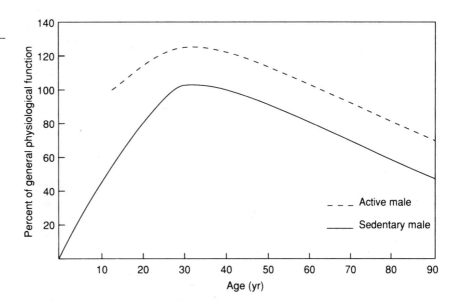

◾ *Figure 4.12*

A hypothetical curve representing physiological function of active and sedentary males over the life span

the key differences between children and adults, as derived from McArdle et al. (2001), Wimore & Costill (1999), and Rowland (1996).

◾ *Changes with Aging*

Objective 4.9   ➤ Physiological maturity and motor performance peak between the approximate ages of 25 and 30 years. In the age span of 30 to 70 years, most physiological functions decline at the rate of 0.75% to 1.0% per year. The rate of decline in some functions depends to some degree on lifelong health practices, including physical activity. The difference between physiological age and chronological age may be considerable. Figure 4.12 shows hypothetical curves of physiological function of active and sedentary males across the life span. Excellent reviews of change with advanced aging are found in McArdle et al. (2001), Shephard (1997), and Spirduso (1995) (see Suggested Readings).

Change in Cardiorespiratory Function

Maximal oxygen uptake follows a clear trend of decline with a drop of approximately 30% between 30 and 70 years of age (see figure 4.3 on page 119). Sedentary persons have nearly a two–fold faster rate of decline in VO_2max as they age. The closely related function of cardiac output, which consists of stroke volume and maximal heart rate, also declines about 30% over this time span. It should be noted that resting cardiac output (stroke volume and resting heart rate) is not affected markedly by age. Parallel to the loss in aerobic capacity is a slightly greater decline in anaerobic power—about 40% by age 70. With this is a slower clearing of blood lactate in older adults, which may partially explain age-related decrements in endurance. Although there is little change in diastolic blood pressure, systolic values may increase significantly. Aging also produces an increased resistance to blood flow due, in part, to a stiffening of the blood vessels and/or fatty deposits on the vessel walls.

Respiratory function, in general, also declines with age. The main outcome of the aging process in terms of lung function is the reduction of the amount of oxygen delivered from the outside air to the arterial blood. Along with changes in the cardiovascular and muscular systems, the effects of aging in the respiratory structures compound the limitations on the ability to perform physical work. Vital capacity may diminish up to 40% while residual lung volume (the amount not expired) increases 20% to 50%. The aging process also has been associated with a decrease in the surface area available for the exchange of gas between the alveoli and capillaries, due primarily to loss of functioning alveoli and the associated capillary network. Perhaps the most significant functional change with aging is a decline in the static-elastic-recoil force of the lung and the decreased resistance of the chest wall to deformation. Under normal conditions of respiratory function, the lung recoils inward and the chest wall expands outward, in balance, at the end of expiration. As the lung expands inspiration, the elastic-recoil force (pressure) increases, thereby assisting in expiration. The loss of recoil force means that less pressure by the chest wall is needed to produce a change in lung volume. In practical terms, this change means that an older individual performs about 20% more work to overcome the elastic resistance compared to a young adult. Loss of pulmonary elasticity also is related to impaired ventilation due to the premature closing of the airways. Figure 4.13 shows pulmonary ventilation values at maximal exercise (keep in mind that ventilation refers to the volume of air breathed per minute). Note the decrease with advanced aging and the slower recovery in older untrained persons.

Change in Basal Metabolic Rate

Closely associated with the decline in work capacity and muscle mass is the decreased ability of the individual to function within the environment. This decline affects basal metabolic rate with a decline of about 10% to 15% during adulthood (see figure 4.7 on page 127).

Change in Muscular Strength

With aging comes a deterioration in muscle mass of approximately 25% to 30%. Accompanying this loss are decreases in the size and number of fibers and the functioning of individual motor units. As this takes place, less contractile force is available when a motor unit is recruited for muscle contraction, and the action potential of the muscle is

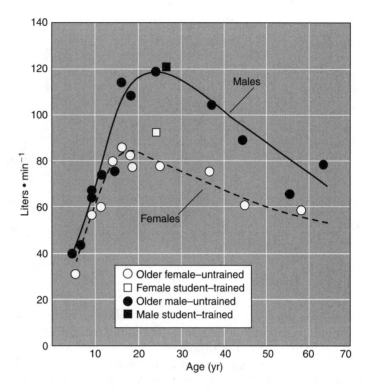

■ *Figure 4.13*

Pulmonary ventilation values at maximal exercise

decreased. In addition, type II muscle fibers, which are associated with strength and power, are lost. These fast-twitch fibers are thought to atrophy because the motoneurons that activate the muscles themselves atrophy, and the muscle fibers die because of the loss of innervation. After the period of peak strength between the ages of 25 and 29, it is not surprising to see muscular force decrease by about 25% to 30% with aging, thus matching the loss in muscle mass.

Change in Flexibility

Flexibility generally declines across adulthood, but after about age 50, the trend appears to be more significant. In specific areas, such as the lower back (extension), significant loss can occur much earlier; Einkauf and associates (1987) found sharp declines between 30 to 49 years (figure 4.14 on page 136). Closely linked to decreased flexibility and range of motion with aging are changes in the joints and muscles and the presence of degenerative joint diseases. The smooth functioning of the body's joints is made possible by the strength and elasticity of the tendons and ligaments and the condition of the synovial fluid. As individuals age, their joints become less stable and their mobility diminishes as collagen fibers and synovial membranes degrade and the viscosity of synovial fluid decreases. As a result, the joints become stiff, which possibly decreases their range of motion.

■ *Figure 4.14*

Decline in lower
back flexibility
(extension)

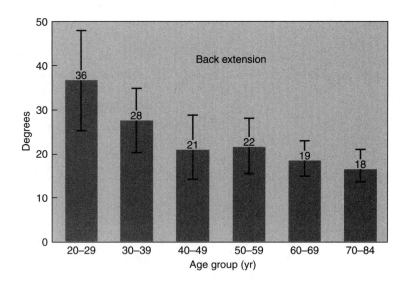

However, there is no conclusive evidence that biological aging inherently causes decreases in flexibility. A considerable amount of research also links loss of flexibility with degenerative joint diseases such as osteoarthritis and osteoarthrosis. Osteoarthritis affects more than 80% of individuals over 65 years of age, more females than males have the disease.

Table 4.4 summarizes selected physiological changes that occur with aging. Table 4.5 is a more comprehensive outline of topics covered in

TABLE 4.4

Summary of Selected Physiological Changes with Aging

Physiological Characteristic	
Cardiorespiratory	
Maximal oxygen uptake	Decreases
Stroke volume	Decreases
Max heart rate	Decreases
Vital capacity	Decreases
Ventilation	Decreases
Functioning alveoli	Decreases
Blood pressure (systolic)	Increases
Blood flow resistance	Increases
Basal metabolic rate	Decreases
Muscular strength	Decreases
Flexibility	Decreases

TABLE 4.5

Summary of Changes with Aging after Peak Maturity (30 Years of Age)*

	Decrease (↓) Increase (↑)	
Cardiorespiratory system		
Maximal oxygen uptake (VO$_2$max)	↓	30%
Cardiac output	↓	
Stroke volume	↓	
Heart rate (max)	↓	
Anaerobic power	↓	40%
Blood pressure (systolic)	↑	
Elasticity of blood vessels	↓	
Blood flow (resistance)	↑	
Respiratory		
General pulmonary function	↓	
Vital capacity	↓	40%
Lung residual volume	↑	20%–50%
Functioning alveoli	↓	
Ventilation	↓	
Basal metabolic rate	↓	10%–15%
Nervous system		
Brain cells	↓	
Synaptic delay	↑	
Motor unit size	↓	
Nerve conduction velocity	↓	10%–15%
Reaction time	↑	slows
Muscle		
Mass	↓	25%–30%
Fiber number/size	↓	
Biochemical capacity	↓	
Strength	↓	25%–30%
Height	↓	
Body weight	↑	↓ after age 60
Body composition		
Body fat	↑	
Lean body weight	↓	
Skeletal (bone loss)	↓	female 30% male 10%–15%
Flexibility	↓	
Joints		
Stiffness of connective tissue	↑	
Accumulated mechanical stress	↑	

*Overall decline of functional capacity approx. 0.75% to 1.0% per year the last three chapters on the effects of aging on various growth and development functions.

Summary

Growth and development of the cardiorespiratory system begin with a single, noncirculating heart tube and the appearance of respiratory buds during the early stages of fetal development. From these beginnings, the system experiences tremendous growth and development prior to birth that continue across the life span.

Maximal aerobic power increases through childhood. Much of the difference between individuals can be explained by variations in body weight. Peak capacity occurs around age 25 and declines steadily thereafter. Anaerobic power also rises steadily to early adulthood.

Heart rate changes with age are described in terms of resting, submaximal, and maximal values. Resting and submaximal heart rate levels normally decrease with age; females have slightly higher levels than males. Maximal heart rate also decreases with advancing age.

Cardiac output is the major indicator of the functional capacity of the system and a primary determinant in maximal oxygen uptake (aerobic power). In general, as heart volume increases with age, maximal cardiac output also increases. The trend is similar to that associated with maximal oxygen uptake; it increases until early adulthood and declines shortly thereafter. Vital capacity tends to increase as body size increases. As with a number of other physiological functions, the measured values of both sexes are similar until after puberty, after which the larger body size of males produces the greater absolute values found.

The production of red blood cells begins by the second week of gestation and increases, with only a slight interruption, throughout adolescence. As body weight increases, comparable increases in total blood volume take place. With this increase come higher numbers of red blood cells and higher levels of hemoglobin, that collect oxygen from the lungs and transport it to the tissues. Systolic blood pressure values rise steadily during childhood with a much faster rate of increase during adolescence. Quantitative differences related to age and size are observable in systolic and diastolic blood pressure. Physical activity can have a marked influence on blood pressure values.

Basal metabolic rate declines continuously from birth to old age; males have slightly higher values at all ages. The gender difference is due primarily to greater levels of fat tissue in females, which is metabolically less active than lean body tissue.

Muscular strength normally increases with age up to a peak that takes place between 25 and 29 years of age. Due largely to higher levels of androgen and larger lean body mass after puberty, males are typically 30% to 50% stronger than females in most muscle groups. Decline in strength after the peak years is closely related to the loss of muscle mass.

The literature on flexibility is perhaps the most inconclusive of all the developmental characteristics discussed. In general, range of motion increases steadily through childhood. Then during early adolescence it begins the continued life-span trend of decline.

After peak physiological maturity between the approximate ages of 25 and 30, functions begin to show a decline at the rate of 0.75% to 1.0% per year between the ages of 30 and 70 years. Although there are wide differences among individuals due to factors such as physical activity, the effects of age are evident. By age 70, substantial losses are observable in cardiorespiratory function, basal metabolic rate, muscle mass and muscular strength, and joint mobility (flexibility).

Think about It

1. What factors contribute to making a great sprinter and long-distance runner (nature/nurture)?
2. Recently, there has been controversy regarding weight training of prepubescent children. What do you suppose is the issue?
3. Take a position that males are as flexible as females. Can you provide proof?
4. Considering all of the changes (regression) that occur with advanced aging, what daily living activities are more likely to be profoundly affected?

Suggested Readings

Bar-Or, O. (Ed.). (1996). *The child and adolescent athlete.* Oxford, England: Blackwell Science.

McArdle, W. D., Katch, F. I., & Katch, V. L. (2001). *Exercise physiology.* 5th ed. Philadelphia: Lea & Febiger.

Rowland, T. W. (1996). *Developmental exercise physiology.* Champaign, IL: Human Kinetics.

Shephard, R. J. (1997). *Aging, physical activity, and health.* Champaign, IL: Human Kinetics.

Spirduso, W. W. (1995). *Physical dimensions of aging.* Champaign, IL: Human Kinetics.

WebLinks

American College of Sports Medicine
www.acsm.org

American Heart Association
www.americanheart.org

International Society for Aging and Physical Activity
www.isapa.org

National Strength & Conditioning Association
www.nsca-lift.org/menu.asp

5 *Factors Affecting Growth and Development*

OBJECTIVES

Upon completion of this chapter, you should be able to

5.1 List and briefly describe maternal factors that can affect prenatal development.

5.2 Identify the principles of teratogenic effects and describe associated environmental agents.

5.3 Discuss the role of nutrition on postnatal development.

5.4 Identify the possible effects of physical activity on growth, development, and motor performance after birth.

5.5 List and briefly describe the possible effects of hormones on growth and development over the life span.

KEY TERMS

teratogen

sensitive periods

fetal alcohol syndrome

low birth weight (LBW)

preterm

growth hormone (GH)

thyroxine

A VARIETY OF FACTORS and conditions may affect the normal course of human growth and development, including motor behavior. Common to the research and discussion in this field of study are the risk factors that are either suspected or have been proven to negatively affect prenatal development. This information is vital to a comprehensive understanding of the genetic and environmental influences on early development, and has profound implications for physical growth and motor behavior. Other factors come into play to affect the growth and development processes after the birth process; the most important of these are nutrition, exercise and physical activity, and hormones.

Prenatal Development

Objective 5.1 ➤ Several factors and conditions can affect the normal development of an unborn infant. Some of these are classified as *internal (maternal) factors* because they are linked with genetic influences or the maternal conditions of the prenatal environment.

Although the fetus is well protected by the placenta, it is not impervious to the outside environment. Through this membrane, the fetus is affected by *external (environmental) factors*—by what the expectant mother eats, breathes, drinks, or smokes. Certain substances are known to penetrate the placenta and cause negative reactions in the form of physical deformities and behavioral dysfunctions. An environmental agent that can cause a birth defect or kill the fetus is called a **teratogen.** Fortunately, about 97% of all babies are born without serious defects or deficiencies; human beings have a strong tendency to develop normally under all but the most damaging conditions.

Principles of Teratogenic Effects

Objective 5.2 ➤ Although the effects on the developing organism vary with the specific teratogen, several general principles appear to apply to most of them (Bukatko & Daehler, 2001; Shaffer, 2002):

1. Teratogens affect prenatal development by interfering with basic biochemical processes.
2. The susceptibility of a developing organism to a teratogenic agent varies with the organism's developmental stage at the time of exposure. In general, once the different body systems have begun to form, each is most vulnerable at the time of its initial growth spurt; this is associated with a sensitive period in development.
3. Each teratogenic agent acts in a specific way on specific developing tissue, therefore causing a particular pattern of abnormal development.
4. Not all organisms are affected in the same way by exposure to a given amount of a specific teratogen. Reaction depends to some degree on

the organism's and the mother's genotype and the mother's physiological state (e.g., age, nutrition, and hormonal balance).

5. In general, the greater the concentration or longer the exposure to the teratogen, the greater the risk of abnormal development.
6. Levels of teratogens that can produce defects in the developing organism may affect the mother only mildly or not at all. For example, some diseases and drugs that have minimal effect on the mother can lead to serious abnormalities in the developing organism.
7. Some teratogens may cause temporary delays in development with no long-term negative consequences, whereas others will cause problems late (sleeper effects) in development.

As you will recall from chapter 1, a basic assumption of this text is that there are **sensitive periods** in human development when an organism is most sensitive to certain environmental influences, such as teratogenic agents. Most experts agree that, in general, the entire prenatal period could be considered a sensitive period. However, it seems that during the embryonic period (weeks 2–8) when most organs and body parts are rapidly forming, the individual is most vulnerable to damage. Once an organ or body part is formed, it becomes less susceptible to harm. However, some organ systems such as the eyes and central nervous system (CNS) can be damaged throughout pregnancy.

The following material discusses selected maternal influences and environmental (teratogenic) agents.

Internal (Maternal) Factors

Maternal Age The age of the expectant mother appears to have some bearing on the ease of the birth process and the general well-being of the child. Females over 35 and under 16 years of age have a higher risk of infant defect, prematurity, and low birth weight. Risks to older women include difficulties in conceiving and delivering, an increased probability of having a child with Down syndrome, and low birth weight. According to the Centers for Disease Control and Prevention (CDC) records, the number of births to women 35 years and older almost tripled from 1980 to 2000 (4.6% versus 13%). More recently, Tough et al., (2002) reported that older women are 20–40% more likely to have low birth weight babies, a condition that may affect later outcome, including motor development. In young women the reproductive system may not be mature and general prenatal care may be poor. The years between 22 and 29 are physiologically the best time to have a baby. However, we still have much to learn about this issue; proper exercise and nutrition may help prolong the efficiency of the reproductive system.

Nutrition The development of the fetus can be affected by the quality of the expectant mother's diet both before and during pregnancy.

Because the mother is the sole source of nutrients for the fetus, an adequate diet is vital. If the mother's diet is deficient in the nutrients the fetus needs, the developing infant may exert such parasitic effects on the mother's body as draining calcium from the mother's teeth. Several studies indicate a relationship between maternal diet deficiencies and low birth weight, prematurity, brain development, skeletal growth retardation, below normal motor and neurological development, and poor mental functioning (Morgane et al., 1993). The first trimester is an especially vulnerable time. However, the last three months also may be critical because this is a time of rapid brain growth. In addition to a well-balanced diet, recommended additives commonly include iron, calcium, and folic acid.

Genetic Abnormalities   Each year in the United States, approximately 125,000 infants are born with a genetic abnormality, which represents approximately 3% to 5% of births.

Down syndrome, one of the most common genetic abnormalities, is caused by the presence of an extra chromosome in the 21st pair of chromosomes; thus the zygote has 47 instead of the normal 46 chromosomes. Individuals with this condition generally have retarded mental and motor development, heart defects, short hands and feet, and distinctively abnormal facial features. This condition is not inherited. The risk that a woman will bear a child with Down syndrome increases markedly with the expectant mother's age, especially after the age of 35. Down syndrome appears approximately once in every 800 live births.

Phenylketonuria (PKU) is a metabolic disorder that is also genetically based. It is a hereditary defect in an enzyme of the liver that the child needs to metabolize phenylalanine, a common protein food product. Without this enzyme the child cannot digest many needed foods including milk products. If the abnormality is not detected and treated soon after birth, substances may accumulate in the blood and damage the brain. Symptoms include irritability, hyperactivity, seizures, and perceptual problems. The condition can be detected with a blood test; treatment generally consists of a scientifically controlled diet.

Other frequently observed genetically related abnormalities include *sickle-cell anemia, Turner's syndrome,* and *Klinefelter's syndrome.*

Sickle-cell anemia is a painful and sometimes life-threatening disease that occurs when harmful genes are passed on from parents to their children. Among Americans it is found primarily in the African-American population; approximately 10% of African-Americans carry the harmful gene. In people with the sickle-cell trait, red blood cells become sickle-shaped and bind together when the level of oxygen is low, for example, during exercise and illness, and at high altitude. These clumps of cells then block the flow of blood through small blood vessels. Depending on the location and extent of blockage, the condition can cause severe pain or death.

Turner's syndrome occurs only in females who have only one (instead of two) X chromosomes. These females lack normal ovarian tissue and do not develop sexually. Symptoms include distinctive physical features such as a short, thick build, webbed neck, and prominent earlobes, as well as spatial perception difficulties. Most children with Turner's syndrome have normal IQs.

Klinefelter's syndrome is the most common of the sex-linked abnormalities associated with males. These individuals have an additional X chromosome (XXY), generally lack sexual development, and tend to be much taller than average. Intelligence levels are generally close to normal. As with mothers of children with Down syndrome, mothers of children with Klinefelter's syndrome tend to be older than average.

Fetal Position   The position of the fetus in the uterus is another internal factor that may affect its development. Pressure on the skeletal structure, specifically on the tips of the bones, stimulates ossification. If the fetus is positioned in such a way that this pressure is insufficient, immature skeletal development may result. Some depressurizing may take place as the fetus relaxes to accommodate to its somewhat cramped quarters.

THINK ABOUT IT

Consider how maternal factors effect postnatal motor development?

Emotional State of the Mother   Today we know that an expectant mother's stress can be transmitted to the fetus. Due to psychological experiences such as intense fear and prolonged anxiety and depression, physiological changes can occur that may affect the developing fetus. For example, fear can produce hormonal changes such as higher levels of adrenaline that restrict blood flow to the uterine area and possibly deprive the fetus of the normal flow of oxygen (Monk et al., 2000; Dunkel-Shetter et al., 2001). Another possible complication of stress can occur during the birth process; an emotionally distraught mother may experience greater difficulty in labor, thus affecting the newborn's immediate adaptation to its new world (Field, 1990).

External (Environmental) Factors

As noted earlier, although the fetus appears safe in its protective membrane, it is not impervious to the external environment. Although the placenta does a good job filtering many contaminants, the fetus still can be affected by disease-producing bacteria and by what the expectant mother eats, breathes, drinks, or smokes (teratogenic agents).

Infection and Disease   Fortunately, several potentially dangerous infections have been minimized through preventive drugs (e.g., rubella [German measles]). However, other viral influences and diseases still can be a danger to the developing fetus including cytomegalovirus disease, diabetes, and toxoplasmosis.

No infections are more common and few are more hazardous than sexually transmitted diseases. *Syphilis* is a potentially dangerous disease that if undetected in an expectant mother can attack the nervous system of the fetus and thus produce complications. The disease has been linked to miscarriages, stillbirth, deafness, blindness, and congenital mental dysfunctions. The signs of damage from syphilis may not appear until the child is several years old. Another sexually transmitted disease that can harm the fetus in a manner similar to syphilis is *genital herpes.*

A condition receiving much attention today is *acquired immune deficiency syndrome (AIDS).* More and more children are born infected as a result of the mother's condition. Aside from causing death during the first few years of life, the effects of AIDS on motor behavior are currently unreported.

Drugs and Chemical Substances   This section addresses the potential effects of tobacco, alcohol, and drugs on the developing fetus. Included in the drug category are over-the-counter remedies, prescribed medicines, and illegal substances.

SMOKING. Prenatal smoking is one of the most preventable causes of low birth weight and fetal growth retardation (Wang et al., 2000). The nicotine from tobacco use has the same effects on the fetus as it does on the mother. But because the same amount of the drug is available to a much smaller body area, the effects of the drug on the fetus are much greater. The carbon monoxide produced while smoking is known to interfere with the oxygen-carrying capabilities of the hemoglobin and, therefore, to increase the risk of hypoxia, or oxygen deprivation. Associated with the infants of mothers who smoke are low birth weight, more muscle tension, and poorer language and cognitive development during early childhood (Chasnoff, 1991; Fried & Watkinson, 1990). Cigarette smoking also has been associated with malformation of the heart and other organs, and deficits in long-term physical growth. Marijuana smoking produces similar detrimental effects on a developing child (Day, 1991). Approximately one quarter of women who are of child-bearing age smoke (National Center for Health Statistics, 1999).

ALCOHOL. Alcohol can have serious direct effects on fetal and neonatal development because the substance can cross the placenta. Because the fetus's liver is immature, the alcohol remains in its system for a long time. The fetus can be very sensitive to alcohol and even in small amounts has been shown to cause abnormalities in development. During the last trimester of pregnancy when brain development is rapid, alcohol may be extremely harmful.

Fetal alcohol syndrome is a condition suffered by some infants exposed to alcohol during the prenatal period. The syndrome was first identified among infants born to pregnant women who drank heavily.

Infants with this condition do not go through the normal catch-up period of growth after birth and exhibit signs of mental retardation and immature motor development. Other commonly found characteristics are low birth weight; facial, limb, and organ defects; and repetitive body motions associated with autistic behavior.

Unfortunately, the long-term outlook for children with fetal alcohol syndrome is not positive. Barr and associates (1990, 2001), using a longitudinal design, found that 4-year-olds whose mothers had consumed moderate levels of alcohol during their pregnancies showed deficiencies in fine motor control and balance. The researchers also reported that alcohol scores from the period prior to pregnancy recognition were the highest predictors of poor motor performance. In a review of this literature, Larroque et al. (1995) note that alcohol exposure is associated with poor motor coordination, weak grasp, and delayed motor development in general. Doctors at one time thought pregnant women could drink moderately without harming the fetus. However, more recent evidence has brought this assumption under serious question with reports suggesting that there may be no safe level of intake during pregnancy. Approximately 20% of women drink during pregnancy (National Center for Health Statistics, 1999).

DRUGS. Many drugs can cross the placenta barrier to have a direct effect on the developing fetus. Substances included in the category of drugs are prescribed medicines such as antibiotics; over-the-counter substances such as aspirin, vitamins, and cold remedies; and narcotics such as heroin, cocaine, amphetamines, and marijuana. Drugs strike the fetus with such force for two primary reasons. First, a small amount of a drug for an adult may be a dangerously huge amount for the tiny fetus. Second, the liver enzymes necessary for breaking down drugs do not develop until after birth. Therefore, just as with alcohol, drugs remain in the body of the fetus.

In recent years, with the increase of narcotic use in our society, pregnant women addicted to heroin or cocaine are giving birth to infants with symptoms of addiction. Cocaine use constricts the blood vessels, reduces the flow of oxygen to the fetus, and increases fetal blood pressure. The number of these cases is growing at an alarming rate in the United States. Along with the life-threatening ordeal of going through withdrawal, these babies are often born premature, underweight, jittery, exhibit impaired motor control, and are fragile. Several studies confirm that cocaine babies from 1 to 3 years of age display delayed motor development and impaired information processing (Arendt et al., 1999; Singer et al., 2001; Swanson et al., 1999).

The full impact of the influence of drugs of any type on fetal development is still being investigated. The general consensus in the medical profession is that expectant mothers should be very cautious about taking *any* medication (including aspirin) that is not prescribed.

THINK ABOUT IT

Advances in science are telling us more and more about what affects prenatal development. Are you suspicious of any other (than the already described) agents that might affect prenatal development?

Radiation   The radiation from X rays and other sources has been linked to harmful mutations of genetic material in the fetus. Exposure to radiation after conception but before the egg implants in the uterine linings is likely to end the pregnancy. Exposure to radiation *after* implantation may affect development in a variety of ways that include deformities of the CNS which may cause the death of the infant soon after birth, malignant tumors, leukemia, stunted growth, mental retardation, Down syndrome, and defects of the skull. Today X rays are seldom taken during pregnancy except in cases of emergency.

As noted earlier, by no means is this discussion exhaustive. Numerous additional environmental agents may have teratogenic effects. Other considerations include specific prescription and nonprescription drugs, and chemicals commonly found in paints, dyes, solvents, oven cleaners, pesticides, food additives, and cosmetic products.

A rather common symptom found among the prenatal influences described is **low birth weight (LBW).** LBW infants are born after a regular gestational period of 38 to 42 weeks but they weigh less than 5.5 pounds (2,500 grams). This condition is the chief contributor to infant illness and mortality and has implications for motor development. Closely associated with low birth weight are deficits in physical growth and motor behavior, due in large part to impaired neurological and skeletal development. Babies born prematurely (**preterm**)—prior to 38 weeks after conception—often are of low birth weight and are high-risk also. Influences mentioned that typically result in low birth weight and physical growth and motor deficits include mother's diet (nutrition), smoking, alcohol, and cocaine use. For example, pregnant smokers deliver infants who, on average, are 200 g lighter than those of nonsmokers. Smoking is associated with a two-fold increase in risk of low birth weight (Hellerstedt et al., 1997). As a general observation, more LBW infants are born to a parent(s) of low socioeconomic status (SES). This suggests that parent education—especially for the mothers—and prenatal care are important factors in preventing low birth weight.

The spectrum of impairments associated with LBW/preterm includes a broad range neuropsychological and cognitive outcomes, including motor behavior (Becker et al., 1999; Hack et al., 1995). These infants are at risk for motor dysfunction and delay. One of the most frequently cited deficits is poor fine- and visual-motor integration (e.g., review by Gabbard et al., 2001). In addition to the direct perceptual-motor development concern, the literature provides a reasonable case that such deficits place this population at increased risk for poor academic performance and difficulties with specific daily living (self-help) activities. Typically, infants and children born with very low birth weight (<1500 g) exhibit more deficits than the LBW group. About 8% of babies are born LBW/preterm.

■ *Figure 5.1*

Low birth weight and preterm birth may seriously affect later physical growth and motor development

■ *Nutrition and Physical Activity during Postnatal Development*

Objective 5.3

➤ The intake of essential nutrients and physical activity play influential and complementary roles in postnatal growth and health-related physical fitness across the life span. Children whose diets are unbalanced or are lacking in proper nourishment generally show below-average physical growth by age 3. Although diets lacking in protein and calories are by far the most common cause of growth failure during infancy and childhood, this problem is relatively rare in the United States and among other economically developed countries. We all know by now that the American diet consists of too much fat, refined sugar, and salt as evidenced by the high incidence of childhood obesity and by the link that has been established between diet and cardiovascular disease in adults (CDC, 2000). According to the CDC (2000), more than half (55%) of U.S. adults are overweight or obese. The Harvard School of Public Health estimates that by the year 2025, this figure will reach 75%. Complementing these figures is the Surgeon General's (1996) report that 60% of adults are not physically active enough to reap any significant health benefits. It has been estimated that physical inactivity and poor diet cause at least 300,000 deaths a year; only tobacco use causes more preventable deaths. Weight-related diseases (often associated with physical inactivity) cost the U.S. economy more than $100 billion every year. A sedentary lifestyle almost doubles one's risk for coronary heart disease, a condition that can begin to develop in childhood. Perhaps not surprisingly, almost one-quarter of children are now obese. This represents a dramatic increase of over 20% in the past decade; overall the percentage has doubled in the last 30 years. A significant portion of overweight children grow up to be overweight adults. Type 2 diabetes, strongly linked to obesity in adults, was virtually unheard of in children a decade ago. Now as many as 300,000 have the disease, which has been linked in part to obesity and low physical activity levels in children (American Diabetes Association, 2000).

A low physical activity level is characteristic of overweight children. Many children watch too much television and are not physically active. The overall trend appears to be increasing, especially among young females (Andersen et al., 1998; Bar-Or et al., 1998). Participation in all types of physical activity declines dramatically as age and grade in school increase. Evidence of this is the observation that nearly 50% of young people from ages 12 to 21 are not vigorously active on a regular basis. This trend results in about 60% of adults not achieving the recommended amount of physical activity. Today, only about 25% of children participate in any type of daily physical education. Daily participation in physical education by adolescents has declined dramatically, from 42% in 1991 to 27% in 1997. For a comprehensive discussion of fitness in Americans, refer to the CDC report (2000) in the Suggested Readings.

Nutrition

Diet is perhaps the most potent environmental influence on growth and development. Regardless of age, individuals must have proper food for growth and for maintenance and repair of body tissues. Exciting research conducted over the last 15 years has revealed that the nutritional practices of infants and children also may have a marked influence on their health as adults. Since no standard for optimal growth ever has been defined and because individuals have varying nutritional needs based upon differences in energy expenditure and bodily functions, it is difficult to determine what would compose the ideal diet for optimal growth.

The term *malnutrition*, in terms of physical growth, generally refers to an inadequate intake of energy in the form of calories or quality protein. A basic symptom of malnutrition is stunted growth. Two extreme examples of protein deficient malnutrition are kwashiorkor and marasmus. *Kwashiorkor* occurs after an infant is cut off from the mother's breast milk, a primary source of protein, due to the arrival of another infant. Some of the main symptoms are edema, skin disorders, loss of hair and appetite, diarrhea, and muscle hypotonicity. *Marasmus*, a wasting away of body tissues in the infant's first year, is related to protein deficiency and an inadequate intake of total calories. Common characteristics of the syndrome include retarded growth and maturation, muscle atrophy, and a loss of virtually all body fat.

Malnutrition and starvation in adults have very little effect on brain mass, but nutritional deficiencies in children during the early periods of growth can result in underdevelopment of the brain. An inadequate intake of nutrients during prenatal development (especially during the last trimester) and in the early stages of life after birth can significantly affect brain weight, brain size, number of cells formed, and amount of myelin developed in the brain, which possibly results in impaired mental and motor behavior. Adequate nutritional intake is critical to sexual maturation and the development of muscle tissue during the pubertal growth spurt. Potential consequences of an inadequate diet are smaller body mass and delayed menarche.

Physical Activity

Objective 5.4

➤ Physical activities are, in essence, the manifestation of the body's motor capabilities. The effects of physical activity on human development and behavior may be described from several perspectives. Two that are of direct bearing on the study of lifelong motor development are (a) the effects of physical activity and exercise on the structural aspects of physical growth and maturation, and (b) the influence of physical activity on the physiological function of the human body.

Most professional educators and researchers would agree that a minimum of physical activity is probably necessary for optimal biological growth and development. However, very little scientific information has been published on the subject, especially with respect to the long-term influence of habitual physical activity on human development. Much of the available information found in numerous dated physical education sources has been speculative. The difficulty in identifying the specific benefits of physical activity to growth and development from a scientific perspective lies primarily in the definition of terms. What is meant by the term optimal growth? And what *level* of activity is most beneficial to optimal growth?

Level of physical activity may be used to describe individuals as active or inactive, to identify those children who engage in play as normal, or to classify individuals who participate in regular physical training programs ranging in intensity from moderate to strenuous. Difficulty also lies in attempting to isolate physical activity in the growth process. An inherent weakness of almost any study of a topic that spans the growing years is how to explain the complex interaction of both genetic and environmental variables. In recent years, a considerable amount of information has been gathered on the specific effects of various types and intensity levels of physical activity on health-related fitness characteristics across virtually all ages. However, much work remains to be done to develop a clear understanding of how much physical activity is required to stimulate normal or optimal growth and development of other biological components.

Selected literature reviews and reports on the subject agree, in general, that a minimum of physical activity is apparently essential for specific aspects of normal growth and development to take place. However, just how much is necessary is unclear. The phenomenon of accelerated maturation and the increased body size associated with secular trend over the last 100 years or so have given little mention to the possible contributions of exercise or physical activity. Instead, explanations speak more to better nutrition, improved health care and health status, and contributing genetic factors. It is probably best to view secular trend as an interactive result of several genetic and environmental factors, including the possible influence of physical activity.

The following discussion concerning the effects of physical activity on biological growth and development was derived primarily from comprehensive reviews reported by Zauner, Maksud, and Melichna (1989), Broekhoff (1986), and Malina and Bouchard (1991). In the context of these reviews, the term *physical activity* refers to practices that are habitual or additional to normal movement or irregular patterns of play and recreation. Included in this definition are regular physical training programs such as physical education in schools, swimming, running, youth sports, calisthenics or aerobics, and weight training.

Stature The vast majority of evidence based on studies using equivalent control groups of preadolescent and adolescent children indicates that regular physical activity has no apparent effect on stature. Although some earlier studies suggested that stature increases with physical activity, reviewers of that research have pointed out that the differences were usually quite small and the experimental procedures questionable. In some studies reporting increased growth in stature due to athletic training, the apparent increase was probably not as much the product of intensity of training as it was early maturity. One study of female swimmers found they were taller than the average in the years prior to the research; apparently they had entered puberty earlier than the reference group with which they were compared. The same problem may have been prevalent among studies comparing young athletes with normal reference data. Note that the evidence does not indicate that training actually *promotes* significant growth in stature. It is clear however, that the training has no *negative* effect on this aspect of physical growth.

Body Mass The existing data are limited for younger and older populations. However they suggest that although body composition changes considerably during normal growth, particularly during adolescence, it can be further modified by habitual physical activity. Regular physical activity is, in fact, an important factor in the regulation and maintenance of desirable body weight. Optimal change, however, occurs when diet also is controlled. Even during the growing years in which an increase in body weight is characteristic, and across the life span as well, individuals who engage in regular training programs tend to have more lean body mass and less body fat than their nontraining peers. Ample evidence exists to verify that carefully designed physical activity programs can be effective in reducing the percentage of body fat in children and adults. The magnitude of change, however, may vary considerably depending on the intensity and duration of the program. Changes in body composition are highly dependent on continued activity.

Evidence also suggests that individuals who maintain a program of habitual physical activity, especially endurance training, throughout adulthood have less tendency for increasing body fat with advancing age. The available information on individuals who began training in older adulthood provides mixed results. In some cases minimal changes occurred in body fat, body weight, or lean body mass, whereas other studies reported significant losses of body fat. Further research is needed to arrive at more definitive conclusions.

Related to the fat cell theory mentioned in chapter 3, the results of a series of experimental studies using rats (Oscai et al., 1972, 1974) indicated that there is a critical time in early infancy in which fat cell proliferation may be enhanced by overfeeding. This results in an abnormal number of cells that remain with the body for life. Evidence suggested that increased physical activity and control of diet initiated in the early stages of development can effectively limit fat cell proliferation and reduce body fatness in later life. These results, although not decisive, have some very practical implications for infant care and weight control.

Body Proportion and Physique   In general, there is little evidence to suggest that physical activity at any level of intensity affects body proportions or overall body shape. Interestingly, although there have been significant increases in the secular trend of height and other dimensions over the last 100 years or so, changes have been approximately proportional. Thus, if any alternation in body proportionality occurs it is minimal. Studies that have focused on this aspect of physical activity and growth also indicate minimal influence due to training.

In one of the more comprehensive longitudinal studies of physical activity and growth, Parizkova and Carter (1976) found that boys engaged in various levels of physical activity, from intense to untrained, over a seven-year span from 11 to 18 years of age, showed no significant difference in the distribution of somatotype ratings among the activity groups. It also was noted that individual ratings changed considerably over the period and occurred in a random manner among the groups, which suggests that such changes cannot be attributed to physical activity. All participants changed somatotype rating at least once, and the majority changed in component dominance.

The short-term benefits of training for muscular development through weight training to increase the mesomorphic component of the somatotype have been verified with numerous studies of teenagers and adults.

Skeletal Growth and Development   Evidence currently suggests that regular physical activity has no apparent effect on skeletal maturity with regard to stature; however, it does enhance skeletal mineralization and density. Data from the Parizkova longitudinal study of change in physique also provide information about the effects of physical activity on skeletal maturation. Findings indicated there were no significant differences among the various groups before, during, or after the study as assessed using ossification ratings of the hand and wrist. Results also revealed that variation was greater within specific activity groups rather than between them. Other longitudinal studies have reported similar findings which suggests that skeletal maturity is not affected by regular physical training.

Numerous studies have suggested that greater skeletal mineralization and bone density and wider, more robust bones are associated with prolonged physical training. Although several of the studies have been conducted with animals, observations on adult humans have indicated similar results. In general, the effects of prolonged activity provide localized results that are activity related. For example, studies involving athletes have indicated that the more actively preferred limb of, for example, a tennis player, pitcher, or soccer player will exhibit greater mineralization and density than the nonpreferred limb. Studies that have observed bone density changes in runners relative to nonrunners also suggest greater values as a result of training. Similar findings have been reported on premenarcheal gymnasts and dancers compared to control groups (Bennell et al., 2000, Nickol-Richardson et al., 2000). The researchers suggested the results were due to the high-impact loading nature of the activities. As noted earlier, it has been suggested that these effects are related to regular physical training over several years' time. The data related to children are limited and perhaps problematic due to the confounding growth factor and lack of a long-term perspective.

The information on training and its effects on bone length is limited. Evidence has been reported indicating increased linear growth in dominant compared to nondominant limbs; however, other studies using animals have reported reduced bone lengths as a result of training. The apparent conflicting results center on the effects of pressure on bone growth plates. Theoretically, the pressure effects of physical activity either can stimulate growth or, in excessive amounts, retard linear growth. The difficulty lies in identifying and defining what is perceived as required, optimal, and excessive pressure. A theoretical notion known as *Wolff's Law* may have implications for bone growth in general. The law simply states that bone structures will adapt to suit the stresses and strains placed on them. Obviously more research and information are needed relative to the effects of varying levels of physical activity on growth plate genesis.

One of the more practical questions this data cannot answer clearly is whether active children have any skeletal advantages over relatively active children in later years. At this time, it appears that a lot more is known about the effect of physical inactivity on bone structure changes than about the effects of varying levels of physical activity.

Sexual Maturation It was pointed out that individuals today mature earlier than people did 100 years ago. The secular trend for onset of menarche has decreased approximately 4 months per decade since 1850. There is no evidence that this trend is linked to changes in physical activity patterns, nor has there been any documentation in recent years that supports the theory that habitual physical activity has a positive influence on sexual maturation of the reproductive system. There have been indications that high-intensity physical training and athletic competition may be factors in delayed menarche, however. A consistent body of evidence indicates that selected athletes (e.g., gymnasts, long-distance runners, ballet dancers, and figure skaters), on the average, experience menarche later than the general population. Observations also indicate that the number of years of training as well as the level of competition, prior to maturation, are linked to delayed menarche. It should be noted that most of the data on this subject are limited, associative, speculative, and do not control for other factors that may have influenced the onset of menarche. It is generally agreed that it is difficult, at best, to design a study in which individuals are randomly assigned to athletic activities and then to isolate the training factor as the primary cause for delayed menarche. However, it is reasonable to suggest that overtraining, which varies in individuals, may play an important role in altering the reproductive system (Rogol, 1996).

Of the proposed theories related to the possible influence of intense physical training on the timing of menarche, one in particular called the *critical-weight theory* (Frisch, 1991) has received considerable attention. The researcher proposed that a critical percentage of body fat (approximately 17%) must be reached before menarche can occur. It also is suggested that a body fat level of 22% is optimal for maintaining regular menstrual cycles. Thus, the association between female athletes who stay lean (i.e., below 17% body fat) throughout their training and the incidence of amenorrhea (irregularity) and delayed appearance of menarche provide the evidence to support this theory. There are indications that a relationship exists between the number of years of training prior to menarche and the time at which it appears. Marker (1981) noted that delayed menarche occurs more frequently in gymnasts (who have the highest mean age), figure skaters, and divers than among other athletes. An inferred relationship can be drawn, since females in these sports usually begin training early in life. Both studies reported mean ages for menarche of slightly above 15 years for those females who had extensive training before menarche; the average for the general population is around 12.5 years. The critical-weight theory has not found universal support, and the mechanisms by which intense strenuous physical training may affect the timing of menarche have not yet been clearly discerned.

Other theories have been proposed. For example, Warren (1980) concluded that along with a low percentage of body fat, an energy drain as a result of the intense training significantly may alter the hormonal processes that affect the set point of menarche. This alternation may result in a prolonged prepubertal phase and induced amenorrhea. A sociological explanation also has been suggested (Hata & Aoki, 1990); females who mature and reach early menarche may be socialized away from sports participation, whereas females who mature late tend to be drawn to sports participation.

In summarizing this literature, Rogol (1996) suggests that to truly understand the phenomenon described, one must consider several factors. In addition to exercise, one should address associated, or prior, nonexercise variables, such as diet, stress, hormone activity, and body weight.

Muscular Development and Strength   The evidence is overwhelming that specific strength training increases muscular force capabilities in adults and postpubertal children. Regular physical activity also results in some degree of skeletal muscle hypertrophy; the degree of hypertrophy varies with the intensity of training. The characteristics that generally accompany muscle hypertrophy are increases in enzymatic activity, myofibrils, contractile substances, and muscular strength. Muscles are strengthened by increasing their size and by enhancing the recruitment and firing rates of their motor units. Both of these processes are involved in the body's response to resistive physical activity, or exercise.

It appears that older males, prepubescent children, and females increase muscular strength primarily by neural adaptation (with some hypertrophy), whereas young males rely more on increases in muscle size. An ongoing debate in exercise physiology is whether resistance training induces the muscle to both increase the number of muscle cells (hyperplasia) and increase the cells in size (hypertrophy). For a long time the consensus was that muscles increased in size only after the hyperplasia period that ends shortly after birth. However, some recent though controversial evidence suggests that as a result of resistance training, muscle fibers may split as a means of increasing cell number. Even with this new hypothesis, it is generally agreed that the primary response to overload stress is muscle hypertrophy. Since the effects of intense (resistance) physical training on muscular development and increases in strength in postpubertal teenagers and young adults are well known, the remainder of this discussion will focus on the young and old.

We learned in chapter 3 that adult men have approximately 10 times the androgens of children and adult women, and that the bulk of this amount is produced during the adolescent growth spurt. At this time the greatest changes in male strength seem to appear and evidence strongly suggests that improvements in muscle force are related to greater testosterone levels. Often asked is whether prepubescent children can make significant gains in strength with training. Several studies confirm that prepubescent children are capable of making significant gains in strength, even though they possess relatively low hormone levels (reviews by Payne et al., 1997; Weltman, 1989).

Evidently, circulating androgens may not be the only primary influencing mechanism for strength development in this case. It is well documented that women, who also have low androgen levels, can make significant gains in strength without appreciable muscle hypertrophy. It appears that increases in strength in prepubescent children are probably the result of neural adaptions, that is, number of motor units recruited and their level of synchronization. It also suggested that the risk of short-term musculoskeletal damage is minimal if training is supervised; the use of hydraulic machines reduces the risk even more. However, more research is needed with regard to the effects of resistance training on articular cartilage. The American Academy of Pediatrics (1990) has published recommendations for weight training children.

With regard to the effects of regular participation in sports, children and adolescents who are involved in youth sports on a regular basis typically are stronger than those individuals who do not participate. Although this result may be an indication of the strength-promoting benefit of sports, it also could be due to a weak comparison between groups because young athletes often mature early and thus are bigger for their age. It is reasonable to assume that any benefits to strength development depend primarily on the specific physical activities associated with a particular sport.

With regard to older individuals, it appears they are not able to improve their strength capacity to the same extent as young people are able to do; however, significant improvement from regular vigorous training can be expected regardless of age. Older persons who stay physically active generally are stronger than sedentary individuals. The reasons for the decrease in trainability with age are not well understood, but it has been speculated that they are due, in part, to the general decline in neuromuscular functions. As with prepubescent children, studies of older individuals indicate their strength increases not primarily by muscle hypertrophy but by increased neural stimulation, or motor unit recruitment. As discussed in chapter 4, a general decrease of strength with age is expected because individuals generally experience a loss of muscle mass followed by a loss of motor unit fibers. A review of several studies suggests that significant gains in muscular strength can be achieved with vigorous training, at least into the ninth decade of life (McArdle et al., 2001). A remarkable testament of this has been reported for individuals in the age group 86 to 96 years (Fiatarone, 1994).

Cardiorespiratory Development   There is little question today that regular vigorous physical activity produces physiological improvements regardless of age. However, just as in the case of muscular development, the magnitude of the potential improvement depends on several factors, including initial fitness level, type of training, and age. With regard to age, the situation is again similar to that describing the effects of training (physical activity) on strength development. Older teenagers and adults who engage in vigorous aerobic activity for 20 minutes or longer at least three times per week are likely to experience physiological changes that include an increase in heart volume and cardiac output, a lower resting heart rate, and a faster return to resting heart rate.

In chapter 4 it was noted that the aging process can decrease general cardiovascular function by approximately 1.0% per year between the ages of 30 to 70. Along with the general decline in cardiorespiratory function as an individual ages, there also appears to be decreased trainability; that is, older individuals are not able to improve to the same extent as young people do.

In the final report of a longitudinal study of active men aged 45 to 65 years, evidence suggested that physical training may delay the decline in maximal oxygen uptake until at least age 65 (Kasch et al., 1990). Instead of the typical decline of 1% per year over the 20-year span, aerobically active men declined an average of only 12% over that time. A similar finding has been reported for men, ages 25 to 70 (Jackson et al., 1995). As noted earlier, sedentary individuals typically have nearly a twofold faster rate of decline in VO_2max as they age, compared to aerobically active persons.

THINK ABOUT IT

This discussion primarily noted the effects of normal habitual physical activity on development. What is your reaction to Olympic-style programs (e.g., 3 to 5 hours daily of swimming and gymnastics) for children?

Skill-Related Fitness   The contention that regular instruction and practice of motor skills result in improved balance, coordination, speed, power, agility, and other skill-related fitness is well supported in the literature (Malina & Bouchard, 1991). Such findings explain why regular participation in physical education programs is emphasized.

In addition to the issue of the extent that habitual physical activity enhances growth and development, is the concern over how competitive sports adversely affect prepubertal growth. Obviously, too much training in any sport could produce adverse effects. Psychological and physical stress (and fatigue) are not uncommon among young competitive athletes. And, as pointed out in the discussion of delayed menarche (sexual maturation), there are considerable individual differences within and between sports. With this in mind, Damsgaard and colleagues (2000) studied groups of competitive athletes from ages 9 to 13 who represented swimming, tennis, team handball, and gymnastics. In addition to considering hours of training, the researchers considered genetic factors, birth weight, and early growth patterns. These factors were compared with the athletes' height, weight, pubertal development, and body mass index. The overall conclusion was that *prepubertal growth is not adversely affected by sport at a competitive level.* However, it should be noted that most of the athletes studied trained less than 18 hours per week. Among top-level young performers in such sports as gymnastics and swimming, 3 to 5 hours per day of training is not unusual. As noted in the introduction, the inherent problem with studying this issue is the difficulty in discerning normal growth patterns from level of exercise or other factors that might influence growth (nutrition, genetics, and individual constitution [e.g., training tolerance]).

■ *Glands and Hormonal Activity*

Objective 5.5   ➤ Hormonal activity has been discussed in terms of its relevance to the adolescent growth spurt. Though it is beyond the scope of this text to detail the endocrine system, a brief review of hormonal activity as it relates to more general growth and development across the life span is appropriate.

Remember from chapter 3 (in reference to the adolescent growth spurt) that the endocrine system consists of several different glands that secrete hormones directly into the bloodstream (see figure 3.4 on page 73). The endocrine glands regulate such vital functions as skeletal and muscle growth, sexual reproduction, metabolism, and the aging of cellular tissues. As with most physiological mechanisms in the human body, aging also affects the endocrine system. Characteristic of these changes are a decrease in the secretion of hormones, diminishing responsiveness of specific cells to hormones, a change in the chemical transmitters that carry hormonal messages into cells, and a change in the levels of enzymes that respond to hormones. Hormones, in general, are highly interactive and affected by numerous factors, many of which have not been identified; consequently, the study of the effects of hormonal activity on growth and development is a complex undertaking. For in-depth discussions of the endocrinology of growth, refer to Tanner (1990) and Malina & Bouchard (1991). An illustration of the general location of major hormonal structures is shown in figure 5.2 on page 160.

Pituitary Gland

The pituitary gland is the master gland of the endocrine system. It produces one of the most important hormones involved in the process of human growth—the **growth hormone (GH).** GH is necessary for normal growth from birth to older adulthood. The only major portion of the body not affected by this hormone, in terms of growth stimulation,

■ *Figure 5.2*

General location of major hormonal structures

Pituitary gland (secretes GH and stimulates other glands)

Hypothalamus (control center for pituitary gland)

Thyroid gland (thyroxine)

Adrenal glands (androgens)

Pancreas (insulin)

Gonads (sex glands: estrogen and androgens)

is the CNS. The fetus has the capacity to synthesize GH by the end of the first trimester. Blood serum levels of the hormone in the neonate are significantly elevated above levels found during childhood. The importance of GH to the adolescent growth spurt is well documented; its relevance to fetal and infant growth is relatively unknown, although it has been determined that normal fetal development does occur in the absence of GH. Interestingly, the maximum production and secretion of GH occurs in association with periods of deep sleep.

As noted in chapter 3, GH promotes the incorporation of amino acids into tissue protein and stimulates the development of muscle and bone rather than fat tissue. Growth hormone also is known to stimulate DNA synthesis and cell multiplication. Its influence on increasing the number of cells in the body lasts from late infancy until adulthood, and its metabolic functions continue until death. The thyroid hormones and androgens interact with GH to perform functions vital to cell multiplication. In recent years, the development and use of synthetic GH

(GH therapy) have been quite effective in boosting the growth rate of children deficient in the hormone (Patlak, 1992).

Although the size and weight of the pituitary gland do not change with age, its blood supply gradually decreases after puberty. After about age 30, secretion of GH tends to decline, which in older adults is responsible in part for the decrease in lean body mass and bone density, and thinning of the skin (Rudman et al., 1990).

Thyroid Gland

The thyroid gland is second only to the pituitary in terms of influence on human growth and development. This gland produces **thyroxine,** which is important to cell multiplication and growth in the fetus and young child. In contrast to GH, thyroxine is essential to CNS development. Its presence is so important that regardless of other hormones, its absence would result in retarded and abnormal growth. Thyroxine is vital to the production of all forms of RNA (ribonucleic acid), and its presence stimulates ribosome production and protein synthesis. Other functions include metabolizing fats and carbohydrates, stimulating the cell's use of oxygen, and, along with sex hormones, facilitating skeletal development through calcium and phosphate absorption. GH is relatively ineffective without thyroxine. In contrast to GH, which has little if any effect on fetal and early infant growth, thyroxine is very influential. Children with too little thyroxine grow at a below-average rate, but with prompt treatment typically catch up to normal size (Tanner, 1990).

As people age, the cells within the thyroid gland undergo several structural changes and collagen fibers appear. With increasing age, the blood levels of thyroxine do not drop even though the thyroid itself produces fewer hormones. The thyroid gland continues to function normally in healthy adults throughout the life span.

Pancreas

The pancreas, which is well developed by the end of prenatal development, secretes a powerful anabolic hormone called insulin. Its primary functions are to metabolize sugars in the diet and increase the transport of glucose (blood sugar) and amino acids across the plasma membrane. Insulin also enhances protein synthesis, although tissue hypertrophy can occur in its absence, and appears to increase the synthesis of DNA (deoxyribonucleic acid) and RNA in muscle and bone tissues. The commonly known disorder of diabetes is a result of an abnormality in the body's ability to metabolize blood sugar. With increasing age, many people experience longer and higher levels of blood sugar as a result of the aging cell's tendency to absorb less blood sugar and decrease its active insulin secretion.

Adrenal Glands

Of the several groups of hormones the adrenal glands produce, the androgens are the most important to a discussion of factors influencing growth and development. Although androgens are secreted by the adrenal cortex in both sexes, they also are produced by the testes in the male; their release is triggered by actions originating from the pituitary gonadotropins.

Chapter 3 discussed the importance of adrenal hormones to the development of muscle tissue and skeletal growth. Other functions include causing the release of epinephrine and norepinephrine to mediate the response to stress, mediating the kidney's absorption of sodium and chloride, and metabolizing fat and carbohydrates. Although a major portion of the adrenal cortex is developed and differentiated by the third fetal month, it does not reach its adult character until about the third postnatal year (Lowrey, 1986).

As the system ages, the production of some adrenal hormones, including androgens, declines. The hormone secretions that regulate fat and carbohydrate metabolism do not decline with aging, although it will take individuals longer to complete this metabolic process as they age. Hormones affecting fluid balance in kidney function remain relatively stable well into old age.

Other Glandular Functions

Closely associated with sex differentiation, physical growth, and sex hormones are the functions of the *gonads* (the testes and ovaries). Adrenal and gonadal tissues originate from similar cells; both are known as *steroid-producing glands*. Exposure of the brain to sex hormones during early fetal development is associated with future reproductive physiology and sex-oriented behavioral characteristics. For example, during the early stages of fetal development, androgens interact with the immature CNS to imprint future male characteristics. Ovarian estrogens in females, like testosterone in males, normally are not secreted in physiologically effective quantities until shortly before puberty.

Hormones secreted by the *parathyroid glands* also play a major role in normal growth and development. At birth the parathyroid glands are similar morphologically to those of the adult. These hormones are responsible for normal skeletal development by regulating calcium and phosphorus metabolism. In addition to its function in skeletal development, these hormones also enhance calcium absorption in the presence of vitamin D. The parathyroid glands, located at the base of the throat, grow heavier until males turn 30 and females reach 50 years of age. After these peaks, their size and rate of hormone production remain stable.

Most experts agree that physical activity probably influences many of the relationships among hormonal activity, growth, and behavioral characteristics. Although exercise of varying levels and types has been shown to affect specific hormone concentrations, the consensus is that it does not significantly influence physical growth beyond that which would occur naturally.

Summary

Several factors may affect the normal course of growth and development throughout the life span. A number of maternal and external factors can have a profound effect on development of the unborn infant. Among the potentially harmful maternal factors are age of the mother, nutrition, genetic-related abnormalities, fetal position, and the mother's emotional state.

Although the fetus appears safe in its protective membrane, the fetus can still be affected by external environmental factors through the placenta. Broadly, external factors can include anything the expectant mother breathes, drinks, eats, or smokes, or the disease-producing bacteria with which she comes in contact. Exposure to harmful agents (teratogens) can cause negative reactions in the form of birth defects and behavioral dysfunctions. Among them are infectious diseases, tobacco, alcohol, drugs, radiation, and various chemicals. In spite of the possible dangers, human beings have a strong tendency to develop in what appears to be a normal manner under all but the most damaging conditions.

The intake of essential nutrients and water are vital to growth and development throughout the life span. In general, infants with malnourished diets (especially diets low in protein and total calories) show below-average physical growth by early childhood. However, the primary concern for children in the United States appears to be the over-consumption of fat, refined sugar, and salt rather than a deficiency of protein and calories.

Although the literature is unclear regarding what level of physical activity is beneficial or harmful to physical growth and development, its effects on specific characteristics have been documented. In general, habitual physical activity has been shown to have a positive influence on body weight, lean body mass, skeletal mineralization and density, muscular development and strength, and cardiorespiratory development. Most of the literature, however, does not claim that habitual physical activity has any significant influence on stature, skeletal maturity, or body proportion and physique. Some research has suggested that intense exercise may be a factor in delayed menarche, but there is no evidence that physical activity has a positive influence on sexual maturation. For the typical young competitive athlete, training does not appear to adversely affect pubertal growth.

One of the most influential factors in physical growth and development throughout the life span is hormonal activity. Hormones, in general, are highly interactive and affected by numerous factors, many of which are unknown.

Think about It

1. Consider how maternal factors effect postnatal motor development.
2. Advances in science are telling us more and more about what affects prenatal development. Are you suspicious of any other (than the already described) agents that might affect prenatal development?
3. What do you think is the greatest problem with children's health: lack of exercise or poor diet? What, specifically, is the solution for an overweight child?
4. This discussion primarily noted the effects of normal habitual physical activity on development. What is your reaction to Olympic-style programs (e.g., 3 to 5 hours daily of swimming and gymnastics) for children?

Suggested Readings

Malina, R. M., & Bouchard, C. (1991). *Growth, maturation, and physical activity.* Champaign, IL: Human Kinetics.

McArdle, W. D., Katch, F. I., & Katch, V. L. (2001). *Exercise physiology* (5th ed.). Philadelphia: Lea & Febiger.

Physical activity and good nutrition, (2000). U.S. Department of Health and Human Services, Centers for Disease Control and Prevention.

Tanner, J. M. (1990). *Fetus into man.* Cambridge, MA: Harvard University Press.

Tough, S., Newburn-Cook, C., Johnston, D., Svenson, L., Rose, S., & Belik, J. (2002). Delayed childbearing and its impact on population rate changes in lower birth weight, multiple birth, and preterm delivery. *Pediatrics, 109*(3), 399–403.

WebLinks

American Academy of Pediatrics (policy statement on strength training by children and adolescents)
www.aap.org/policy/re0048.html

American Academy of Pediatric Committee on Nutrition
www.aap.org/visit/cmte25.htm

American College of Sports Medicine
www.acsm.org

Centers for Disease Control and Prevention (Health and fitness statistics)
www.cdc.gov/nchs

Centers for Disease Control and Prevention (Physical activity and health: A report of the Surgeon General)
    www.cdc.gov/nccdphp/sgr/sgr.htm

March of Dimes
    www.modimes.org

KidsHealth, (Provides health and development information about children from before birth through adolescence)
    http://kidshealth.org/parent/growth/senses/sensenewborn.html

National Association for the Education of Young Children
    www.naeyc.org

National Strength & Conditioning Association
    www.nsca-lift.org/menu.asp

Perception and Information Processing

PART THREE takes a developmental perspective to focus on the way people perceive and act upon sensory information from the external and internal environments. This general process is called **information processing.** From a motor behavior perspective, information processing involves both *perception* (monitoring and interpreting sensory information) and *motor response* (deciding upon and organizing response activity). Figure 6.1 illustrates the information-processing, or *perceptual-motor process*, model. The model contains four primary components: sensory input, reception of information, interpretation of information and decision making, and overt motor response.

The processing stage will be studied in two separate chapters. Chapter 6 focuses on the developmental aspects of the perceptual systems with regard to receiving, monitoring, and interpreting sensory data. Chapter 7 covers the developmental aspects involved in processing and acting on the information. It gives special emphasis to attention,

c h a p t e r s

6   Perceptual Development

7   Information Processing and Motor Control

memory, processing speed, motor programming, and theories of motor control. Chapters 6 and 7 together provide a framework for studying the complex processes involved in the central issue of the text understanding

> *Perception* → *Action*
> (motor response)

6 *Perceptual Development*

OBJECTIVES

Upon completion of this chapter, you should be able to

6.1 Diagram the information-processing model (perceptual-motor process) and briefly explain the four primary components.

6.2 Explain the terms *sensation* and *perception*.

6.3 Briefly describe the basic visual process and structural changes that occur over the life span.

6.4 List and describe the nine basic functional aspects of the visual modality and the changes associated with visual development.

6.5 Explain the term *kinesthesis*.

6.6 Outline the basic function and structure of kinesthetic perception.

6.7 Distinguish between kinesthetic acuity and kinesthetic memory, give an example of each, and describe their developmental characteristics.

6.8 List the five components of basic movement awareness associated with the kinesthetic modality and describe how they function and change over time.

6.9 Discuss auditory perception in terms of its basic function, structural change over time, and developmental characteristics.

6.10 Describe tactile perception and identify the significant events that take place in its development.

6.11 Provide a general definition of perceptual integration and discuss the specific visual-auditory, visual-kinesthetic, and auditory-kinesthetic intermodal relationships.

6.12 Describe the major changes that occur in perception with aging.

6.13 Discuss *Gibson's ecological perspective* and its role in understanding *perception to action*.

KEY TERMS

information processing

perception

visual acuity

object permanence

A-not-B error

embodiment

perceptual constancy

spatial orientation

figure-ground perception

depth perception

field of vision

coincident timing

visual-motor coordination

kinesthesis

body awareness

spatial awareness

directional awareness

vestibular awareness

rhythmic awareness

tactile perception

perceptual integration

intermodal perception

Gibson's ecological
perspective

affordances

THE ESSENCE OF HUMAN BEHAVIOR and motor performance is based on the ability to receive and interpret sensory information. Human beings live in a vast sea of sensory information, yet they thrive rather than drown because of an elaborate network of perceptual systems. The human perceptual system, in fact, has a constant need to receive sensory input from the external world and from its own internal environment. When sensory input is reduced or eliminated, the system reacts negatively. This same negative reaction also can occur when the system is overloaded by too much sensory input. This happens when you try to carry on a telephone conversation while reading a paper, or when a beginner in dance class tries to stay in step with the teacher's instructions during a fast-paced song.

Objective 6.2

➤ **Perception** refers to the processes used to gather and interpret sensory information from the external and internal environment. The two related processes of sensation and perception enable the body to receive stimulation and organize it for further processing.

Sensation refers to the stimulation of sensory receptors (figure 6.1) by physical energy received from the internal and external environment. The retina of the eye, for example, reacts to light rays (sensory input) and translates the message into nerve impulses (reception). The nerve impulses then are transmitted via the perceptual modality to the brain,

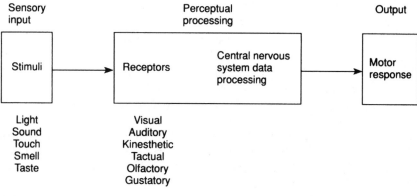

Sensory input · Perceptual processing · Output

Stimuli → Receptors · Central nervous system data processing → Motor response

Sensory input	Perceptual processing
Light	Visual
Sound	Auditory
Touch	Kinesthetic
Smell	Tactual
Taste	Olfactory
	Gustatory

▪ *Figure 6.1*

The general information-processing (perceptual-motor) model

which reacts to the stimulation in various ways. At this point perception occurs. Basically perception involves the monitoring (reception) and interpretation of sensory information. The interpretation given to the information is based on past experience (memory) and cognitive analysis (judgments) of the information. Intertwined with interpretation is the ability to discriminate among various types of sensory stimuli with varying degrees of precision—the similarities or differences, arrangements, and organization.

Another complex function of the brain in this process is to integrate information coming from different perceptual modalities. This information provides the basis for formulating a motor response, which completes the information-processing cycle. This sequence may be thought of as the information-gathering segment of the general information-processing model.

Of the six perceptual modalities, perhaps the two that provide the most relevance to the study of motor behavior are *vision* and *kinesthesis.* This is not to minimize the importance of audition and tactile information; these modalities will be discussed briefly along with system integration. However, human movement is universally described in terms of its spatial-temporal characteristics—the spatial coordinates and timing of the body with moving stimuli, as well as internal rhythmic awareness. Although individuals can move in the environment without visual information (as the blind do), this modality is crucial in determining reference points and judging the movement of objects. The visual modality provides spatial-temporal information about the external environment, and the kinesthetic system may be described as the body-knowledge network that provides information about the body's movements without reference to auditory or visual cues.

Visual Perception

Objective 6.3

➤ In many ways, vision is the dominant perceptual modality. For human beings, the visual world is the richest source of information about the external environment. Experts estimate that approximately 80% of all sensory information derived outside the body is channeled through the visual system. In terms of movement, visual input provides a primary source of information from which motor behavior is organized and carried out. Visual information is used to formulate a motor program, monitor movement activity, and provide the feedback that allows for immediate correction. Visual input is such a dominant source of information that people tend to rely on it even though other sensory information may be more useful.

Most of the available data on this subject focus on infants and children during the growing years. Until about 25 years ago, it was believed the newborn infant was incapable of processing information meaningfully. Today most experts agree the visual system of the newborn is relatively well developed at birth and the neonate demonstrates considerable visual ability. On the other end of the lifelong developmental continuum several deficits attributed to aging have been documented, though the information on perceptual changes during adulthood and old age is sparse.

The Visual Process

Three basic functions occur in the course of visual perception. First, the eyes receive light and generate messages through nerve impulses about that light. Second, visual pathways transmit those messages through the optic tract from the eye to the visual centers of the brain. Finally, the visual centers interpret those messages.

Light enters the eye through the pupil, passes through the lens and chambers, and terminates in the retina. The retina is a complex structure consisting of numerous photosensitive receptors and other cells that assist in optic transmission of visual nerve impulses. After nerve impulses are transduced from light energy in the retina, they are transmitted over the optic nerve. The optic nerve from each eye resembles a cable that contains approximately 1 million wires and acts as a huge communication line. The optic nerves must input all of the visual information that comes into the brain for neural processing. Optic nerves from the two eyes pass backward to unite at the optic chiasma and from there project posteriorly even further as the optic tracts. Fibers from these tracts make synaptic connections with several subcortical structures in the brain. Signals then enter the visual projection areas located in the occipital lobes, at which point impulses are dispersed in various directions to the association areas where interpretation, or perception, takes place.

Developmental Change in Visual Structures

Every structure in the visual system undergoes some early postnatal change. Although all of the visual structures are intact at birth, several are immature in terms of myelinization and synaptic potential. There is also great variability in the growth rate of different parts of the eye. The size of the eye approximately doubles between birth and maturity.

The newborn retina, the part of the eye that turns light into nerve signals to the brain, is similar in structure to that of the adult but is thicker and has no distinct fovea. The fovea is the area in which central visual images are formed. Without this structure, the processing of spatial resolution is poor in the central retina; thus the ability to see images clearly is relatively weak in comparison to the mature structure. Development proceeds rapidly. By the end of the first year the major structures of the retina are like those of the adult.

The part of the nervous system that relays visual impressions between the retina and the cortex of the brain also develops quickly and reaches a large part of its ultimate efficiency during the first 11 to 12 months. In the visual cortex, dendritic development at the ends of the nerve cells forms more branches, and by 4 to 5 months of age, the myelinization process is almost complete. At about 2 months, the infant's visual cortex begins to process visual stimuli.

Compared to that of the adult, the newborn's eyeball is short, and the distance between the retina and the lens is reduced. This results in a temporary form of farsightedness. Many infants also will have astigmatisms (difficulty in focusing) during the first year because their cornea is not yet symmetrical. Another developmental difference between the neonate and the adult is in the strength and control of eye muscles. Because of weak ciliary muscles attached to the lens, few newborns can change the shape of the lens to accommodate to the shifting plane of focus for visual targets, as occurs in the adult eye. Until the end of the first month, infants can adjust their focus only for targets between 5 to 10 inches away. By 4 months of age, infants can accommodate to shifting planes of focus as well as adults. Figure 6.2 on page 174 illustrates a comparison of the adult and newborn eye.

Developmental Change in Visual Functions

Objective 6.4 ➤ **Visual Acuity** **Visual acuity** refers to clearness of vision and the capacity to detect both small stimuli and small details of large visual patterns. From a motor behavior perspective, visual acuity often is classified as static or dynamic. *Static visual acuity*, the most common form of assessment, is concerned with the ability to detect detail in a stationary object. *Dynamic visual acuity* refers to the ability to perceive detail in a moving object.

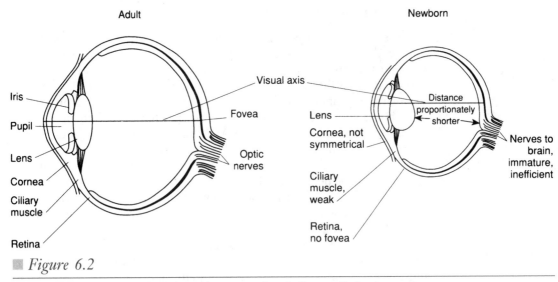

Iris
Pupil
Lens
Cornea
Ciliary muscle
Retina

Visual axis
Fovea
Optic nerves

Adult

Newborn

Lens
Cornea, not symmetrical
Ciliary muscle, weak
Retina, no fovea

Distance proportionately shorter
Nerves to brain, immature, inefficient

■ *Figure 6.2*

A comparison of an adult and newborn eye that indicates limitations of the infant's visual system

At birth the neonate can see; however, it is not known with what degree of clarity. It was once assumed the newborn could not see more than a blur until 3 or 4 weeks of age. Researchers now know that soon after birth a baby can focus on a near object and respond visually to a moving light. By 3 months a baby can focus quite well, but not with good clarity.

Using Snellen values as a reference, a newborn's acuity has been estimated between 20/200 and 20/600. This means an individual sees an object 20 feet away as if it were 600 feet away. The 20/600 value is about 30 times lower than adult visual acuity (20/20). By 6 months, the baby's acuity has improved significantly, to about 20/100. By the end of the first year, the baby sees about as well as an adult.

Although these comparative figures might lead one to speculate that a young infant cannot see well, it should be noted that infants are far from blind. Banks and Salapatek (1981) suggest that though the young infant's visual window is quite limited, it can detect the contours of many common objects. For example, young infants can see the contrast between hair and skin on a parent's face and can detect large objects at close range.

The perceptual component of dynamic visual acuity reflects the ability of the central nervous system (CNS) to estimate the direction and velocity of an object, and the ability of the ocular-motor system to catch and hold its image on the fovea long enough to permit resolution of its detail. Different estimates of age-related acuity levels have been reported. It is quite evident, however, that static visual acuity matures before dynamic acuity and that the ability to focus on a moving object is a function of the speed at which it is moving (i.e., efficiency decreases as speed increases). Dynamic acuity increases gradually during childhood with notable periods of improvement from 5 to 7 years, 9 to 10 years, and 11 to 12 years. Efficiency remains relatively stable from 12 years of age to the beginning of middle-age adulthood. Males demonstrate superior abilities in static and dynamic acuity over females at all ages.

As noted earlier, among the primary factors that affect visual acuity are development of the fovea, degree of myelinization, number of neural connections in the visual cortex, shape and structure of the eye, and strength of the ciliary muscles. There is also some indication that the quality of visual acuity coincides with the development of binocular vision (the ability to use both eyes together and fixate on an object), which is evident by 2 months of age.

Object Permanence The realization that objects continue to exist when they are no longer in view is **object permanence.** This ability is considered one of the more notable achievements in sensorimotor development. Young infants typically rely heavily on vision and movement to derive information about an object. When an attractive (distinctive) object is shown then hidden from view, babies (from 1 to 4 months) typically lose interest, as though the object did not exist (figure 6.3). This observation was noted frequently in Piaget's (1952) early work. Between the ages of 4 to 8 months, when infants can successfully reach for objects, they continue to be disinterested unless the object is partially

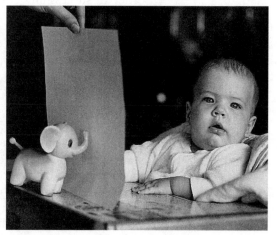

■ Figure 6.3

A baby shows no sign she knows the toy is still there

visible. Between the ages of 8 to 12 months, signs of object permanence begin to emerge. However, at this stage they will typically search for a hidden object *where they first found it,* rather than where they saw it last (when the location is switched). This phenomenon is known as the **A-not-B error,** a classic (hide-and-seek) experimental design introduced by Piaget and used with variations in contemporary research. Between the ages of 12 to 18 months, this ability improves significantly; infants search for the object *where they last saw it.* However, infants still have difficulty perceiving invisible displacement and programming a reach response. Between the ages of 18 months and 2 years, infants are capable of making this integration. Using a more sophisticated but similar paradigm (i.e., four doors), Berthier et al. (2000) found results consistent with the Piagetian view. Among children who were 2, 2½, and 3 years of age, only the older children reliably chose the correct door. This suggests that the ability to integrate memory with motor ability develops slowly over the first years of life. It appears that developmentally infants have difficulty integrating knowledge (perceptual information about an object) with action, which requires a certain level of cortex maturation that may not be present until after the first year (Bell & Fox, 1992; Diamond, 1998).

THINK ABOUT IT

Consider child's play. How is it related to embodiment?

The phenomenon of the A-not-B error continues to be a highly studied and debated issue in child development. In fact, the basic concept provides a key experimental vehicle by which contemporary researchers are studying the notion of **embodiment** (e.g., Thelen et al., 2001), that is, the role of motor behavior in higher cognition such as memory and decision making. The underlying hypothesis is that perceptual and motor abilities are inseparately linked and together form the basis for cognition, emotion, and language. Supporters point out that in order to successfully complete the reaching task in the A-not-B setup, the infant must perceive, remember, create a plan of action, and reach. Although critics of the theoretical claims remain, few would disagree that the experimental task provides an excellent study of the infant's ability to perceive and act on information. Similar arguments that there is a bodily basis to thought, such as in music and language, have drawn attention to the role of movement in human development (Cassell et al., 2001; Seitz, 2000).

Perceptual Constancy Of the various aspects of **perceptual constancy,** the one most closely related to the study of motor behavior is the perception of size constancy. Other constancies include shape and color. When an object becomes known to an infant, it becomes recognizable as that specific object regardless of the angle or distance from which it is observed. The object has constancy because it remains the same form even though the retinal image changes. Hence, the ability to perceive constant size is referred to as perceptual constancy.

Another way of describing constancy is the notion that the perceived size is scaled. That is, one unit of measurement is converted, or scaled, into another (perceived size). Road maps, for example, typically include scales that transform inches into miles; theoretically, the visual system contains a mechanism that scales an image into object size.

Sekuler and Blake (2002) provide an excellent example of how constancy seems to occur automatically. Hold up both thumbs side by side with nails facing you, approximately 8 inches (20 cm) from your eyes. At this point both thumbs look identical in size. Next, extend one arm until the thumb is about 16 inches (40 cm) away. At first glance the two thumbs should continue to appear identical in size, even though the image size of the closer thumb is now twice that of the farther one. This is perceptual constancy.

Another example is perceiving that the airplane on the ground before takeoff is the same object that, minutes later, is several thousand feet in the air. The importance of constancy is that it represents perceptual stability and underlies the ability to interpret the environment consistently and accurately.

In the past, researchers thought this ability did not appear until 4 to 5 months of age, but it seems that even newborns know something about an object's size (Slater et al., 1990). Important stimuli for perception appear to be kinetic cues noted as an object approaches and recedes. This ability steadily improves; maturity is reached between 10 and 11 years of age. As noted earlier, the ability to understand the constancy of objects is essential to motor development, especially when the infant explores *affordances* in the environment.

Spatial Orientation Perception of **spatial orientation** refers to the ability to recognize an object's orientation or position in three-dimensional space. Closely associated with this visual ability is a component of kinesthetic perception known as *spatial awareness*. This is the internal awareness of the position (orientation) of objects and of the body in three-dimensional space. This discussion concentrates primarily on the visual perception of objects rather than on aspects of internal awareness of spatial orientation and movement in the external environment.

It is important to recognize the differences in spatial orientation of objects. Most older children and adults have the ability to immediately notice these differences, whereas young children do not have this facility. Young children first must learn to recognize the spatial characteristics of objects before they can ignore irrelevant information. In some everyday tasks and motor skill activities it is important to recognize an object even if it is upside down, rotated, or angled to one side. In the case of recognizing letters such as d and b, and p and q, proper identification of spatial orientation is critical. Successfully performing certain target projecting tasks, gymnastic events, and game activities by recognizing boundary lines and designated spaces also necessitates the accurate perception of spatial orientation.

By 3 to 4 years of age, children are aware of most basic spatial dualisms such as over/under, high/low, front/back, in/out, top/bottom, and vertical/horizontal. However, until these characteristics become commonplace and perceptually refined in their spatial worlds, children are likely to get things reversed, inverted, and confused. It also has been observed that children appear to master spatial dimensions in a fairly orderly sequence—vertical to horizontal, then to diagonal or oblique. Although 3- and 4-year-olds have some ability to distinguish vertical from horizontal, they still lack the ability to effectively perceive mirror images (left-right reversals) and oblique lines and diagonals. By 8 years of age, most children can perceive the spatial orientation of objects, although some individuals continue to have problems with right-left or mirror image reversals.

Figure-Ground Perception **Figure-ground perception** refers to the ability to distinguish an object from its surrounding background. This ability, as with most meaningful motor behavior tasks requires an individual to concentrate on and give selective attention to a visual stimulus. Examples of figure-ground perception include the ability to track and/or intercept objects in sports such as softball, golf, soccer, and ice hockey. To catch a softball hit into the sky, the outfielder must first focus on and track the ball (figure) against the backdrop (ground) of white sky or lights (if at night).

Figure-ground perception appears to improve rapidly between the ages of 4 and 8. Evidence also suggests that the refinement of figure-ground perception continues to improve between the ages of 13 and 18. Individuals at all ages are more proficient at identifying familiar figures embedded in distracting backgrounds than they are at perceiving unfamiliar figures from similar backgrounds.

Depth Perception **Depth perception** is the ability to judge the distance of an object from the self. This automatic occurrence takes place every time an individual judges the distance to other vehicles when driving or attempts to shoot a basketball. Reacting quickly to such tasks requires the individual to know where the object is located in three-dimensional space.

Depth perception is referred to in absolute distance and relative distance. Absolute distance refers to a precise judgment of the space from the person to an object. For example, a short-stop attempting to throw out a runner at first base must judge the distance between himself and the base. An infant attempting to place a cap on a bottle and an adult reaching for a cup of coffee are other examples of judging absolute distance.

Relative distance refers to the estimation of distance between one object and another or between different parts of a single object.

Examples include discriminating the distance between two rattles or determining whether an opponent or partner is closer to the goalpost. The ability to judge relative distance is much more precise than the detection of absolute distance.

The perceptual system uses two types of cues to detect depth: oculomotor cues and visual cues. The development of each is tied to independent perceptual systems (i.e., visual and kinesthetic). Oculomotor cues are kinesthetic in nature, which means cues are derived from the kinesthetic receptors located in the muscles and joints. An example of this is evident in the absolute distance task of using the arm and hand to reach for a glass of water. Visual cues, in contrast, provide good relative depth information but also might offer additional information about absolute distance. Information is gathered through visual perception either with binocular cues (using both eyes) or monocular cues (using one eye). The independent development of kinesthesis (kinesthetic sense), monocular vision, and binocular vision all have developmental implications for the individual's ability to judge distances.

It is generally agreed that depth perception is absent at birth. *Most sources indicate that by the age of 6 months, children are capable of judging depth with fair accuracy.* However, a number of studies of infants as young as 2 months of age suggest they are aware of and perceive to some degree the spatial dimensions of depth. As a result of studies in which objects were dropped toward an infant's face (protected by a sheet of glass) to evoke defensive blinking, researchers have suggested that some aspects of depth perception are developed by the age of 2½ to 3 months (Pettersen, et al., 1980). Supporting evidence for the presence of depth perception in this age range is based on the fact that true binocular vision, a primary component of accurate depth perception, appears at about 2 months. This suggests the basis for refinement of the ability. Binocularity continues to improve from ages 2 to 6 and is closely tied to improvements in depth perception. By the age of 6 or 7, children can judge depth as accurately using monocular cues as binocular cues.

A simple observation of 4-month-old infants in grasping objects reveals they have some degree of depth perception. When an object is placed within grasping range, most infants will attempt to grasp it; when the item is placed out of reach infants rarely grab for it.

The classic study of depth perception in children involved the use of a visual cliff (Gibson & Walk, 1960). The apparatus consisted of a table several feet high covered with a heavy sheet of glass. On one side of the table (runway), a checkerboard pattern was fixed just beneath the surface of the glass. On the other side, the same checkerboard pattern was set 3½ feet below the surface of the glass, thus creating a visual cliff. Infants were placed on the shallow side and beckoned by their mothers to cross the glass over the cliff. The investigators found that infants as young as 6 months of age clearly paid attention to depth cues

THINK ABOUT IT

Can you think of ways to modify the visual cliff experiment to study other aspects of depth perception?

Confronting the
visual cliff

and would not crawl to their mothers over the deep end, even when
coaxed (figure 6.4).

The data suggest that depth perception capabilities are present to
some extent in infants as young as 2 months, and improvement proceeds
rapidly up to 6 months. Refinement (especially of absolute distance) continues until approximately age 12.

Field of Vision   Also known as *peripheral vision*, **field of vision** refers
to the entire extent of the environment that can be seen without changing the fixation of the eye. References to peripheral vision frequently are
described in terms of lateral and vertical capabilities. Most animals can
visually take in the majority of their surroundings all at once. In contrast, humans have a rather limited field of vision. Humans can compensate for this relative limitation by adjusting where the eyes are
directed (e.g., looking both ways before driving through an intersection).
According to Sekuler and Blake (2002), normal adult lateral peripheral
vision is approximately 90 degrees from straight ahead, which creates a
visual field of about 180 degrees. In contrast, vertical peripheral vision
in adults is approximately 47 degrees above and 65 degrees below the
visual midline.

Information on the development of peripheral vision, especially the
vertical aspects, is quite limited. At 7 weeks, lateral peripheral vision is
about 35 degrees, roughly 40% of adult capability. According to a
review by Cummings et al. (1988), most sources indicate that by the
end of the first postnatal year, visual field extension is still immature.
Only after age 5 are visual fields equivalent to those of adults. A person's lateral field of vision is at its peak at about age 35. Although the

role of peripheral vision in children's motor performance is not clear, its importance in sports at the adult level is evident. In activities that involve quick responses and numerous visual cues (e.g., basketball, tennis, hockey, and soccer), central and lateral peripheral vision are essential for spatial orientation.

Perception of Movement   One of the most important and complex perceptual abilities related to motor behavior is the detection, tracking, and interception of moving objects. Many more demands are placed on the perceptual system when objects begin to move in space and individuals are confronted with dynamic rather than static conditions. Just a few of the difficulties are evident when one considers the differences between static (stationary) objects and dynamic visual acuity, and the perception of depth in reference to moving (dynamic) objects in comparison to stationary objects.

In addition to the functional aspects of these perceptual abilities, the developmental dynamics of eye movement changes are also factors that influence the ability to perceive moving objects. *Saccadic eye movements* are rapid movements between one point of visual fixation (i.e., focusing one's gaze on something) and another. These movements are slower and more numerous in young infants than in older children and adults. At maturity (approximately 12 years), a saccade moves the eye about 90% of the distance to the visual target, but in infants several saccades are required to reach their visual target. An infant's eyes also move less smoothly in tracking a moving object and tend to refixate frequently, or focus first on one spot and then another. It is difficult for the newborn to focus both eyes on the same point (convergence) and thus to see only one stimulus.

By 48 hours after birth, most infants can track a slow-moving object. This response is uneven, however, and focus is easily lost (Haith et al., 1993). Smoother, more accurate tracking is evident by 2 months. By 4 months the more complex task of tracking and predicting the path of a slow-moving object is within most infants capabilities. By 4 to 5 months the infant has reached an unrefined visual-motor stage and exhibits approaching movements with the upper body as if attempting to receive the object.

A comprehensive review of the subject by Williams (1983), which includes much of the researcher's own work, suggests the ability to accurately perceive moving objects continues to develop through the childhood years until relative maturity at approximately 12 years of age. However, between the ages of 6 and 11, a number of developmental trends have been observed. When asked to judge the speed, direction, and interception point of a moving object, children 9 to 11 years of age judged the flight of the moving object with significantly more accuracy than the younger children did. Although the younger children generally responded quickly to the object, they were not able to effectively integrate the available sensory information about its flight path with their motor behavior. It appears the upper elementary school years are a period of transition during which the ability to integrate the visual and motor mechanisms increases. By the sixth grade, older children make judgments much faster and more accurately about moving objects than younger children do. This behavior suggests that the visual-motor processes are nearing maturity.

Coincident timing, another aspect of tracking and intercepting objects, also appears to improve with age. Coincident timing tasks are commonly used in sport activities that involve the ability to coordinate visual and motor behavior to a single coincident point (interception) such as in catching a ball, kicking a moving ball, and passing a ball to a running player. An important determinant in coincident timing performance is the relative direction of the moving object. In general, the ability of the individual to time movements to an interception point with a moving object improves with age up to young adulthood (e.g., Fischman, et al., 1992; Keogh & Sugden, 1985). And, as might be expected, accuracy tends to decrease as velocity increases. Proficiency is generally achieved during the early teenage years.

Other than the fact that coincident timing abilities seem to improve with age, the specific developmental mechanisms involved are not well understood. A more recent longitudinal study that tracked the coincident timing abilities from ages 6 to 12 years has noted an interesting finding (Kuhlman & Beitel, 1997). For both sexes, the amount of time spend playing sports (e.g., soccer and softball) and video games was a better indicator of ability than age. This ability is an excellent example of complete information processing; much more is involved than the simple perception of moving stimuli. Coincident timing involves a complex interplay between visual-perception proficiency and motor control. The discussion of motor performance provides a more complete treatment of visual-motor abilities.

Visual-Motor Coordination The ability to coordinate visual abilities with movements of the body is **visual-motor coordination.** This aspect of movement combines both visual and kinesthetic perceptions with the ability to make controlled and coordinated bodily movements that usually involve eye-hand or eye-foot integration. Development of these actions generally follows the proximodistal (midline to periphery), cephalocaudal (head to toes), and gross-to-fine motor order. Much of the contemporary research on this topic involves reaching, which will be discussed in greater detail in chapter 8. Briefly, eye-hand coordination emerges during the first 6 months of life, as evidenced by reaching to objects reasonably well by 4 months. By 7 months of age, the trajectory

TABLE 6.1

Selected Fine Visual-Motor Characteristics of Children 3 to 8 Years Old

AGE (YR)					
3	**4**	**5**	**6**	**7**	**8**
Uses hand constructively to direct visual responses	Makes visual manipulation; does not need support of hands	Understands horizontal and vertical concepts	Easily performs copying tasks	Prefers pencil over crayons	Copies a diamond shape
Makes skillful manipulations	Makes discoveries in depth perception	Copies squares and triangles	Prints fairly well	Makes uniform size letters, numbers, etc.	Attempts cursive writing
Draws lines with more control	Laces shoes	Increases fine finger control		Draws a person more accurately	Aligns letters uniformly
Copies circles and crosses	Buttons large buttons	Colors within the lines			
Stacks 1-inch cubes	Orients movements from center of periphery	Cuts fairly accurately			
Handles utensils like adults do	Draws a recognizable picture with some detail	Draws a recognizable person			
Strings beads					
Cuts with scissors					

of most reaches is more adult-like, due in large part to better use of visual information. At approximately 14 months, the infant's form for reaching and grasping is more adult-like. In fine motor tasks such as lacing shoes or writing, the small muscles of the hand or foot are synchronized and, in turn, are coordinated with vision. Table 6.1 presents a selection of fine visual-motor behaviors characteristically exhibited by children during the developmental period of 3 to 8 years of age. The development of gross-motor abilities that require visual-motor coordination will be discussed in subsequent sections. Table 6.2 summarizes visual perception milestones.

TABLE 6.2

Summary of Visual Milestones

Aspect	Basic Function	Adult-like
Visual acuity (static)	3 mo can focus	12 mo
	6 mo 20/100	
Object permanence	8–12 mo	2 yrs
Field of vision	12 mo	5 yrs
Spatial orientation	3–4 yrs	8 yrs
Perceptual constancy	4–5 mo	10–11 yrs
Depth perception	6 mo	12 yrs
Perception of movement	4 mo	12 yrs
Figure-ground	<4 yrs	13 yrs>
Visual-motor coordination	(highly dependent on task)	
(reaching)	7 mo	14 mo
(fine-motor)	3–8 yrs	

Kinesthetic Perception

Objective 6.5

THINK ABOUT IT

What motor skill activities require a high degree of kinesthetic ability?

➤ Often referred to as the sixth sense, kinesthetic perception is a comprehensive term that encompasses the awareness of movement and body position. The word **kinesthesis** derives from two Greek words meaning to move and sensation. It involves the ability to discriminate positions and movements of body parts based on information that derives from the individual's internal environment. Unlike the visual, auditory, and tactile perceptual modalities that receive sensations from outside the body, the kinesthetic system receives sensory input from receptors located in muscles, tendons, joints, and the vestibular (balance) system. Although kinesthetic information is not the exclusive determinant of the way movement patterns are organized, it provides body and movement knowledge without reference to visual and verbal cues. This modality is basic to all movement and, along with the visual modality, dominates the learning and acquisition of motor skills.

Structure and Function of the Kinesthetic System

Objective 6.6

➤ In spite of several years of inquiry on the subject, kinesthesis is not fully understood either physiologically or psychologically. Its complexity is due, in part, to the fact that kinesthetic perception is not a single sensory system. Rather, the kinesthetic system consists of several different sensory receptors.

The group of kinesthetic receptors are associated with the *somatosensory system* that handles sensations from the body. Somatic receptors are located in the skin, muscles, joints, and the vestibular apparatus of the inner ear. Somatic receptors may be further subgrouped into cutaneous receptors and *proprioceptors*. Cutaneous receptors are located near the skin and perceive touch, pressure, temperature, and pain. The sensations these receptors pick up come primarily from outside the body and do not appear to play a primary role in motor behavior. However, because there is such a strong relationship between the two perceptions, they often are referred to as tactile-kinesthetic perception. Collectively the proprioceptors of the muscles (spindle receptors), joints, tendons (Golgi), and inner ear (vestibular apparatus) form the perceptions known as kinesthesis (kinesthetic perception). All are sensitive to stimuli arising from movement.

As noted in chapter 2, spinal tracts are the major pathways for transmitting signals from these receptors via the periphery to the specific brain interpretation centers. Spinal tracts are located alongside the vertebrae that make up the spinal column. Input to the CNS, except for kinesthetic input from the structures in the head (vestibular apparatus), comes through roots (nerve bundles) that collect and guide the input to the spinal cord at each segment, which serves a specific region of the body. One of the most important concepts concerning kinesthesis is the understanding that any one of the kinesthetic receptors in isolation from the others is generally ineffective in signaling information about the movements of the body. The various receptors are often sensitive to a variety of aspects of body motion at the same time.

Development of Kinesthetic Perception

Objective 6.7 ➤ The developmental aspects of kinesthetic perception may be measured and described in terms of their basic physiological qualities and in their applied context involving knowledge of the body and movement awareness.

Keogh and Sugden (1985) discuss what may be described as two basic physiological aspects of kinesthetic perception: *kinesthetic acuity* and *kinesthetic memory*. *Kinesthetic (discrimination) acuity* refers to the ability to proprioceptively detect differences or match qualities such as location, distance, weight, force, speed, and acceleration. Examples include the ability to discriminate the difference between two objects of slightly different weights when placed in the hands while blindfolded (weight discrimination), and the ability to detect when blindfolded which arm has been raised slightly higher than the other (location).

If the stimulus is removed after presentation, then *kinesthetic memory* is involved. Tests of kinesthetic memory usually involve a reproduction of movements. For example, a blindfolded individual is asked to move one hand to a distance of choice or at a measured speed and, after a pause, to reproduce the movement. In another passive variation, the experimenter moves the subject's limb and then asks the subject to reproduce the movement. The subject has less motor information in the passive situation.

A review of the studies on this topic suggests that kinesthetic acuity improves faster and earlier than kinesthetic memory. The ability to discriminate kinesthetic information approaches adult levels by age 8, whereas the mature stage of kinesthetic memory generally is not reached until after 12 years of age. Although very little information is available on young children, research findings note substantial yearly decreases in performance errors after age 5 up to the age of 8.

Objective 6.8 ➤ Several different descriptors may be found in the literature concerning the more applied developmental aspects of kinesthetic perception. Some sources use single descriptors such as body knowledge, body awareness, or spatial awareness, whereas others have identified several subcategories. All of these terms have been used to identify movement awareness (both cognitive and motor) abilities theoretically associated with kinesthesis and one's internal awareness of various movement parameters. The following basic movement awareness components are related to kinesthetic perception: body awareness, spatial awareness, directional awareness, vestibular awareness, and rhythmic (temporal) awareness. These awarenesses are closely interrelated and are inseparable in most movement conditions. The components have been identified to aid in categorizing the various kinesthetic abilities based on the notion that presenting the parts to such a complex process will produce a better understanding of the whole.

Body Awareness Sometimes referred to as body concept, body knowledge, or body schema, **body awareness** involves an awareness of body parts by name and location, their relationship to each other, and their capabilities and limitations. As children age, they become increasingly more aware of their body parts in reference to the aspects described. With this basic movement knowledge they gradually improve their ability to perform desired movements efficiently.

The knowledge of body parts and their functions is one of the most basic aspects of kinesthesis and one of the more researched topics. At birth the newborn is not capable of true conscious body awareness. However, during the first month a relatively crude awareness appears to emerge that the body is distinct from the surroundings. With growth, the infant then becomes increasingly aware of the capabilities of various body parts in moving the eyes, head, trunk, arms, and legs. By the end of the first year or so, correct reactions to verbalizations of body parts become more evident. Even though infants at this age cannot identify specific parts verbally, they are capable of indicating a few body parts (tummy, nose, ears, eyes, and feet) correctly when given verbal cues. They can do this first on their own bodies and then later on other people. As their body-part vocabulary increases, so does their accuracy at physically touching and verbally identifying specific body parts. At age 5 or 6, the majority of children can accurately identify the major parts. By age 7 the ability to distinguish the minor parts (ring finger, wrists, heels, ankle, and elbows) also has been mastered.

The ability to identify various body parts depends heavily on both conceptual and language abilities, as well as other sensory perceptions. For example, a response to "Where is your left ankle?" involves both auditory memory and the ability to plan a motor response. If a series of responses to such commands such as "Touch your right elbow to your left knee" is required, the demands of the situation are increased significantly. It is reasonable to assume that children who have been tutored in body-part identification will show superior abilities in comparison to the norm described.

Spatial Awareness As noted earlier, the spatial awareness aspect of kinesthetic perception interplays with the visual perception of spatial orientation. Both perceptions involve the ability to recognize objects in three-dimensional space. The two differ in that **spatial awareness** involves the ability to draw inferences in relationship to self space or position *as well as* object recognition. In essence, it is the sense of the location of one's body in space in relationship to the environment. This aspect of kinesthesis also has been viewed in the developmental psychology literature as the general sense of direction required for spatial mobility.

Spatial awareness may be described in terms of *egocentric localization* and *objective localization*. Egocentric localization refers to the ability to locate objects in space in reference to the self, which is characteristic of younger children. Objective localization generally follows egocentric perception; it is the ability to locate objects using something other than the self as a reference. Such behavior is exhibited by older individuals who can locate an object relative to its nearness to other objects. Knowledge of the spatial environment and of the body is necessary for an individual to formulate a motor program (plan) and project the body effectively.

Before individuals can effectively project their bodies into space they must have a sense of where objects are located. The ability to make such perceptions is based somewhat on the frame of reference used. This general sense of direction, as it is sometimes called, may include several perceptions in addition to kinesthesis—visual, auditory, tactile, and even smell (olfactory). For example, an individual might perceive or learn the location of an object relative to him- or herself (e.g., second base is directly in front of me when I am batting) to demonstrate the use of an egocentric frame of reference, or egocentric localization. If an objective frame of reference or objective localization were in use, the individual might learn the location of second base relative to various landmarks in the area (e.g., second base is between first and third; or second base is next to shortstop). The strategy used in objective localization is quite similar to that required in map reading and orienteering.

Typically, adults have the ability to use and exercise both egocentric and objective frames of reference. For example, an adult may learn a new pathway through a mountain bike course in an egocentric way ("Go to the first sign and turn right, then go straight ahead until you get to the fork and turn left, etc."). In other situations, however, the cyclist may use objective localization in checking out the possibility of a shortcut on the second run or in looking at a map and then using his or her sense of direction to proceed. Apparently, young infants under 12 months of age do not have the ability to use objective frames of reference and are restricted to egocentric orientation. Objective localization appears sometime between the ages of 12 and 16 months and seemingly is used with increasing frequency through childhood.

One interesting study (Thomas et al., 1983) investigated the strategies children 4 and 9 years of age used to recall spatial locations and distances in their environment while jogging. As one might expect, the older children recalled both spatial location and distance better than the younger children. However, both groups had difficulty recalling distance even after cues were presented. Approximately 30% of the 9-year-olds used a strategy like counting steps to judge distance, whereas the younger group in general did not exhibit such maturity. These researchers also found that children 5 to 12 years of age can be taught to effectively use a strategy to recall jogging distances. Interestingly, tutored 5-year-olds were as good as 9-year-olds and only slightly less proficient than 12-year-olds who were not provided with instruction.

Directional Awareness In theoretical terms, **directional awareness** is that aspect of kinesthetic perception assumed to be an extension of body and spatial awareness. Directional awareness refers to the conscious internal awareness of two sides of the body *(laterality)* and the ability to identify various dimensions of external space and project the body within those dimensions *(directionality)*. The term *lateral preference*, which involves hemispheric control and preferential use of one eye, hand, or foot over the other, also is associated with directional awareness and will be discussed in chapters 8 and 9 in reference to asymmetries.

Laterality is the basis for directional awareness and the ability to identify the dimensions of space and project the body purposefully through those dimensions. The internal awareness that the body has two sides and that those sides can be differentiated as right or left is thought by many to be the essential foundation on which the delineation of other spatial dimensions are derived. The first observations of laterality may be noted early in life. During the first six months of postnatal life, babies exhibit this perceptual distinction by using their hands independently and in a coordinated manner. For example, they may use one hand to hold a cube and the other to explore it, then interchange the function, or even use both hands. Seemingly, babies recognize they have two limbs that can perform independent functions or work together.

Refinement of this awareness continues with other body parts as the child realizes that, though a number of these parts comes in pairs, each part of the pair can be positioned and moved independently. This awareness continues to improve steadily until approximately 4 to 5 years of age when the understanding that the body has two distinct sides is well developed. Around this same time period, a more advanced form of laterality begins to emerge—the ability to label specific body parts as right or left (i.e., left-right discrimination). As this aspect of laterality develops the child clearly moves from the perceptual-motor phase of development to the conceptual-cognitive phase. Children at this age may realize that right and left are opposite sides of the body. But they may not perceive which is which, or they will oftentimes reverse the two. Although there is a wide variance among individuals, children younger than age 5 are likely to give correct responses to right-left discrimination questions only by chance. By the age of 8 most children can respond accurately to questions regarding the left-right discrimination of specific body parts.

From a theoretical perspective, *directionality* is the motoric expression of laterality and the perception of spatial orientation. Along with the understanding that the body has two distinct sides that work independently and in unison, the identification of the dimensions of external space are prerequisite to purposeful movement in the environment. In the discussion of spatial orientation we learned that by 4 years of age children are aware of the most basic spatial dualisms (also referred to as *locatives*) such as over/under, high/low, front/back, in/out, top/bottom, and vertical/horizontal. It also was noted that children appear to master spatial dimensions in a fairly orderly sequence: from the vertical to the horizontal, to the diagonal or oblique. At this age children still lack the ability to effectively perceive mirror images and oblique lines and diagonals. Although most children by age 8 have the basic ability to effectively perceive the spatial orientation of objects, some individuals continue to have problems with right-left or mirror-image reversals.

The perception of objects and spatial dimensions is a basic prerequisite to moving purposefully within the environment, but the ability to discriminate and move correctly in response to verbal cues concerning spatial dimensions is a much more complex function. By 3 years of age a high percentage of children can position an object in front of or behind their bodies, but a great many of them experience difficulty placing objects in front of or behind another object. Shortly after, most children can effectively identify front and back on objects external to the body and can perform the more difficult task of placing an object to the side. It is important to understand that positional relationships between objects and oneself, using the self as a reference point, appear to develop prior to positional interrelationships among objects in space. In other words, in most instances children must become aware of the concept in relation to themselves before they can detect the same qualities in objects external to the body. Remember that although most 5-year-olds realize left and right are distinct and opposite sides of the body, it is not until about the age of 8 that children respond accurately to questions regarding the left-right discrimination of their specific body parts.

Refinement of directionality continues to about age 12, when this aspect of kinesthetic perception approximates adult behavior. Some mature characteristics are present as evidenced when the child begins to use a natural reference system (e.g., "The sun rises in the east").

Vestibular Awareness The successful performance of virtually all motor skills depends on the individual's ability to establish and maintain *equilibrium* (balance). The general description for this component is **vestibular awareness.** The newborn must establish equilibrium before achieving any of the early developmental milestones of maintaining head position, sitting, and standing. Remember, the vestibular apparatus is the part of the kinesthetic modality that provides the individual with information about the body's relationship to gravity and its head position. In a general sense balance, which depends primarily on information from the vestibular apparatus, refers to the ability to maintain equilibrium in relation to the force of gravity. Regardless of how the term is defined, it is clear that balance involves the successful integration of several anatomical and neurological functions (e.g., the skeletal, muscular, sensory, and motor systems).

Typically, balance is subdivided into three types: postural, static, and dynamic. *Postural balance* refers to the relatively unconscious level of basic reflex functioning that enables one to maintain upright posture, hold the head erect, sit, and stand (to be discussed in greater detail in chapter 8). *Static balance* is the ability to maintain a desired body posture when the body is relatively stationary. Common testing procedures include standing on one foot and balancing on a stabilometer or balance board. *Dynamic balance* refers to the body's ability to maintain and control posture while in motion. This type of equilibrium is used in numerous motor skill activities; it usually is evaluated based on the ability to walk on balance beams of different widths and heights. Although these definitions may appear somewhat simple and relatively clear, balance tasks are complex. The assessment of balance at any age is related to the specific task used to measure it. Thus balance is better described as a set of specific characteristics or components that describe the task to be performed, rather than as a single, unitary ability.

Specificity of the task appears to be a major determinant in the exact pattern of change. For example, improvement for a group of children on some tasks may be significant and steady over a number of years;

TABLE 6.3

Selected Balance Abilities

Type of Balance	Task	Approximate Age
Static	Balances on one foot (3–4 sec)	3 yr
	Balances on one foot (10 sec)	4 yr
	Supports body in basic inverted position	6 yr
Dynamic	Walks on straight line (1-in. line)	3 yr
	Walks on beam using alternating steps (4 in. wide)	3 yr
	Walks on circular pattern (1-in. line)	4 yr
	Walks on beam using alternating steps (2–3 in. wide)	4½ yr
	Hops proficiently (traveling)	6 yr

performance on other tasks may change very little, not at all, or decline. A review of several studies also indicates that across a wide range of ages and tasks there are few, if any, differences between males and females in general balance performance. Table 6.3 shows selected balance abilities of young children in approximate developmental order.

In addition to the relatively simple balance tests such as standing on one foot and walking across a beam, researchers now use an array of sophisticated measurement techniques to better determine the specific mechanisms involved. Typically, these techniques involve a moving surface to momentarily destabilize the person, with focus given to postural sway and/or specific muscle group activation (electromyography [EMG] responses). Figure 6.5 on page 192 provides an example. Although refinement with specific tasks may continue across the lifespan, a review by Shumway-Cook & Woollacott (2001) indicates that by 7 to 10 years of age, postural responses are similar to those of adults. From a dynamic systems perspective, as with other motor skills, success with balance is based on the individual's ability to adapt (self-organize) his or her motor abilities to the characteristics of the changing environment—that is, to integrate at times very complex, perceptual information with the motor system.

The ability to maintain and control equilibrium is widely acknowledged as a fundamental motor component. It is included in almost all motor assessment batteries, especially those that focus on the abilities of young children. In fact, some evidence suggests strongly that the balance performance of young children is more closely related to maturational level than to chronological age (Erbaugh, 1984). Other indications are that balance ability is a good predictor of overall

■ *Figure 6.5*

Example of experimental setup used to study postural control (muscle activation with movements)

fundamental gross motor skill performance in children 3 to 5 years of age (Ulrich & Ulrich, 1985). Further discussion of balance ability is presented in chapter 8 (rudimentary behavior) and chapter 11 on adult motor performance.

Rhythmic (Temporal) Awareness All motor activities consist of spatial-temporal characteristics (i.e., movement takes place in both space and time). Coincident timing, one aspect of temporal awareness that already has been discussed, involves the ability to gauge one's position relative to the changing position of an object or another person. Another aspect of the internal awareness of time is *rhythmic awareness*. As with other kinesthetic perceptions, considerable interplay exists among the various aspects of temporal awareness.

   Rhythmic awareness refers to creating or maintaining a temporal pattern within a set of movements. The temporal pattern may be initiated from within by the individual or may be matched with some external pattern. Even young infants seem to be born with the tendency to make rhythmic movements with parts of their bodies. These movements appear within a predictable time during the first year and seem to be triggered by an internal awareness (i.e., an internal drummer) rather than in reaction to any observable external stimulation (Thelen, 1979). Examples of rhythmic awareness are found in such activities as keeping time to music, tapping the hands or feet to stay in rhythm with a sound or light, reproducing a pattern from memory, and creating a rhythmic beat or pattern without external stimulation. Two major differences between this aspect of temporal awareness and coincident timing are evident. Coincident timing occurs primarily in unpredictable situations (i.e., with moving stimuli) and requires visual information for effective completion.

THINK ABOUT IT

Is there any practical application of the information on movement awarenesses?

Little information is currently available on the individual's ability to initiate rhythmic movements without an external stimulus. The absence of criteria by which to make judgments and the strong possibility that most rhythmic responses are not original but are derived from past experiences or memory make this a difficult question to answer experimentally. However, there have been several reports related to the ability to keep time. One study observed the ability of children (from 2 to 5 years) and adults to keep time to piano music played at several different tempos when walking and beating time with their hands (Jersild & Bienstock, 1935). The accuracy rate of the 5-year-olds about doubled that of the 2-year-olds (which was about 21%), and the adults' values were almost double those of the 5-year-olds. These data suggest that children between 2 and 5 years of age improve considerably in their ability to keep time to a rhythmical stimulus and that periods of improvement continue to adulthood. Another interesting note is that better accuracy scores were recorded at faster rather than slower tempos. This type of behavior also has been observed in coincident timing tasks. One could speculate from these observations that the body's rhythmic mechanism responds more effectively to an external stimulus in which the tempo falls within a range of quite fast and quite slow. Keogh and Sugden (1985) concluded from their review of this topic that the ability to keep time to an external stimulus improves significantly around age 6 and continues at a rather steady rate up to adolescence or early adulthood.

■ *Auditory Perception*

Objective 6.9 ➤ The importance of auditory cues is obvious, although they generally are not as vital to motor behavior as visual and kinesthetic information. Very few sport activities are learned or carried out without auditory information and verbal cues. As with all the perceptual modalities, auditory perception derives from a complex system that involves the ability to detect, discriminate, associate, and interpret auditory stimuli. Commonly addressed aspects of auditory perception include auditory localization, auditory discrimination, and auditory figure-ground perception. The following is a brief discussion of the basic structures and functions associated with auditory perception and the general developmental characteristics that take place to maturity.

Structure and Function of the Auditory System

The portion of the ear primarily responsible for sound detection is the *cochlea*, which is located in the inner ear. The inner ear receives auditory sensations and transmits them to the brain for interpretation. Of the major parts of the hearing apparatus, which includes the external, middle, and inner ears, the inner ear develops first. Its essential gross parts are well defined by the second and third prenatal month. At birth, the growth of the bony structures of the ear are near completion and change little thereafter. The middle ear, which collects sound waves and processes them to the inner ear, is practically adult size at birth, although the drum membrane is usually smaller and more oblique. The external ear (canal) consists primarily of cartilage at birth and is much shorter than that of the adult. At birth, both the external canal and eustachian tube are shorter than the adult structures.

Development of Auditory Perception

An infant's sense of hearing is functional prior to birth. Immediately following birth, however, hearing usually is impaired because the auditory canals are filled with fluid. Normal hearing function usually is restored within a few days, and hearing improves rapidly. Young infants have been observed at birth to turn their eyes in the direction of the source of sound, even though they seem unable to locate the exact position from where the stimulus originated. Although the ability is unrefined, newborns are able to make crude discriminations among different pitches. Eisenburg (1976) notes that low-pitch sounds have a calming effect on newborns, whereas high pitches tend to elicit stress reactions. Shortly after birth, the neonate can differentiate sounds of different duration, which is critical to processing spoken language. After four months most new sounds (as opposed to ambient sounds) stimulate searching activities in the infant, an aspect of auditory localization. These activities may include head turning, reaching, and movement toward the sound. Some evidence also suggests that by 6 months of age, infants are almost as sensitive to sounds as adults (Berg & Smith, 1983).

The ability to localize distant auditory stimuli occurs around 12 months and continues to improve. By age 3, children can localize, or determine, the general direction of sounds quite effectively. The ability to discriminate auditory sounds also continues into childhood. There is significant improvement by 8 to 10 years of age and refinement that extends to at least the early teens. Little information is available on the developmental characteristics of auditory figure-ground perception, other than the observation that some children have more difficulty than others separating irrelevant stimuli (background) from the primary task (figure). As with the other aspects of auditory perception, auditory figure-ground perception is closely associated with the ability to selectively attend to the stimuli in the environment.

In summary, although mastery of basic auditory skills is evident by the age of 3 years, refinement continues steadily until approximately 13 years of age when near adult levels are reached.

■ *Tactile Perception*

Objective 6.10 ➤ **Tactile perception** (touch) refers to the ability to detect and interpret sensory information cutaneously (of or on the skin). Most textbooks give little if any attention to tactile perception, perhaps because relatively little information is available on its developmental characteristics and because most aspects of this ability are not closely related to the study of motor behavior. Most information on tactile perception discusses the individual's ability to perceive pain, light, and temperature differences. However, from a motor behavior perspective, several considerations warrant a brief treatment. As we learned in an earlier section, the first phase of motor behavior is the reflexive phase. Several of these initial movements (e.g., grasping, rooting, and Babinski foot reflexes) are elicited through touch stimulation and are dependent on the infant's ability to detect tactile sensations. In conjunction with kinesthetic perception, often referred to as the tactile-kinesthetic system, the individual receives vital information in a movement context with regard to the position of the body in space. For example, a competitive gymnast walking across a balance beam relies primarily on tactile input through the feet and depends relatively little on visual or auditory information. Individuals who are blind depend heavily on tactile input to get feedback for organizing their movements.

Many different neural receptors for heat, cold, pain, pressure, and vibration contribute to tactile perception. Tactile sensations are picked up by numerous receptors and are transmitted to different areas of the brain for interpretation. With growth, increasing numbers of receptors are found in the skin over a wider area and in closer proximity.

The first responses to touch are elicited in the facial area of the fetus, specifically the lips. The general trend of sensitivity to tactile stimulation during the prenatal stage follows a cephalocaudal progression (i.e., head, trunk, and limb). The first prenatal reflex, elicited by tactile stimulation around the mouth, is opposite-side neck flexion at about seven and a half weeks after conception.

Newborns are sensitive to mild and strong tactile stimulation. The most sensitive parts at this time are the lips, eyelashes, soles of the feet, skin of the forehead, and the mucous membrane of the nose. The available information suggests that the development of touch discrimination and localization, as determined by a one-point tactile stimulus, is well developed by 5 years of age. By 8 years of age, children consistently are able to reproduce designs that have been drawn on one of their body parts such as the back of their hand. Interestingly, evidence also suggests that infant and adult females tend to be more sensitive to touch than males.

One of the most researched aspects of tactile perception is the ability to recognize objects (e.g., letters and shapes) through tactile manipulation. Observations indicate that young children generally go from tactile to visual recognition of objects, which suggests that tactile perception may develop before the ability to visually identify objects. In the context of learning, this type of behavior is quite evident in infants and their first responses to something hot, cold, or sharp. The infant learns by touch, places this in memory, and from that time is able to recognize the characteristics of similar items by sight (e.g., fire or a red stove burner). After the age of 4, however, visual recognition of objects is consistently superior to the use of tactile manipulation.

Perceptual Integration

Objective 6.11 ➤ The discussion thus far has focused on the perceptual modalities as independent systems. The description of developmental characteristics and improvements within individual sensory systems is referred to as *intrasensory development.* The perceptual and perceptual-motor processes, however, frequently involve the simultaneous use of more than one system (i.e., *intersensory*). This process is known as **perceptual integration.** This type of functioning is commonplace in motor skill settings. For example, a skill such as hitting a baseball requires the interaction of visual, tactile, and kinesthetic information. The normal academic task of learning to read aloud requires vision and auditory integration. As the dynamic system develops and the individual experiences the environment with various affordances, this ability increases uniquely to the individual.

Closely associated with this ability and one of the most studied aspects of perception is **intermodal perception,** the ability to translate (perceive) information from one sensory modality to another. It is generally acknowledged that intermodal perception is partially functional at birth and improves with increasing age beyond the childhood years. Crude forms exist in newborns as evidenced by their turning their eyes and head toward the general location of a sound.

The next level involves the recognition of a specific stimulus or the features of a stimulus as the same or equivalent (match) when they are presented to two different perceptual modalities. For example, after being allowed to manipulate an object tactually (without use of vision), a child can recognize the object as the same item when permitted to use the visual modality. This level of functioning is often referred to as *cross-modal equivalence.* Evidence clearly indicates that after the newborn stage, this ability emerges in infants and, with experience, improves significantly throughout childhood.

One of the difficulties in interpreting any improvements in intersensory development is isolating improvements in *intrasensory* functioning, which may help improve perceptual integration. Researchers also have found it very difficult to explain how intersensory functioning affects the development of motor behavior. Despite these and other related problems, perceptual integration generally appears to increase with age through childhood as the person gains valuable experience. In subsequent pages we will discuss the effect of experience (that is, nature) on perceptual development as viewed by prominent theories, namely Gibson's ecological perspective. The following briefly describes the development of intermodal perception.

Visual-Kinesthetic Integration

As with visual-auditory integration, the visual and kinesthetic perceptual modalities appear to have some integrative characteristics in the very early stages of infancy. In fact, the abilities associated with visual-kinesthetic integration seem to become refined before those of visual-auditory integration. Information on this topic usually includes mention of tactile integration due to its interrelation with kinesthetic awareness.

The research findings on this aspect of intermodal perception are relatively consistent; most sources note an improvement with increasing age through childhood, up to about 11 years of age. Some of the first indications of visual-kinesthetic integration (cross-modal equivalence) have been observed in children as young as 2 to 3 weeks of age. Meltzoff and Moore (1977) found that babies at this age were able to imitate the mouth and tongue movements of adults. This is quite impressive considering they could not see (and probably never had) their own matched movement. Gibson and Walker (1984) reported that babies only 1 month old could recognize by sight (match) objects they had sucked previously. In these instances, the infants translated visual input into an equivalent body movement, thus exhibiting kinesthesis.

THINK ABOUT IT

Think of a few examples of sport activities that have a high degree of perceptual integration.

By 6 months of age there are numerous studies indicating that children who explore an object with their hands alone can recognize it by sight alone (e.g., Pineau & Streri, 1990). This type of cross-modal equivalence appears to be nearly mature by the age of 5, with slight improvement until about 8 years (Williams, 1983). Evidence also suggests that, among the visual, tactile, and kinesthetic types of perception, visual-tactile integration abilities are the most advanced in 5-year-olds. Hence, the refinement of visual-kinesthetic integration appears, in general, to lag behind visual-tactile integration. The interweaving process that occurs between the visual and kinesthetic modalities is still somewhat of a mystery, as is the way in which intersensory integration affects the development of motor behavior. How experience affects the total process is perhaps as intriguing.

Visual-Auditory Integration

Although unrefined, visual and auditory perceptual abilities appear to be integrated at birth. A common observation upon which many research studies have been developed is that infants will orient their eyes in the direction from which sounds originate. For example, Clifton et al. (1981) observed that newborns turn their eyes and head toward the sound of a voice or rattle. By 4 months infants can link auditory and visual information in a relatively coordinated manner. When shown a film of a bouncing toy monkey on one screen and a bouncing kangaroo on another, infants preferred to observe the film of the animal that bounced in rhythm with the sound track (Spelke, 1987). Thus, they apparently were able to identify the way in which the visual information matched the auditory stimuli. In similar fashion, Soken & Pick (1992) reported that 7-month-olds could match a happy or angry voice with the correct face of a speaking person. In a somewhat more sophisticated study (Wagner et al., 1981), the researchers found what has been suggested are quite remarkable abilities for young children 9 to 13 months of age. The children were presented with pairs of visual and auditory stimuli that matched each other abstractly. For example, a visual pair of a broken line and a continuous line was matched with an auditory pair of a pulsing tone and a continuous tone. The researchers determined that the infants were able to perceive similarity (i.e., match) in three of the eight stimuli sets. This was considered quite remarkable because infants typically are not exposed to these kinds of events.

In general, visual-auditory integration abilities are quite functional by 4 months and continue to improve markedly up to approximately 12 years.

Auditory-Kinesthetic Integration

Compared to the amount of information on visual-kinesthetic abilities, data on auditory-kinesthetic integration are limited. However, the available information suggests there is a natural compatibility between the auditory and tactile kinesthetic modalities. In a frequently used testing procedure, the tester tells the child the name of an object or shape. The child then is asked to select the item tactually from a number of items to create an auditory-tactile/kinesthetic match. Consistent development differences have been reported between individuals 5, 6, and 8 years old in this aspect of sensory integration (Temple et al., 1979; Williams et al., 1978). The evidence also suggests that older children are markedly less variable as a group than younger children. Therefore, although only scant information on a small age range is available, evidence indicates that auditory-kinesthetic/tactile integration improves during childhood. Although intermodal perception is basically functional by the end of childhood, other forms of perception integration continue to improve throughout adolescence, with experience a significant influence.

▪ *Changes with Aging*

Objective 6.12 ➤ As most people begin their middle-age years, the perceptual systems generally become less responsive to stimulation. However, most of these changes do not significantly interfere with everyday functions until the later adult years. Aside from the basic performance decrements associated with the visual and auditory perceptual modalities, little is known or understood about the effects of aging on the perceptual processes. This is especially evident with the various aspects of kinesthetic perception.

Visual Perception

A loss of visual abilities is one of the most noticeable changes in perceptual functioning as the body passes its peak performance level. Most people begin to notice changes in visual acuity between 40 to 50 years of age. Although there are individuals in their seventies and eighties who have 20/20 acuity, only about 25% of 70-year-olds and 10% of 80-year-olds exhibit this level of clarity. By age 85, individuals experience an 80% loss of the acuity they had in their forties. The loss of acuity is especially severe at low levels of illumination and for moving objects.

Closely related to loss of acuity with age is the condition known as *presbyopia*. This is the reduction in the elasticity of the lens of the eye to the point where the lens can no longer change its curvature sufficiently to allow accommodation for nearsightedness (close vision). By age 60, this condition can greatly affect the eye's ability to focus on objects at close distance (Schieber, 1992). As the eye ages, the lens also becomes thicker and less transparent, thus reducing the transmission of light through the lens.

Sensitivity to light is important to optical functioning; it is a major consideration with the elderly. As a result of increased density and yellowing of the lens, the amount of light that enters the eye is reduced; thus, older adults are less able to see in low levels of illumination. Closely associated with this is the ability of the eyes to adapt to dim light. Sensitivity decreases after 20 years of age; this is particularly evident after age 60. Another form of light sensitivity that appears to affect older individuals, especially after age 60, is glare. This also is attributed in part to age changes in the lens that affect the scattering of light over the retinal surface. This, along with problems related to deteriorating acuity, has some practical implications for older individuals who attempt to function in reduced light conditions. One obvious suggestion for minimizing the effects of these changes is to increase the light levels in environments where older adults live and participate in leisure activities.

The information related to aging and its effects on depth perception suggests little or no change up to 60+ years. Yekta et al. (1989) found no difference in depth perception (in stereopsis) in a study of subjects 10 to 65 years. As noted earlier, lateral field of vision reaches a peak at approximately 35 years of age and gradually decreases until about 60 years of age when the decline continues at a much more rapid rate. In addition to associative changes within the visual modality, age-related changes in facial structure (i.e., upper eyelid, and orbital eye sockets) also have been linked to the decrease in field of vision (Shephard, 1978). Another important note related to motor behavior is the observation that older persons require a significantly longer time to process visual information. Williams (1990) estimates that older individuals are about 33% slower in processing than younger persons.

Auditory Perception

With aging comes a gradual loss of hearing that begins around the mid-thirties and continues to progress at least into the eighties. The most common type of age-related hearing loss is associated with the gradual deterioration and hardening of the auditory nerve cells. As a result of this condition, the sensitivity to high-frequency tones is impaired earlier and more severely than the loss of sensitivity to low-frequency tones. The term used to describe this kind of hearing loss is *presbycusis*.

Beginning at about age 40, there are marked sex differences in auditory perception, with females having much better hearing than men at higher frequency levels (Schieber, 1992). There is some suggestion that hearing loss is due in part to environmental noise stress, especially in male-dominated occupations. Hearing loss at higher frequencies becomes more apparent after age 50, especially in males. For age groups over 60, hearing loss progresses to affect the lower frequencies, so that hearing in the elderly is generally impaired for a wide range of tones.

Kinesthetic Perception

Most of the research on kinesthetic perception is grouped under the heading of somesthetic senses. Recall that the word *somatosensory* refers to sensations from the body, which in this context also includes tactile perception. Except for functioning of the vestibular system (balance) and tactile perception, little is actually known about the effects of aging on the kinesthetic receptors and the individual's sense of body position. As with the other perceptual modalities, it might be expected that people approaching middle age would have diminished somesthetic function, that would result in a reduced awareness of bodily orientation, movement, and touch. However, research findings on age differences in somesthetic sensitivity have not provided clear-cut evidence of this parallel. Although structural and functional age effects have been found, no overall deterioration across modalities in the somatic domain are evident (Whitbourne, 1985). This should be considered a preliminary evaluation of the somesthetic domain, however, since documentation of many of these areas is sparse or absent.

Perhaps the most abundant information available about age effects on somesthetic sensitivity is in tactile perception. Some evidence suggests that elderly persons frequently suffer a loss in sensitivity to touch; however, the degree of loss varies widely among individuals and differs for various parts of the body. For example, Corso (1987) has observed that, with advancing age, touch sensitivity of the lower extremities is more impaired than that of the upper body. Caution should be taken in interpreting results such as these, for impairments observed might be related to factors other than age, such as disease, injuries, or circulatory problems. The primary age-related factors responsible for diminished touch sensitivity have been fairly well established. For example, there are cross-sectional age reductions in the number of touch receptors (i.e., Pacinian corpuscles and Meissner's corpuscles) in the skin.

Malfunctioning of the vestibular system, as evidenced by decreased performance on balance tasks, dizziness, and vertigo, are common characteristics among older adults. From approximately 40 years of age a gradual deterioration of vestibular nerve cells takes place. Sensory cell loss may begin as early as the fifth decade in the semicircular canals. It may be quite marked in the saccule and utricle as well after the age of 70 (Rosenhall & Rubin, 1975). As in the case of the cochlear nerve fibers, evidence suggests that the loss of fibers is due to the accumulation of bony material around the opening through which the nerve fibers pass. Apparently, as the holes become smaller, the nerve fibers compress and gradually degenerate. Although decreasing balance performance points to vestibular malfunction in older adults (as one factor), the underlying mechanisms responsible for this response have not been defined clearly. Chapter 11 will discuss balance in greater detail.

As noted earlier, currently little is known about sense of body position (kinesthesis) in the elderly. Although older persons generally show a decrease in the ability to discriminate weight (e.g., held in hands while blindfolded), there are some indications that no major changes occur in active joint-movement (body positioning) sensation (Meeuwsen et al., 1992; Williams, 1990; Spirduso, 1995). For example, Meeuwsen and colleagues reported no significant differences in young and older adults in their ability to blindly compare upper limb body position by location and extent (degree of change). More important, however, the researchers suggest that age-related declines in the elderly cannot be generalized to all perceptual systems.

Table 6.4 summarizes selected perceptual changes due to aging.

THINK ABOUT IT

Describe the impact of regression of perceptual abilities on daily living activities in the elderly. Consider the impact on playing a simple game of softball.

TABLE 6.4

Summary of Selected Perceptual Changes with Aging

PERCEPTUAL CHARACTERISTIC		
Visual Perception	**Auditory Perception**	**Kinesthetic Perception (Somesthetic)**
Acuity (decreases)	Sensitivity to high and low frequencies (decreases)	Touch sensitivity (decreases)
Sensitivity to light (decreases)		Sense of body position and movement (no major change)
Depth perception (little change)		Weight discrimination (decreases)
Visual information processing (decreases)		Balance (decreases)
Perception of movement (decreases)		

■ *Gibson's Ecological Perspective*

Objective 6.13 ➤ Although the role of nature-nurture in children's perceptual development represents one of the classic debates in developmental psychology, most contemporary theorists view the process from an interactive perspective. That is, they believe changes in the ways human beings perceive the world reflect a fundamental interplay between nature (maturation) and nurture (experience and learning within their cultural context). Thelen and Smith introduce the importance of this body of information profoundly by suggesting that "movement as perception, is the critical role of movement in development" (1994, 193).

The perceptual theory that has had the greatest impact on our understanding of how infants perceive and act on that information in the form of movement is **Gibson's ecological perspective,** proposed by Eleanor and James Gibson (Gibson, 1979, 2001). An important characteristic of this theory is the assumption that infants can directly perceive information that exists in the environment. Perception is an active cognitive process in which each individual selectively interacts with a richly varied field of perceptual possibilities. This ties in with our earlier discussion of intermodal perception. According to this perspective, infants actively explore for *invariant features* of the environment—that is, features that remain stable in a constantly changing perceptual world. They search for features that stand out, then they explore their internal characteristics. In this exploration, over time, the infant makes finer and finer distinctions about the feature. This process is *differentiation* (hence, another name for this perspective is differentiation theory). This perspective is in contrast to the traditional (constructivist) view that rather

THINK ABOUT IT

In the Perception→
Action model, where
and how does
Gibson's ecological
perspective fit?

than being able to directly perceive information in the environment, individuals have to make a construction based on sensory input and past experience. In other words, the environment has no meaning without experience. With ecological theory, perceiving is experiencing. The child is an active explorer in the process, where perception and action are coupled (Thelen, 2000).

Movement plays a critical role in this perspective because it provides the infant with means of exploration and a diverse sampling of environmental stimuli. Central to this notion is the observation that infants constantly *explore* ways in the environment that afford opportunities for action. The environment provides *affordances* that invite and challenge the infant to perceive and act on information (invariant features). **Affordances** are opportunities for action that objects, events, or places in the environment provide (e.g., toys, stairs and dance class) (Stoffregen, 2000). This is a major concept in the study of motor skill development today. How the infant acts on the affordance depends on its:

1. Developmental level
2. Past experiences
3. Present need
4. Cognitive awareness of what the object might be used for

The notion of affordances emphasizes there is an *ecological fit* between the individual and the situation. Two examples apply to our study of motor development.

First is the concept of graspability, that is, whether an object is the appropriate size and shape, and within reach. By exploring the object, the infant learns a great deal. A considerable body of research suggests that infants as young as 3 months actually perceive graspability before they are capable of successfully performing the action. That is, after viewing objects that are and are not graspable, they show indications of reaching for those that are the appropriate size and distance for grasping, and simply track the others (Bower, 1989).

THINK ABOUT IT

Identify some
typical affordances
in the environment
that challenge the
pre-walking infant.
What motor skills
do they trigger?

Perhaps more interesting is research conducted by Karen Adolph and her colleagues (Adolph et al., 1993a, 1993b). In one study, they observed two groups of infants, 14-month-old walkers and 8½-month-old crawlers, as they moved up and down ramps sloped at varied degrees (figure 6.6). The researchers predicted that older infants would react more carefully to the inclines due to prior experience with walking; that is, they would perceive the affordance of falling. Their prediction was correct. Older infants confidently walked down gentle slopes and negotiated steeper inclines by sliding down (some went down backward!). In comparison, the young group of infants, regardless of slope difficulty, tried to crawl down (mothers were there to catch them) and never attempted alternative ways of descent. In essence, the older group, due to experience and perceptual ability, found a fit between their abilities and the environment (slopes). Other researchers consider this a form of

■ *Figure 6.6*

Like the other 14-month-olds in Karen Adolph's study, Lauren perceives that a gently sloping ramp (a) affords walking and confidently descends it. When later confronted with a steep slope (b), Lauren, like the other experienced walkers in the study, perceives the affordance of falling, and consequently slides down the slope. (c) This is in marked contrast to the inexperienced 8-month-olds who, like Jack, try to descend every slope, no matter how steep, by crawling, and sometimes end up in a nose dive.

context-specific learning, a notion that will be discussed in more detail in chapter 7. Overall, the ecological perspective provides us with one idea of how *perception and action* work, perhaps the most relevant question in the study of motor development.

■ *Movement-Based Approaches*

Several perceptual-motor programs introduced during the 1950s and into the early 1970s received considerable attention in the educational and research communities (e.g., Barsch, 1965; Delacato, 1966; Kephart, 1971). Underlying most of these theories was the assumption of a strong direct link between perceptual-motor functioning and cognitive functioning. Deficiencies in cognitive performance, such as reading and spelling, were attributed primarily to poor sensory integration. Perceptual shortcomings were seen to be remediable through perceptual-motor training activities requiring those perceptual judgments. For example, some theorists believed that participation in activities involving eye-hand coordination, laterality, directionality, and balance could enhance cognitive and motor functions. Other theories proposed it was critical that the neurological organization of the brain exhibit a dominant hemisphere. That is, if an individual is right-eyed, right-handed, and right-footed, he or she is considered to be neurologically wired to facilitate intellectual development. A proposed method of rewiring was to have an individual perform movement patterning activities such as crawling and creeping.

Although some proponents of these theories still exist, little general support from the scientific community can be found (Salvia & Ysseldyke, 1991; Seefeldt, 1974). Convincing evidence of a true link between perceptual-motor skills and cognition has not been presented. Most studies have reported little or no relationship among perceptual-motor development, perception, and intellectual performance. Kavale and Matson (1983) conducted a sophisticated study of 180 scientific reports designed to research the efficacy of perceptual-motor programs. The researchers concluded that perceptual-motor intervention appears to be ineffective and noted that, compared with other forms of educational intervention, the effects of such programs are negligible. Further, Salvia and Ysseldyke state "There is a tremendous lack of empirical evidence to support the claim that specific perceptual-motor training facilitates the acquisition of academic skills or improves the chances of academic success. Perceptual-motor training will improve *perceptual-motor* functioning" (1991, 322). This in itself is a reasonable goal in motor development programming, especially during the childhood years.

Its is interesting to note that with the recent findings in early brain research and the effects of stimulation on development (chapter 2) dramatic claims for training effects have emerged. Claims are being made, for example, that music and movement activities for infants and young children enhance intellectual abilities. For example, the Mozart Effect theory suggests that exposing young children to classical music may boost their brainpower. It was reported in a major national newsmagazine in 2001 that balancing activities improve learning of math. One trademarked national program claimed that "specific exercises . . . improve reading, writing, and overall academic achievement."

First of all, as discussed in chapter 2, there is little doubt that early stimulation positively affects brain development. However, there is little evidence to suggest that structural change relates to change or improvement in specific functional behavior. Bigger is not necessarily better.

As a final word at this time, the National Academies convened a group of the top developmentalists to address this issue. In the final report *From Neurons to Neighborhoods* (National Academies, 2000), it was noted that while early stimulation and relationships are critical to development, *"there are no special programs that are guaranteed to accelerate early*

THINK ABOUT IT

How would you present the position that movement-based activities are important to child development?

learning during infancy. Despite the proliferation of materials that claim to raise babies' IQs, there is lack of hard scientific evidence on how enrichment activities affect early brain development. For example, the so-called Mozart Effect, has never been studied in young children."

Summary

Both perception and the perceptual-motor process are related to information processing, which involves monitoring and interpreting sensory information, and deciding on and organizing a motor response. Of the six perceptual modalities, the two that provide the most relevance to the study of motor behavior are vision and kinesthesis.

Visual perception, considered to be the dominant modality, undergoes several structural and functional changes across the life span. Significant structural differences between the newborn and adult are accompanied by functional changes in visual acuity, object permanence, perceptual constancy, the perception of spatial orientation, figure-ground perception, object permanence, depth perception, field of vision, the perception of movement, and visual-motor coordination.

Kinesthetic perception, often referred to as the sixth sense, encompasses the awareness of movement and body position. It involves the ability to discriminate positions and movements of the body based on information derived from sensory receptors in the body. The various aspects of kinesthetic perception may be described with regard to their physiological and more applied characteristics. Five interrelated movement awareness components show developmental change: body awareness, spatial awareness, directional awareness, vestibular awareness, and temporal awareness. Each of these components theoretically involves information relative to knowledge of the body and its spatial-temporal characteristics (i.e., position and movement).

Although they generally are not considered as vital to motor behavior as visual and kinesthetic perception, the auditory and tactile modalities provide important cues to successful movement responses.

Though discussions of perceptual development usually focus on the various modalities as independent systems (denoting intrasensory change), the actual perceptual-motor process frequently involves the simultaneous use of more than one system (perceptual integration). A much studied aspect of this ability is intermodal perception that is partially functional at birth and improves with increasing age beyond the childhood years.

Although most people experience some form of regression in perceptual function beginning in middle age, most changes do not significantly affect everyday activities until old age. Most noted among the forms of regression are losses in visual acuity, sensitivity to light, hearing, and a loss of balance.

Gibson's ecological perspective provides insight into our understanding of how infants perceive and act on information in the environment. In the past and even today, there have been claims that specific movement-based perceptual-motor programs directly affect academic skills. But they have received little support from the scientific community.

Think about It

1. Consider child's play. How is it related to embodiment?
2. Can you think of ways to modify the visual cliff experiment to study other aspects of depth perception?
3. What motor skill activities require a high degree of kinesthetic ability?
4. Is there any practical application of the information on movement awarenesses?
5. Think of a few examples of sport activities that have a high degree of perceptual integration.
6. Describe the impact of regression of perceptual abilities on daily living activities in the elderly. Consider the impact on playing a simple game of softball.
7. In the Perception→Action model, where and how does Gibson's ecological perspective fit?
8. Identify some typical affordances in the environment that challenge the pre-walking infant. What motor skills do they trigger?
9. How would you present the position that movement-based activities are important to child development?

Suggested Readings

Birren, J. E., & Schaie, K. W. (Eds.). (1996). *Handbook of the psychology of aging.* 4th ed. San Diego, CA: Academic Press.

Gibson, E. (2001). *Perceiving the affordances.* Mahwah, NJ: Erlbaum.

Sekuler, R., & Blake, R. (2002). *Perception.* 4th ed. New York: Alfred A. Knopf.

Spirduso, W. W. (1995). *Physical dimensions of aging.* Champaign, IL: Human Kinetics.

Stoffregen, T. (2000). Affordances and events. *Ecological Psychology* 12:1–28.

WebLinks

PE Central (Information on perceptual-motor activities)
    www.pecentral.org/adapted/adaptedmenu.html

International Society on Infant Studies
    www.isisweb.org

Mayo Clinic Vestibular Rehabilitation Program
www.mayo.edu/vest-rehab/

National Eye Institute
www.nei.nih.gov

Society for Research in Child Development
www.srcd.org

The Vestibular Disorders Association
www.vestibular.org

7 *Information Processing and Motor Control*

OBJECTIVES

Upon completion of this chapter, you should be able to

7.1 Discuss the roots of information-processing theory.

7.2 Diagram the information-processing model and describe its four basic components.

7.3 Describe the functional and developmental aspects associated with attention.

7.4 Discuss memory with regard to definition, structures, processing strategies, and changes across the life span.

7.5 Discuss the various processes and developmental characteristics associated with information-processing speed and movement time.

7.6 Define *programming* and explain its relationship to schema theory.

7.7 Discuss three features of developmental biodynamics associated with motor control.

7.8 Briefly describe the possible effects of aging on the various aspects of information processing.

KEY TERMS

attention

reaction time

memory

contextual learning

processing speed

programming

schema

motor program

coordinative structures

dynamic systems

neuronal group selection

Information PROCESSING is involved in virtually all forms of human behavior. Whether from the perspective of cognitive psychology or the acquisition and performance of a motor skill, the ability to process information is a major contemporary issue in human development.

Chapters 6 and 7 provide a general framework for studying the complex processes involved in Perception→Action. Chapter 6 focused on the developmental aspects of the perceptional systems and provided insight into how individuals act on information in the environment (Gibson's ecological perspective). Chapter 7 extends our quest to understand the issue by underscoring two critical factors in the perception to action process: *programming* a motor plan and *theories of motor control* (that is, executing the plan via the motor system). The topics of *attention*, *memory*, and *processing speed* also are covered, given their developmental significance in the formulation and execution of a motor plan.

Objective 7.1

➤ Information processing is an approach to understanding human development and behavior that became established during the 1970s with the mass popularity of computers. The roots of the information-processing approach are in the fields of computer science (manipulation of symbols), communications theory (information coding and channel capacity), and linguistics (language). As long ago as 1949 psychologists compared human processing to basic computer functions in which information is encoded, stored, transformed, retrieved, and acted upon (Shannon & Weaver, 1949). During these early stages of information theory, mathematical models were developed to make quantitative predictions about human behavior. Of the numerous traditional and contemporary theories of human development, information processing now dominates the field of cognitive psychology.

Objective 7.2

➤ One of the popular approaches to studying the execution of a motor response has been to conceptualize the process in terms of an information-processing model. Motor developmentalists are concerned with the way individuals use information in perceiving, making decisions, and organizing activity in relationship to the demands the environment places on them. Four basic components have been identified in the simplified model of information processing in figure 7.1: sensory (afferent) input, reception of information through the various perceptual modalities, interpretation and decision making (processing), and an overt motor (efferent) response.

As individuals progress toward adulthood they are able to process more information in a shorter period of time. This concept is relatively simple. Yet the structural and functional aspects of information processing to which it refers are complex and in several instances remain in the little black box of the unknown or highly theoretical.

THINK ABOUT IT

Reflecting back on chapter 6, how does the information presented here fit the introductory information processing model (figure 6.1 on page 171)?

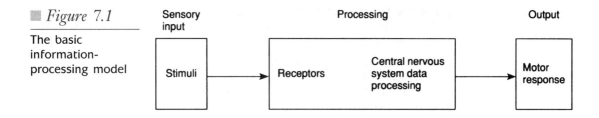

■ *Attention*

Objective 7.3   ➤ **Attention** usually is considered the core of information-processing models. And there is convincing evidence this aspect of information processing changes across the life span. More than a century ago James, one of the earliest and most renowned experimental psychologists, described attention as the "focalization, concentration, and of consciousness" (James, 1890). Although several definitions have been proposed since James's work, two features inherent in his statement are still prominent today. First is the notion that attention is *limited* (an individual capacity exists) so that an individual can attend to only one thing at a time, or think only one thought at a time. From a motor behavior perspective, this statement suggests an individual's capacity could be exceeded if too much activity were attempted. Second, attention is apparently performed in a *serial* manner, which suggests that individuals attend to one thing and then another and that it is difficult (sometimes impossible) to combine certain activities.

While attention is a key component in information-processing models, it is also a strong factor in the successful performance of a motor task. Three basic concepts associated with attention and motor behavior have been identified: (a) attention involves alertness and preparation of the motor system to produce a response; (b) attention is related to individuals' limited capacity to process information; and (c) the successful performance of a motor task requires selective attention, the ability to select and attend to meaningful information. The following pages will discuss the functional and developmental aspects associated with these concepts, and give particular emphasis to capacity and selective attention. For detailed discussions of attention theory see Magill (2001), Schmidt and Lee (1999) and in the Suggested Readings.

Alertness

Alertness and preparation of the perceptual-motor system prior to any initiated motor task are vital aspects of attention and successful movement response. These conditions are evident in the softball batter preparing for the incoming pitch and the sprinter in the starting block before the gun. The level of perceptual alertness and physiological preparation immediately preceding the pitch or the starter's signal are critical to the outcome of these events.

A large portion of the research on this aspect of attention has dealt with individuals' ability to exhibit alertness and response preparation by assessing their ability to detect a visual or auditory signal in a predetermined fashion. Researchers have typically used **reaction time (RT)** experiments to test these abilities. Reaction time is the interval of time between the onset of a stimulus and the initiation of a response. It is important to note that reaction time does not include the physical movement; movement time combined with reaction time is the *response time*. This topic will be discussed in greater detail in a subsequent section. However, an example of alertness is relevant.

In the case of the sprinter, RT is the period of time from the moment the auditory stimulus (gun shot) was received by the auditory receptors to the point just prior to the first motor response. The RT phase includes attention (alertness) to the stimulus, motor system preparation (body position and muscle tension), reception and transmission of the stimulus, interpretation of the information, and organization of a motor program with which to execute the response. Numerous sophisticated functional characteristics are performed within the general alertness and preparation stages. Successful athletes, such as the softball batter, learn to anticipate upcoming conditions by being alert.

Divided Attention

Another aspect of attention that has strong implications for motor performance is the concept of limitations in the capacity to handle information from the environment. This aspect of attention represents the concept of *divided attention*. Basically, if a specific movement activity requires attention, then some (or all) of an individual's limited capacity must be allocated to its performance or control. Because capacity is believed to be limited, interference will occur if another activity requires these resources. Interference could result in the following: (a) a loss of speed or quality in the performance of one of the activities; (b) both activities could be affected; or (c) the second activity could be ignored.

The operational definition of attention generally includes the notion of interference. However, it is possible to perform two tasks simultaneously as long as the total amount of processing capacity is not exceeded. The amount of the capacity resources required for any task or tasks depends on the activity and the individual. Examples of divided attention are abundant in everyday life as individuals try to handle several cognitive tasks at once, sometimes unsuccessfully. The act of driving a car while conducting a conversation may not be difficult if both conditions are relatively light and undemanding. However, if the road conditions deteriorate or the conversation turns to something complex or emotional, processing capacity may become overloaded and performances may suffer.

Numerous studies of the processing capacity of attention have used the dual-task paradigm in which subjects are observed as they perform two tasks simultaneously. Typically, under this method, individuals are presented a primary task and secondary task separately and then are asked to perform the tasks simultaneously. Presumably when the tasks are executed simultaneously, any differences between the events indicate where and how individuals allocate their capacity resources. Younger children most often allocate their available attention somewhat equally between two tasks, whereas older children appear to recognize the significance of the primary task, attend to it, and perform better on it.

The dual-task paradigm experiment also has implications for selective attention, the ability to attend to relevant information in the environment. Wickens and Benel (1982) note that capacity allocation (time-sharing efficiency) improves with age and that developmental differences in attending to dual tasks primarily are due to *automation* and *attention deployment skills*. In the context of this research, automation is a possible source of age-related improvement in which the performance on one task remains the same with less attention used, thus freeing up processing resources for performing a concurrent task. Attention deployment skills are strategies used to process additional information.

Other evidence also suggests improved efficiency of capacity allocation in the dual-task paradigm is linked to age-related improvements in cognitive processes and the ability to adopt strategies (Manis, et al., 1980). Manis and associates found that, from second graders to adults, the capacity allocated to process simple and complex tasks decreased. The underlying notion is that the cognitive processes involved in a task compete for limited central processing capacity. Therefore, as children grow older they become more adept at controlling the allocation of their attention (through the use of strategies) and require less of the capacity resources.

A much debated issue on the topic of processing ability is whether improvements are due primarily to structural increases (actual capacity) or control operations (e.g., the use of strategies). However, it is quite likely that change is a result of structural changes in the central nervous system (CNS) as well as qualitative alterations due to experience.

Selective Attention

Selective attention, although closely related to alertness, response preparation, and processing capacity, is a distinguishable characteristic of attention. Selective attention is the processing of relevant information and nonprocessing of irrelevant information. A frequently used generalization is the cocktail party phenomenon (Cherry, 1953). During a large gathering such as a party or sporting event, an individual can attend selectively to a conversation with one person even though a number of other conversations and noise are taking place around them. Furthermore, if during that personal conversation someone in the crowd mentions the individual's name, his or her attention is immediately diverted to that person in the crowd.

This phenomenon is related closely to another perceptual characteristic mentioned earlier—visual figure-ground perception. Under these conditions, the individual might also attend selectively (visually) to the relevant information in the environment (the figure) and set it apart from its background. Selective attention, however, may involve more than one sense; for example, an individual catching a fly ball must separate relevant information (the ball) from an environment that may be filled with trees, clouds, and crowd noise.

Evidence suggests that children as young as 4 months of age have impressive selective attention abilities (Bahrick et al., 1981). Although infants at this age exhibit impressive skills, refinement appears to continue during the childhood years. In general, older children show better control of selective attention by processing more stimulus features relevant to a particular task and by not processing those that are irrelevant. In contrast, younger children tend to select features of a task that stand out or are salient. And, as noted in the dual-task paradigm studies, older children are more organized and strategic in their processing abilities.

Based on observations of children viewing a visual display that contains relevant and irrelevant features, Ross (1976) proposes that the development of selective attention abilities occurs in three stages. During the approximate period from 2 to 5 years of age, children most often pay exclusive attention to one stimulus in the display; this is termed the *overexclusive mode*. Observations of younger children also suggest they are more easily distracted than older children. For example, while watching television they are more likely to play with toys, look around, and talk with other people during the viewing. The second stage spans the period from about 6 to 11 years of age; it is referred to as the *overinclusive mode*. In this stage children characteristically attend to several features in the display, some of which are irrelevant. The final stage, *selective attention*, is attained by early adolescence when individuals become capable of attending to relevant stimuli in displays of varying complexity (simple to complex). Ross's basic observations, which have been verified by others, demonstrate that older children are much more likely to ignore information that is irrelevant or that distracts from the central activity than younger children are.

As with the other aspects of attention, age differences in selective attention abilities are attributed primarily to experience and the refinement of operational functions (i.e., the use of strategies). Through experience adolescents and adults learn which stimuli are relevant to a particular situation and which are not. They then adopt a strategy to

THINK ABOUT IT

Name some sport activities that require considerable selection attention. Rank the order by complexity and explain why you ranked them as you did.

address the situation. For example, the experienced softball batter knows from past events at what approximate point in the pitcher's delivery the ball will be released. The batter selectively attends to the point of release and follows the ball exclusively to the anticipated point of contact. In contrast, the young, inexperienced batter's attention may be diverted to crowd noise, words from opposing players, and unfamiliar actions of the pitcher. Since the past experiences of younger children likely will be limited, the use of selective attention strategies likely will be restricted. Several studies have noted that children can be taught to resist irrelevant cues and acquire selective attention strategies.

■ *Memory*

Objective 7.4

THINK ABOUT IT

Do you perceive general memory and the ability to recall movements (motor memory) as different from each other?

➤ The study of *memory* and its various systems is vital to understanding information processing and motor performance. Up to this point in the text, various discussions have focused on the developmental aspects of the way information is selected and perceived by the CNS in preparation for a meaningful motor response. However, at some point in information processing, data entering the system must be retained or stored for future use. There have been numerous structural and operational definitions proposed for the term *memory*. In a broad sense, **memory** refers to the retention and subsequent retrieval of information. Some operational definitions also use the term synonymously with *remembering*. In a more global treatment, Tulving describes memory as the "capacity that permits organisms to benefit from their past experiences" (1985, 385). Relevant to our discussion of memory from a developmental perspective are the two primary types: recognition and recall memory. *Recognition* memory involves noticing whether a stimulus is identical or similar to one previously experienced. In contrast, *recall*, the more advanced form of memory, involves remembering a stimulus that is not present.

Most evidence suggests that developmental differences in memory system effectiveness derive primarily from functional refinement *(control processing strategies)* rather than structural (capacity) increases. A basic knowledge of the various memory structures and their capacities is important to a more detailed understanding of developmental differences.

Memory Structures

To use a contemporary analogy, the operational relationship between the structural and functional components of memory is like that of a computer; the structure is similar to computer hardware, while control processes (strategies) are similar to software. Although numerous computerlike schematics and models have been developed and a vast array of terminology used to explain the concept of memory and its elements,

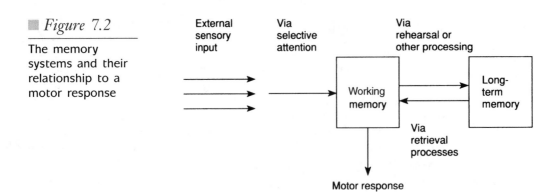

■ *Figure 7.2*

The memory systems and their relationship to a motor response

the two-component model is mentioned most often in contemporary literature (e.g., Baddeley, 2000). According to this view, memory consists of two components: *working memory* and *long-term memory*. A theoretical representation of these systems and their relationship to a motor response is shown in figure 7.2.

Working Memory   *Working memory* is the concept of short-term memory as a place for mental work—that is, a workbench that allows individuals to manipulate and assemble information. This component incorporates characteristics and functions traditionally associated with sensory, perceptual, attentional, and short-term memory processes involved in processing information. It also serves as a processing center to transfer information to long-term memory (Magill, 2001). This system has a small and limited capacity with a storage duration of generally not more than 30 seconds. Evidence of the way this workspace and moment of attentional focus come into play appears in numerous everyday situations. For example, an individual looks up a telephone number, closes the phone book, and by the time he finds the change for the call, forgets the number. Or, picture being introduced to three or four people at a meeting. You could remember the names immediately after introductions were made. But if you conversed for a minute or two and could not rehearse the names, you easily may have lost them.

The working memory system has a capacity of only about 7 ± 2 items. For experimental purposes, the term *item* also has been used to designate the capacity of the system to hold single words or digits. Separate items grouped in some way to make larger collections is a process known as *chunking*. This technique, along with *rehearsal* (repeating the information one is trying to retain), significantly increases the number of items that can be retained; however, without practice or rehearsal, the capacity limit is about five to nine items.

The capacity of working memory is commonly determined using the *memory span* technique in which an individual is presented with a list of digits or words at a given rate (usually one item per second) and asked to repeat the list. The number of items in the list is increased after each perfect recall. Memory studies using this technique are described in subsequent pages. With regard to working memory for motor skills, Ille and Cadopi (1999) reported that after 12- and 13-year-old gymnasts were shown a sequence of discrete movement on video tape, the more skilled group demonstrated a recall of six movements and the less skilled a capacity limit of five. In general these findings support the capacity limit of 7 ± 2 range evidenced with a wide range of verbal tasks.

The question of whether verbal and motor working memory are separate features of the memory system is yet to be resolved. Speculation suggests, however, there is one memory system that adapts to the unique requirements of verbal and motor skills (Magill, 2001).

Long-Term Memory When items are rehearsed, they are transferred in some manner from short-term memory storage to long-term storage where they can be held on a more permanent basis. Both the storage duration and capacity of *long-term memory* are seemingly unlimited. Storage can span hours, days and with several items, years. Perhaps the most often cited examples of long-term motor memory are the ability to ride a bicycle and swim after several years without any intervening practice. One thing that is clear is that long-term memory depends on what control processes and strategies people use when they are learning and remembering information such as rehearsal, coding, decisions, and retrieval strategies.

The following brief overview discusses the development of memory abilities most relevant to the study of motor development.

Memory Abilities

Early Processing Abilities The identification and extent of processing strategies and abilities infants use is difficult to determine. However, there are indications that primitive forms of *recognition memory* are present shortly after birth. Evidence of this phenomenon has been gathered primarily through observing *habituation*. A stimulus is presented to an infant and its responsiveness is monitored (e.g., time and quality of gaze). If the stimulus is repeated, reaction declines and habituation is said to have occurred; but if another stimulus is substituted, responsiveness generally increases. Theoretically the renewed responsiveness to a new stimulus (referred to as *dishabituation*) can be viewed as evidence for recognition memory. Given adequate familiarization and relatively simple stimuli, memory in the form of dishabituation has been observed in newborns (e.g., Gibson & Spelke, 1983). For this type of behavior to occur, it appears that even newborns actively attend to the environment and encode information from it. Habituation improves dramatically throughout the first year, with 5- to 12-month-olds exhibiting the ability quite well (Bornstein & Sigman, 1986; Fagan, 1984).

■ *Figure 7.3*

The technique used in Rovee-Collier's investigation of infant memory. The mobile is connected to the infant's ankle by the ribbon and moves in direct proportion to the frequency and vigor of the infant's kicks.

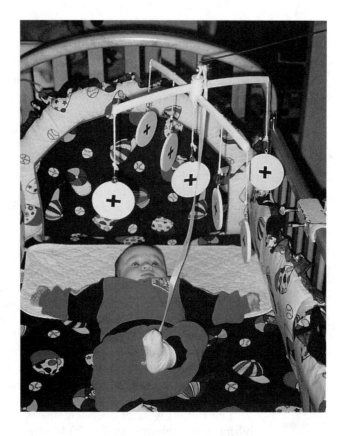

In general, the available evidence suggests that adultlike conscious *recall memory* emerges in the second six months of life (Mandler & McDonough, 1995). This form of memory is more evident by age 2, as exhibited on memory span tests. However, in a remarkable set of experiments conducted by Rovee-Collier (2001 review) with infants 3 and 6 months of age, *cued recall (long-term!) memory* has been shown—that is, a recollection prompted by a cue associated with the setting (context) in which the recalled memory originally occurred. This phenomenon also is associated with **contextual learning,** a much studied topic in memory today. Perhaps most intriguing about these studies is the experimental setup, which is presented in a motor domain. Infants are placed on their backs in a baby crib, with one of their ankles attached by a ribbon to an overhead mobile (figure 7.3). The infants learn within a few minutes that by kicking their leg, the mobile moves; the faster and harder they kick, the more the mobile jiggles and fascinates them with sights and sounds—a spectacle they truly enjoy. Before each training (learning) session begins, the number of kicks is recorded with the ribbon not attached (the infant simply views the interesting mobile). These data are used as the baseline for comparison with learned (attached)

behavior in various conditions. Three-month-old infants typically double or triple their rate of kicks with a few minutes of training. After the ribbon is detached, the number of kicks decreases to baseline level. Then, as a test of immediate recognition, the ribbon is again attached and the rate of kicks compared to the previous attached behavior. Delayed retention (cued recall) of up to 42 days was measured by comparing original kick rate with the same or a novel mobile (ribbon attached). The prediction was that kick rate would be immediately similar within the same context and significantly less when compared to the novel condition.

The findings? Three-month-old infants exhibit perfect retention 3 to 4 days after the training session—convincing evidence for (cued) long-term memory. At 6 months, another very interesting phenomenon occurs—the infants can discriminate with detail differences between the training mobile and the novel task for up to 2 weeks. In the training session for the older infants, the lining of the crib had a distinctive bumper pattern, which they apparently remembered, as evidenced by a significantly lower kick rate in a novel (different pattern) context. Several researchers consider this evidence for contextual learning and suggest that a unique and distinctive context serves as an effective retrieval cue. Researchers once thought infants were not capable of encoding information about where events occur; however, these results suggest otherwise. It also is suggested that this type of information is picked up and encoded in 3-month-old infants.

Working (Short-Term) Memory Abilities   Evidence of working (recall) memory ability as shown by memory span research suggests that it improves markedly up to early adolescence, with the largest changes occurring from about 3 to 7 years (Dempster, 1981). Memory span increases from about two digits in 2- and 3-year-olds to about five digits in 7-year-olds. And interestingly, from age 7 to adulthood the increase is only about two and a half digits (to a maximum of seven and a half digits).

A common method for testing short-term memory within a motor context is the use of an arm-positioning task in which the subject is asked to reproduce the location and distance of a movement. The general findings suggest individuals are most successful in recalling location and that, in comparison, distance information seems to decay rather quickly.

An interesting study (Thomas et al., 1983) produced similar results in a field environment. The working memory of children (from age 4 to 12) was studied by asking them to reproduce location and distance after jogging through a predesigned course. The researchers suggested that all the children encoded location before distance information. They also found that the ability to recall distance improves with age as does the apparent use of processing strategies such as rehearsal.

Overall, working memory increases with age. Children and older adults experience more difficulty with working memory than young adults do (Swanson, 1999). One of the explanations often cited is that as individuals age, they become more *efficient information processors* (Case, 1992; Hale et al., 1993; Kail, 1991). With increasing age, they are quicker to recognize relevant information and more skilled at performing cognitive operations that tie to motor acts. As a result of practice or experience, children become more efficient at using their working memory space (Bjorklund, 1995; Flavell et al., 1993). Another explanation that has gained attention is the general capacity hypothesis, which suggests that age-related changes primarily (but not exclusively) are related to processing capacity. Swanson (1999) drew this conclusion after comparing a large sample of 9 age groups, from ages 6 to 76 years. Subjects performed a series of verbal and visuospatial working memory tasks. Results indicated that children and older adults experience a generalized lower level of performance due primarily to processing capacity constraints. Perhaps most important, age-related differences were not isolated to specific processes or strategies.

It appears the questions remains: Are age-related differences due to process capacity or to efficiency? The extent of each is perhaps in need of continued debate, but no doubt, optimal performance is dependent on both.

Long-Term Memory Abilities   By age 2, children can recall interesting events that happened months ago and even relate them in the form of a story (Howe & Courage, 1993). However, their ability to do this is far from that of older children. Limitations are primarily in control processes and strategies related to coding, rehearsal, decision making, and retrieval of information.

As children become older, they begin to engage in more formal memory strategies, such as *rehearsal*. Although evidence suggests that children as young as 5 and 6 years of age are able to rehearse and memorize information successfully if they are aided, they generally do not begin to independently rehearse on memory tasks efficiently until approximately 10 years of age (Flavell et al., 1993). Children below 8 years of age also exhibit weak encoding and recoding ability compared to young adults.

The organization of material in long-term storage determines the sequence in which the items are recalled. It would be difficult to recall the months of the year alphabetically because it is likely they have been organized sequentially in time. As with their ability to rehearse, children 10 and 11 years old group information rather well, but younger children are still relatively weak in their use of this strategy. However, evidence also suggests that compared to fourth graders (9 and 10 years old), adults tend to organize information in ways that make retrieval much easier (Liberty & Ornstein, 1973).

Retrieval processes pertain to finding information located in long-term storage. The process requires both the ability to search the memory and decide the appropriate information has been retrieved. Differences between children and adults are evident in the retrieval process. The developmental pattern for retrieving ability is similar to that of rehearsal—that is 10- and 11-year-old children are likely to use elaborate strategies to retrieve information from long-term storage but 5- and 6-year-old children are not (Kreutzer et al., 1975). Apparently, older children are better at conducting a thorough and systematic search of the memory store and selecting appropriate material.

With regard to general long-term memory performance and effective use of the control processes, most development appears to occur between the ages of 5 to 12 years. Younger children exhibit more deficiencies than older children do.

Due perhaps to methodological problems associated with studies of memory over long periods of time, little information about long-term motor memory, particularly in children, is available. However, as evidenced by the Rovee-Collier (contextual learning) studies, memory for perceptual-motor actions can be substantial. General observations suggest that for well-learned *continuous motor skills* (i.e., skills with no recognizable beginning or end) such as riding a bike and swimming, long-term motor memory loss is minimal.

With regard to *discrete motor tasks* (i.e., skills with a recognizable beginning and ending) such as kicking and throwing, however, evidence suggests that forgetting can be considerable. For example, Neumann and Ammons (1957) used a stimulus-matching task to test adult retention levels after periods of 1 minute, 20 minutes, 2 days, 7 weeks, and 1 year. The researchers found some loss in performance after only 20 minutes; losses increased as more time passed. After 1 year, performance indicated an almost complete loss of memory. Speculation regarding why there is a difference between continuous skill and discrete task recall has produced a number of hypotheses. Schmidt (1988) suggests that discrete skills generally have more verbal-cognitive components, and these characteristics are more quickly forgotten than motor components. In a review of discrete tasks that are highly motor in nature, Schmidt proposes that retention (loss) is similar to that found in the Neumann and Ammons study, which suggests there is more to the difference than the motorness of the task.

> **THINK ABOUT IT**
>
> Why can we recall how to ride a bicycle (and do it) after years of not practicing, but forget what we wore to class last week?

Not a great deal is known about how individuals code information for long-term storage so it might be retrieved several years later (e.g., how to ride a bicycle or swim). One possible explanation from a motor behavior perspective is that the specific patterns of a movement are not stored, but rather a motor program is formulated based on schemata placed in long-term storage. The functional relationship between long-term memory and the use of schema has broader implications for motor performance. Schema theory is discussed later in this chapter.

Knowledge and Metamemory   It is a widely accepted notion that the knowledge an individual possesses probably contributes to memory abilities. In an interesting study that compared adults and children on memory for chessboard displays, it was found that children had significantly better recall than adults (Chi, 1978). Initially this result seems unusual. But the children were skilled chess players, whereas the adults were novices. It is suggested that due to the children's advanced knowledge base, they used chunking strategy to be more proficient at grouping items of information. It also could be assumed that because of their familiarity with the game, their processing was more efficient. Evidence such as this provides strong confirmation of the power of the effects of knowledge on long-term memory.

Metamemory may be defined as the knowledge or intuitions people have about memory and about themselves as memorizers. Or, more simply perhaps, it may be described as knowledge of one's own memory. An important facet of metamemory is knowledge of how to monitor memory during the course of learning (for example, when you know you have studied enough to be sure you can accurately recall particular information). Metamemory has been shown to improve with age and be more adult-like in children 10 years of age and older (Schneider & Pressley, 1997). With experience, older children undoubtedly learn to discover why various strategies can aid remembering.

■ *Processing Speed and Movement Time*

Objective 7.5 ➤ **Processing speed** is the rate of speed at which information is processed. Although not all cognitive or motor tasks require information to be processed at a fast rate, processing speed may account for many performance differences between children and adults. In a movement setting, there are numerous instances when the ability to recognize a stimulus and process information quickly are critical to an effective motor response (e.g., catching a ball or playing Ping-Pong or badminton). Successful motor performance is based on a combination of perceptual recognition (attention), speed of memory functions, and neuromuscular response time.

Reaction time (RT) is the basic measure of processing speed. As noted in earlier discussions of perception and attention, RT refers to the interval of time between the onset of a stimulus (e.g., light, buzzer, or shock) and the initiation of a motor response (e.g., lifting a finger off a button). When the individual being tested is asked to respond to only one stimulus, the task is referred to as *simple reaction time. Choice reaction time* tasks are more complex and involve a greater information load because more than one signal requires discrimination in a more unpredictable setting. For example, a red light may mean move one way, blue another, and yellow another. A well-known concept related to processing speed, information load, and complexity is *Hick's Law:* Reaction time increases linearly as information load increases. That is, as the complexity of the

■ *Figure 7.4*

Reaction time and movement time as a function of age

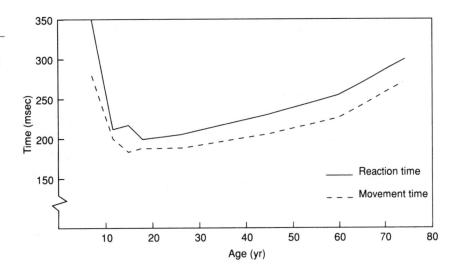

THINK ABOUT IT

As future teachers and coaches, is there any practical value to this information—we (as adults) are about twice as fast with processing and reaction as a 5-year-old?

processing task increases, so does the time it takes to process that information.

The time required to complete motor response is referred to as *movement time*. Movement time combined with the reaction time is known as *response time*. Reaction time usually is calculated as the amount of information (or bits) processed per second.

A comprehensive review about age differences in information-processing rates (Cerella & Hale, 1994) and performance on speeded tasks (Kail, 1991) suggests that differences are large and remarkably consistent. Speed of processing, as determined by reaction time, improves with age up to the early adult years and then remains stable until about age 60 (Hodgkins, 1962; Wilkinson & Allison, 1989). The period of greatest improvement appears to occur between the ages of 6 and 15 (figure 7.4). Similar age trends were reported by Kail and Salthouse (1994) among 6- to 80-year-olds on perceptual speed tests.

More specifically, Hale (1990) found that on a simple reaction time task, 10-year-olds were about twice as slow compared to young adults, whereas 12-year-olds were approximately 1.5 times slower. However, the processing speed of a group of 15-year-olds was about the same as the young adults. Adding to this, Surwillo (1977) estimates that it takes a 5-year-old nearly three times as long as a 17-year-old to process one bit of information. This estimate was based on differences between simple and choice reaction times. It has been suggested that the slower processing speed of children is due primarily to central processing factors, such as attention and speed of memory processes.

It was alluded to in the earlier discussion of memory storage that children and adults differ in their ability to process information into memory. It is also apparent there is a difference in the speed with which these memory functions are performed. Along with the greater difficulty they have in searching for and retrieving information, children appear to take longer than older individuals to encode information into memory (Chi, 1977a, 1977b).

Most discussions of reaction time also include movement time, particularly within the context of motor behavior. The close or, in most conditions, inseparable association between the two phases of a movement response time has been discussed (see figure 7.4). Movement time usually is defined as the interval from the initiation of the movement (or the end of RT) to the completion of the movement.

A well-known law of motor behavior closely associated with movement is *Fitts's Law* (Fitts, 1954). This law also is referred to as the *speed-accuracy trade-off*, which means that when performers attempt to do something more quickly, they typically do it less accurately. That is, under most movement conditions, as speed increases, accuracy decreases. Exceptions are those conditions in which moving too slowly is not conducive to motor efficiency that can affect accuracy (e.g., striking a fast-moving object).

Other factors such as task complexity and movement distance also can affect an individual's movement time. Movement time often is described as the capacity of the motor system to use an amount of information per second. Within this definition, capacity is expressed as the index of difficulty divided by the movement time; it is evidenced when movement times become faster (lower) for a specific information load.

Using a lifespan approach to the study of rapid aiming arm movements, Yan and colleagues (2000) report data relevant to the concepts of processing speed and Fitt's law. The researchers examined four age groups of 6-, 9-, 24- and 73-year-olds. As you would predict, young children and older adults were slower, more variant, and less smooth in their movements than the other groups were. Much of the difference was related to task characteristics involving movement accuracy demands and response uncertainty. In general, the younger and older groups performed in a similar manner. However, the younger group's performance is improving over time, whereas the older adults' performance is regressing. The researchers concluded that the lower performances for the two groups was due in large part to their making more on-line movement adjustments, as opposed to movement under central (programming) control.

Programming

Objective 7.6   ➤ Perhaps the most sophisticated mental operation is programming. In a broad sense, **programming** is cognitive processing that results in the formulation of a thought, cognitive expression, or *motor program.*

Depending on the task, several factors are involved in these functional operations. For example, attention, perceptual awareness, and information stored in the working and long-term memory systems all influence programming. You may recall from the general information-processing model that individuals collect information from the external and internal environments through the various perceptual modalities, interpret that information, decide whether a motor response is appropriate and, if so, generate that response. Obviously it is also possible to generate a thought or motor program in the mind without perceptual information. But in most cases, an overt expression requires additional environmental information.

Cognition is a major psychological determinant in the ability to program. This term generally refers to any mental process that results in the generation or obtaining of knowledge. It is also known as the means by which individuals can think. Cognition is an integral part of perceiving, recognizing, conceiving (i.e., generating information), decision making, reasoning, and varying any of the perceptual-conceptual processes. One of the most popular theories of cognitive development was noted in chapter 1 in reference to Piaget's work. Some of the theorist's original ideas can be linked to contemporary notions regarding verbal and motor skill learning theory. In the context of this discussion, three of Piaget's ideas are applicable. Piaget postulates that humans characteristically systematize and organize mental processes and the content of knowledge into coherent systems; this is referred to as *organization*. It was also his belief that individuals use *adaptation*—that is, people use cognitive processes to change experiences into a cognitive form that can be used later in addressing new situations.

The third notion, the formulation of **schema,** has direct relevance to programming. Piaget was not the originator of the term (Bartlett, 1932; Head, 1926) but he popularized the concept of schema as important to a comprehensive theory of cognitive development. In Piaget's framework, organization and adaptation combine to produce cognitive structures called *schema.* Schema was defined as a number of ideas or concepts organized into a coherent plan (program), or outline, that indicates the relationship between concepts. The definition of schema that perhaps best fits contemporary motor learning theory is described by Schmidt and Lee in reference to Bartlett's (1932) thoughts: "For Bartlett, the schema is an abstract memory representation for events or skilled actions, thought of as a rule, concept, or generalization" (1994, 483).

Richard Schmidt, a renowned motor behavior scientist and the originator of the schema theory of motor skill learning (Schmidt, 1975, 1988), notes that at the heart of schema is the notion of the *generalized motor program* (GMP). Schmidt describes the **motor program** as a memory representation of a class of actions responsible for producing a unique pattern of motor activity if the program is executed. For a person to produce a specific action, the person must retrieve the appropriate program from memory and then add movement-specific parameters such as force, duration, and movement pattern that must be used to perform the skill. The emphasis and application of the motor program concept are the core of schema theory.

Schema Theory

Briefly, schema theory offers an explanation of the way individuals learn and perform a seemingly endless variety of movements. The theory suggests that the motor programs stored in memory are not specific records of the movements to be performed; rather, they are a set of general rules, concepts, and relationships (schemas) to guide performance in keeping with the concept of a GMP. Basically individuals store past movement experiences in memory. Storage of movement elements and the relationship of these elements to each other is called *movement schema*. Individuals call up the schema for programming or, in a sense, they piece together desired movements.

An example of the theory in practice is the performance of an individual playing shortstop in baseball or guard in basketball. The shortstop can field a ball from numerous positions, many of which are unpracticed, and still get the ball to first base, just as the basketball player can shoot successfully from almost any position on the court.

There are two control components: the GMP and the motor response schema responsible for dictating the specific rules governing an action. Thus, the motor response schema provides parameters to the GMP.

The motor schema (concept) for a general skill area (e.g., throwing and jumping) is bounded by dimensions related to space, time, and force. Each dimension represents a continuum that, depending on experience, may be limited or diverse. Theoretically, the greater the variety of experiences produced by the individual, the more diverse the schema becomes and the greater the capacity to move. The motor schema enables the individual to select the appropriate level from each dimension to program a task that may be known or novel. In shooting a basketball, for example, the child calls upon a program consisting of a relationship among distance the ball has to travel, required muscular force, arm speed, and angle release—all of which may change from one attempt to the next.

A major prediction of schema theory is that increasing *variability in practice* on a given task will result in increased transfer to a novel task of the same movement class. The strength of the schema is a positive function of the amount and variability of practice of responses within a movement class.

Most studies have tested these predictions by manipulating the variability of practice factor. It is predicted that subjects exposed to a high variability of practice regime but who never experience the test condition will perform as well or better than subjects who practice only on the test condition relevant to a final observation on that test condition. In addition, it is predicted that the high-variability group will outperform the specificity group on transfer to novel tasks. Numerous studies supporting the variability hypothesis have been generated using children and adults as subjects and a gross motor skill as the task (e.g., Kelso & Norman, 1978; Kerr & Booth, 1978; Moxley, 1979; Wulf, 1991).

For example, Carson and Wiegand (1979) found that young children (from ages 3 to 5) with more variable practice experience had greater overall success when throwing a beanbag of a new weight at a target on the floor and at a relocated target attached to a wall. The variable-practice group also maintained its performance level in all conditions after a period of two weeks, in contrast with a loss in performance by the control, low-variability, and specific-practice groups. The findings of Carson and Weigand demonstrated that young children can establish a movement rule or relationship, use it, and retain it for later use.

According to a review by Shapiro and Schmidt (1982), one conclusion that emerges from the literature when comparing studies using adults and children is that children's motor skills apparently are affected more easily by variability in practice. This observation suggests that the schemata of children are easily developed, whereas adults already may have developed schemata for the relatively simple tasks used in the investigations. The authors also note that various rival theories (e.g., Adams, 1971) cannot explain how performance on variations of a task leads to essentially the same transfer performance in adults as practicing the criterion task itself. Nor can they explain why varied practice for children was consistently more effective than practicing the criterion task itself.

Variability in practice is predictably more effective for children, especially young children (Yan et al., 1998), than for adults simply because young individuals have considerably more to learn. Typically, children learning to read are taught to recognize letters, then parts of words, then complete words, and finally sentences. Children studying mathematics learn to solve problems after they have grasped the basic functions of numbers and signs. When a child learns to play a musical instrument, he or she studies the scale before attempting a song. In physical education or a youth sport setting, however, children frequently are taught games and dances before they are able to perform prerequisite skills. Generally, schema theory supports variability in practice and problem solving (within the same class of movements and rules) during early years rather than instruction in specific sport skills.

THINK ABOUT IT

As a physical education teacher for children, how would you use this information for teaching—for example, the manipulative skill of throwing?

Developmental Theories of Motor Control

Objective 7.7 ➤ Although it is generally accepted that the control of motor behavior is under the direction of some type of generalized motor program, what the program actually controls and how control develops have been two of the most active areas of contemporary motor development research.

Under the heading of *developmental biodynamics*, as discussed in chapter 1 (Lockman & Thelen, 1993; Thelen, 2000), this general approach to the study of perception and action is based on the general hypothesis that motor coordination and control emerge from continual and intimate interactions between the nervous system and the periphery, the limbs and body segments (in essence, the brain and body). From this multifaceted approach, three ideas have emerged that have exciting implications for better understanding the processes and mechanisms involved in motor development (Perception → Action): *coordinative structures, dynamic systems,* and *neuronal group selection.*

Coordinative Structures   The general consensus in past years was that the individual muscles were given instructions by the commands produced in the motor program. Bernstein (1967) challenged this notion. He argued there are too many independent operations for the motor program to control them all simultaneously. In more recent years researchers have supported Bernstein's initial concern (e.g., Thelen, 2000; Turvey, 1990; Vereijken, 1991). They find it difficult to consider that the nearly 800 muscles and 100 mobile joints of the body are under the control of the CNS in all the possible degrees of freedom (i.e., controlled action of an independent joint movement). Bernstein suggested that motor programs control groupings of muscles instead of individual muscles. These groupings of muscles with associated joints have been termed **coordinative structures,** dynamic structures, and *synergies.* The commands generated by the motor program are said to be directed toward the specific coordinative structure that, is constrained to act as a single functional unit. For a simplified analogy consider the actions of a puppeteer who controls several degrees of freedom (e.g., the action of the whole arm of the puppet) with a single finger. From this general notion, a new definition of the term *coordination* has been proposed. It is the process by which an individual constrains, or condenses, the available *degrees of freedom* into the smallest number necessary to achieve a goal (Rose, 1997).

The actual nature of how the motor program controls movement patterns is not yet clear. However, the existence of coordinative structures has been verified (e.g., Gentilucci et al., 1992; Kelso et al., 1984; Saling et al., 1998). It has stimulated considerable inquiry in developmental research, much of which as been associated with the dynamic systems perspective.

Dynamic Systems   In chapter 1, we saw that the **dynamic systems** perspective seeks to provide an understanding of how movement and control emerge or unfold developmentally. Based on highly complex principles from theoretical physics, theoretical mathematics, and ecological psychology, this theory proposes that qualitative changes in motor behavior emerge out of the naturally developing dynamic properties of the motor system and coordinative structures (Kugler, et al., 1982, 1980).

The following features of dynamic systems should be noted (as interpreted from Thelen & Smith, 1994):

1. Movement appears to emerge from *self-organizing properties* of the body. Individuals are composed of several complex and cooperative systems (e.g., perceptual, postural, muscular, and skeletal), with each developing at different rates; thus the intricacy of coordinated movement. Even the simplest skill requires a cooperative effort, with each system providing critical input. For example, muscular strength of the legs and postural control are critical controllers for walking. Supposedly, there is a rate controller for each skill that organizes the system or systems needed to execute the task.

2. Another assumption is that movement is determined not only by muscular forces, but also by mechanical interactions (e.g., body segments and joint reaction forces). The contribution of these forces may be influenced by speed of movement, body position, length and mass of body segments, and the intentions of the movement. Research in this area seeks to examine the developmental characteristics associated with the generation and apportionment of forces and the timing-based control system.

3. With regard to the question of continuity or discontinuity, the dynamic systems perspective suggests that in the transition from old movement patterns to new ones, referred to as a *phase shift*, disruptions (discontinuities) occur in performance. The major challenge is to account for these characteristics from processes that are inherently continuous.

4. In addition to the biological contexts of dynamic systems, the nature of the environment and demands of the task influence development.

Using the dynamic systems perspective in motor behavior, inquiries have begun unfolding the developmental picture of how interlimb coordination emerges. Specifics from some of these studies will be described in chapter 8, with the discussion of early movement behaviors (e.g., stepping, cruising, reaching, and walking).

This line of developmental research shows great promise for providing a more comprehensive understanding of motor control and performance across the life span. Of utmost benefit will be the identification of factors that both facilitate and constrain development. It is hoped that future studies will complete the picture of lifelong development by observing the effects of aging on the coordinative structures of older adults. Since the presence of dedifferentiation and other neurological losses are assumed sometime during late adulthood, there is likely some accompanying effect on the coordinative structures. For a more detailed discussion of dynamic systems theory refer to Kelso (1995) and Thelen & Smith (1994).

Neuronal Group Selection The dynamic systems perspective provides a glimpse into self-organizing properties of developing and mature motor systems, but it does not identify specific underlying neural mechanisms. The theory of **neuronal group selection** (Edelman, 1989, 1987) holds such promise and is tied to the theory that the emergence of coordinated movement is tied closely to the growth of the musculoskeletal system and development of the brain. A key issue is how changes in brain circuitry-controlling synergies (coordinative structures) become matched to developmental changes in the musculoskeletal system and the environment of the organism.

According to Sporns & Edelman (1993), during the early stages of development, neuronal circuits are not precisely wired to execute specific skills. Instead the brain contains variant circuits (structural variability) with dynamic properties. That is, those circuits selectively form *neuronal groups*, localized collections of hundreds to thousands of interconnected neurons. Neuronal groups are arranged in the brain in neural maps that represent the body surface. Though they are separated in regions of the cortex, they are linked anatomically through long-range neural connections and thus allow for global mapping. Theoretically these selected neuronal groups temporarily share functional properties to accommodate the desired task.

THINK ABOUT IT

Summarize the issue of prewired versus self-organized motor development.

In essence, the theory of neuronal group selection accounts for the brain's organization of synergies as functional units of motor control (coordinative structures). One of its merits is that it accounts for the spontaneous adaptability of coordinative structure in response to biomechanical and environmental changes. Therefore, as with the dynamic systems perspective, neuronal group selection supports the contextualist approach to the study of motor development. Refer to Hadders-Algra (2000) for additional information on this attractive theory.

A commonality among all three theoretical notions and Gibson's ecological perspective is the suggestion that the brain and body are not prewired for skilled movements; rather, they have amazing adaptable self-organizing properties that adjust for biological and environmental contexts. In this dynamic process, exploration and selection are critical factors. To illustrate this observation and summarize contemporary theory, Case-Smith (1996) describes the following dynamic events to explain how infants acquire new movement skills.

Foremost, there is a *coupling of perception and action*. This notion suggests perception and movement continually interact in learning. As described earlier in reference to Gibson's ecological theory (chapter 6) and the concept of environmental affordances, infants coordinate their movements with concurrent perceptual information. The infant derives meaning from the environment through a continuous input of multisensory information. Change is driven primarily by the infant's need and desire to select and explore specific features of the environmental context.

With exploration of the environment there is *development of adaptable and functional movement synergies*. Basically, motor control progresses from movements of great variability to more restrictive functional motor synergies. Complementing our previous discussions of neuronal and muscle group selection, this idea suggests the basic units of motor behavior are functional synergies or coordinative structures rather than the actions of specific muscles. These synergies are highly adaptable to meeting the demands of the infant's changing movement patterns to complement the challenges of the environment.

And, as the infant progresses from one level of skill to the next, *there are phase shifts in which new movement patterns are explored and selected.* During this transition movement is typically quite variable and performance unstable. The infant may experiment with a wide variety of movement patterns that are driven primarily by exploration and the need to find a solution(s) to the new task. Goldfield (1995) describes this phase of development as beginning with an assembly of early movements, followed by a tuning to establish the more desired stable pattern. All of this illustrates the adaptive and self-organizing properties of the dynamic system.

A truly remarkable example that helps summarize this concept and section on the development of motor control is the phenomenon of *conjoined twins*. Extremely rare, these identical twins have separate necks, heads, and hearts, and their nervous systems are distinct. They are joined together at the chest. Perhaps most remarkable, they share one set of upper and lower limbs. In the case reviewed, 6-year-olds share motor acts; one controls the right side and the other the left (figure 7.5). Although coordination does not come easy, these are

THINK ABOUT IT

Using the theories and discussion from chapters 6 and 7, how would you tell the story of Perception→Action?

■ *Figure 7.5*

Tied together
Abigail controls the right hand; Brittany, the left.

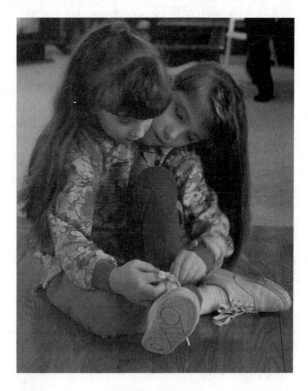

THINK ABOUT IT

What explanation is there for how conjoined twins learned to swim?

among their amazing feats: they learned to walk at 15 months and now can swim and ride a bicycle (as reported by Wallis in Time, March, 1996). How can two separate brains coordinate such complex functions? Although researchers contend that specific answers are out of reach presently, one could speculate that the self-organizing dynamics of control are truly at work. For a more detailed account of perception to action, see Bertenthal and Clifton (1998) in the Suggested Readings.

Changes with Aging

Objective 7.8 ➤ The discussion of the effects of aging on brain structures noted that not only does a significant loss of neurons occur, but other possibly debilitating changes occur within neurons themselves (e.g., senile plaques, vacuoles, and tangles). However, even with these conditions, it is believed that the brain may lose only a small portion of its ability to function.

Attention

As a general observation, as long as the two competing tasks (divided attention) are relatively easy, younger and older adults perform in a similar manner. However, as task difficulty increases, younger persons do better (Stine-Morrow & Soederberg Miller, 1999). Explanations focus on reduced amounts of processing capacity and the notion that the total amount of capacity stays constant across age but that older persons require more capacity to perform elementary functions. Thus, less space would be available for higher-level processing operations. Although these views are somewhat different, both suggest that capacity (i.e., total or space capacity) is affected by older age.

With regard to selective attention, Plude et al. (1994) report an increase throughout young adulthood, followed by selective preservation in later years. It seems that when appropriate environmental supports are available (e.g., distinctive features), differences are minimal in filtering out irrelevant stimuli. However, if speed is a requirement, older adults are slower than young persons.

Working (Short-Term) Memory

In general, working memory declines during the late adulthood years (Oberauer et al., 2001; Swanson, 1999). A study by Botwinick and Storandt (1974) found that memory span remained relatively constant from the twenties through the fifties, then dropped only about one item following those years. However, greater comparative deficits between young and older adults have been found on other tasks, such as math problems and the linear ordering of items. Once again, is the age difference due to processing efficiency or capacity (refer back to the discussion regarding children on pages 219–220)?

One explanation for any age difference is that, compared with young adults, older persons are slower in searching or scanning short-term memory (Fisk & Rogers, 1991). From another perspective, the difference is a result of information-processing abilities growing less flexible with age, a loss of information during reorganization (encoding), or a diminished ability to process the encoded information (Perlmutter, 1983; Walsh, 1983). In addition to this processing deficit explanation, the hypothesis that older adults have a storage capacity deficit compared to young persons also has been supported by research (Swanson, 1999). In short, it appears that the deficit with age is both a hardware and a software problem.

Long-Term Memory

Older adults often exhibit significant deficiencies on memory tasks that involve the transfer of information between short- and long-term stores. In general, older adults are less able to recall details of past events. This deficiency likely is due to the difficulty that elderly people have with both encoding and retrieving information from the long-term store. Older adults, like young children, apparently do not engage as frequently as young adults in deep elaborate encoding strategies. However, wide individual differences are normal. A study by Till (1985) found relatively small deficits on long-term memory tasks among well-educated, elderly individuals. Long-term memory in older adults has been shown to improve with instructions to use imagery and when plenty of time is provided for the task.

Metamemory and Knowledge

Interestingly, older adults may use metamemory to compensate somewhat for limitations in encoding and retrieving information. A number of studies suggest that with age, adults maintain or increase their understanding about the memory system. A separate but related consideration is how knowledge of materials influences memory. Just as knowledge of materials positively can affect age differences in children, it also can override age differences in adults.

Although there is no doubt that a tremendous base of knowledge is accumulated throughout childhood, there is little evidence that basic knowledge shows a similar decline in late adulthood. Tests of common, factual knowledge typically show no decline from young adulthood to old age (Perlmutter & Hall, 1985).

■ *Figure 7.6*

Age-related
increase in
processing speed
(response time)
with increase in
complexity

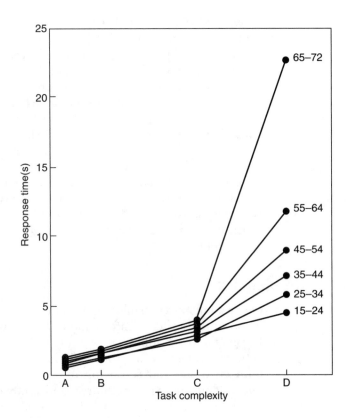

■ *Figure 7.6*

Age-related increase in processing speed (response time) with increase in complexity

Processing Speed and Movement Time

A consistent finding in the study of aging is a decline in processing speed as measured by reaction time and other manipulative tasks. Overall, processing speed of many types reaches a peak in young adulthood (twenties) and declines slowly thereafter (Cerella & Hale, 1994; Yan et al., 2000). If it takes a 20-year-old 200 milliseconds to perform a reaction time task, the same task will take a 60-year-old about 250 milliseconds, and an 80-year-old over 300 milliseconds (see figure 7.4 on page 223). In contrast, a 6-year-old typically performs the task in just under 350 milliseconds. Welford (1984) estimates that older adults may decrease 20% to 50% in processing speed depending on the complexity of the task (figure 7.6).

Apparently, with advancing age, there is little change in the speeded performance of single, discrete arm/hand actions and simple repetitive tasks that can be programmed in advance (Welford, 1977). However, much greater decrements among older persons have been found on timed (speed) tasks that involve decision making based on perceptual information and the programming of movement sequences. This is partially evidenced by large performance decreases on complex sequential tasks that require a series of different movements, particularly when speed is a critical factor (Lupinacci et al., 1993; Williams, 1990). Overall, older adults are capable of demonstrating accurate motor performance on well-rehearsed tasks when speed is not a critical factor (Yan et al., 2000).

THINK ABOUT IT

Do you suppose the rate of psychomotor slowing in the elderly can be controlled? If so, how?

The general slowing of the body with advanced aging constitutes a universal phenomenon referred to as *psychomotor slowing*. Although the mechanisms responsible for this condition remain unexplained, Cerella (1990) contends that slowing is attributed to numerous factors associated with advanced aging (e.g., neuron loss, synaptic delay, decrease in excitability, and decrease in nerve conduction velocity), which causes disruptions of connections within the neural network. Supposedly each disruption increases the time to process information. Other researchers also agree that, although neuromuscular factors contribute to slowing with age, most of the decrement can be attributed to central mechanisms (i.e., CNS). The topic of psychomotor slowing will be discussed in greater detail with performance examples in chapter 11.

Programming

Welford (1984) suggested that the major limitations of older adults in the performance of a motor task are their ability to make decisions based on perceptual input and to program movement sequences. Evidence also suggests that older adults learn new motor and cognitive tasks more slowly than young individuals. One may speculate that while the schemata of older people can be complete for skills learned in past experiences, the ability of the mind to form new schemata diminishes somewhat with age.

Recall from the discussion of processing speed and Fitt's law (Yan et al., 2000), while studying lifespan differences in rapid arm movements, noted that older adults were slower, more variant, and less smooth than young adults. Much of the difference was attributed to the older group making more on-line movement adjustments as opposed to movement under central (programming) control, especially when confronted with accuracy demands and response uncertainty. In essence, it was speculated that older adults lacked programming control. However, when accuracy was not critical and practical trials were provided, older adults performed much better. Fisk and Rogers (2000) reported similar findings after a comprehensive review of research—that is, older adults can learn (program) new skills with practice, but they are slower than younger persons. This conclusion applies to relatively simple and more complex tasks.

A summary list of selected information-processing changes with aging is presented in Table 7.1. A general observation is that young children and older adults have several characteristics in common.

TABLE 7.1

Summary of Selected Information-Processing Changes with Aging

Information-Processing Characteristic	
Attention	Declines
Working memory	Declines slightly
Encoding and retrieval abilities	Decline
Long-term memory	Declines
Metamemory and knowledge	No apparent change
Processing speed	Slows
Movement time	Slows slightly
Response time	Slows on tasks requiring that movement sequences be performed quickly
Programming	Ability to learn new motor tasks and program movement sequences (no apparent change)

Summary

The four basic components of the information-processing model are sensory input, reception through the various perceptual modalities, interpretation and decision making (programming), and overt motor response. Information processing can be discussed under the general topics of attention, memory, processing speed, and programming. Although much about information processing is unknown and highly theoretical, it generally has been observed that as individuals progress toward adulthood, they are able to process more information in a shorter period of time.

The core of most information-processing is attention. The primary importance of attention to motor behavior involves alertness and the ability to select and attend to meaningful information. The developmental trend in selective attention appears to move from young children, who primarily attend exclusively to one stimulus (and are easily distracted), to older children who may attend to too much information (some of which is irrelevant), and finally, to the early adolescent who shows the more adultlike ability to attend to relevant information in complex conditions. Age differences in this aspect of information processing are attributed primarily to experience and the refinement of strategies.

The two primary types of memory are recognition and recall. The two basic memory systems are working memory and long-term memory.

Evidence that primitive forms of recognition memory are present in the newborn is found in the observation of habituation. There are also indications that young babies learn to remember (cued recall memory) using contextual information. In addition to age differences in some aspects of storage capacity, differences between young children and adults also can be found in coding, searching and retrieving, and recalling information. Other functional abilities that have developmental implications are rehearsal and chunking. An individual's knowledge or intuition about memory and himself or herself as memorizer is known as metamemory.

The rate at which information is processed, as reflected by an individual's reaction time, improves with age up to the early adult years, then remains relatively stable until later adulthood. Though not all motor tasks require information to be processed at a fast rate, processing speed may account for many age-related performance differences. This appears to be especially evident when comparing young adults to young children and the aged.

Programming is considered one of the most sophisticated operations in information processing. With regard to the development of a theoretical base for motor programming, the concept of a *schema* has received considerable attention as a result of the schema theory of motor skill learning.

The notion of some form of motor program generally has been accepted, but does not explain the link between brain on body (motor control). Three aspects of the developmental biodynamics perspective offer some insight: *coordinative structures, dynamic systems,* and *neuronal group selection.* A commonality among these ideas is the suggestion that the brain and body are not prewired for skilled movements; rather, they have adaptable self-organizing properties that adjust for biological and environmental contexts.

It is fairly well accepted that changes in the brain structure with advancing age produce some degree of regression in information-processing abilities. A general observation is that the abilities of the old approximate those of children; both perform below the level of the young adult.

Think about It

1. Reflecting back on chapter 6, how does the information presented here fit the introductory information processing model (figure 6.1 on page 171)?
2. Name some sport activities that require considerable selection attention. Rank the order by complexity and explain why you ranked them as you did.

3. Do you perceive general memory and the ability to recall movements (motor memory) as different from each other?
4. Why can we recall how to ride a bicycle (and do it) after years of not practicing but forget what we wore to class last week?
5. As future teachers and coaches, is there any practical value to this information—we (as adults) are about twice as fast with processing and reaction as a 5-year-old?
6. As a physical education teacher for children, how would you use this information for teaching—for example, the manipulative skill of throwing?
7. Summarize the issue of prewired versus self-organized motor development.
8. Using the theories and discussion from chapters 6 and 7, how would you tell the story of Perception→Action?
9. What explanation is there for how conjoined twins learned to swim?
10. Do you suppose the rate of psychomotor slowing in the elderly can be controlled? If so, how?

Suggested Readings

Bertenhal, B., & Clifton, R. (1998). *Perception to action.* New York: John Wiley & Sons.

L. W. Damon (Ed.). Handbook of child psychology: Vol. 2. Cognition, perception and language: 51–102. New York: Wiley.

Kelso, J. A. (1995). *Dynamic patterns.* Cambridge, MA: MIT Press.

Lockman, J. J., & Thelen, E. (1993). Developmental biodynamics: Brain, body, behavior connections. Special feature. *Child Development* 64:953–1190.

Magill, R. A. (2001). *Motor learning: Concepts and application* (6th ed.). Dubuque, IA: Wm. C. Brown. (undergraduate)

Schmidt, R. A., & Lee, T. D. (1999). *Motor control and learning.* 3rd ed. Champaign, IL: Human Kinetics. (graduate-upper undergraduate)

Spirduso, W. W. (1995). *Physical dimensions of aging.* Champaign, IL: Human Kinetics.

Thelen, E., & Smith, L. (1994). *A dynamic systems approach to the development of cognition and action.* Cambridge, MA: MIT Press.

WebLinks

Esther Thelen's Infant Motor Development Laboratory at Indiana University
    http://php.indiana.edu/~gormleyf

National Association for Sport & Physical Education: www.aahperd.org/naspe/

International Society on Infant Studies: www.isisweb.org

Society for Research in Child Development: www.srcd.org

part four

Motor Behavior across the Life Span

IN THE STUDY of motor development, researchers gather information related to *growth* (change in size), *development* (change in level of functioning), and *motor behavior* (performance) across the life span. The text up to this point primarily has addressed the growth and development aspects of the various dynamic systems of the human body and the factors that can affect them. Part Four builds upon this foundation by documenting observable movement characteristics that typically occur within the phases of motor behavior.

In essence, motor behavior is the movement expression of the human body with regard to its physical size, neurological and physiological functioning, information-processing abilities , and self-organizing properties. For the study of motor development, the information provided so far serves as the basis for understanding why characteristic movement abilities within each phase are feasible and what factors of change are responsible for the transition across phases. For example, what factors are responsible for the regression of

chapters

8 Early Movement Behavior

9 Motor Behavior during Early Childhood

10 Motor Behavior during Later Childhood and Adolescence

11 Motor Behavior in the Adult Years

motor performance? What characteristics account for the peak performance generally found between 25 and 30 years of age? What factors account for the transition from reflexive behavior to voluntary movement? These questions are the foundation of motor development inquiry.

Part Four is divided into four chapters; each chapter describes those movement characteristics associated with one or more of the phases of motor behavior. Chapter 8 describes the reflexive, stereotypic, and rudimentary behaviors that span the prenatal stage through infancy (2 years of age). Chapter 9 documents the development of fundamental movement patterns and manipulative behaviors characteristic of the early childhood years (approximately ages 2 through 6). Chapter 10 presents information related to motor behavior during later childhood and the adolescent years (age 7 to 18) in which individuals generally exhibit sport skill abilities and rapid periods of physical growth and development. Chapter 11 deals with the characteristic behaviors of the adult years, which normally feature peak motor performance and the inevitable course of regression.

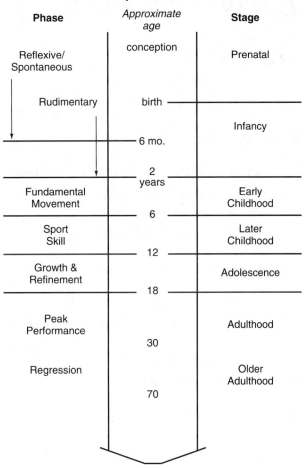

The Developmental Continuum

Phase	Approximate age	Stage
Reflexive/ Spontaneous	conception	Prenatal
Rudimentary	birth	Infancy
	6 mo.	
Fundamental Movement	2 years	Early Childhood
Sport Skill	6	Later Childhood
Growth & Refinement	12	Adolescence
Peak Performance	18	Adulthood
	30	
Regression	70	Older Adulthood

8 *Early Movement Behavior*

OBJECTIVES

Upon completion of this chapter, you should be able to

8.1 Discuss reflexes with regard to definition, control, relevance, and developmental characteristics.

8.2 Identify the three general types of reflexes and provide examples of each.

8.3 Explain the various theoretical views of reflex behavior.

8.4 Describe the developmental characteristics of spontaneous movements (stereotypies).

8.5 Provide a brief overview of the rudimentary phase of motor behavior.

8.6 Outline the developmental milestones associated with basic postural control and rudimentary locomotion.

8.7 Describe the developmental characteristics involved in manual control during the first two years of life.

8.8 Discuss the theoretical views associated with motor asymmetries.

KEY TERMS

reflexes	creeping
primitive reflexes	walking
postural reflexes	prehension
locomotor reflexes	manipulation
spontaneous movements	manual control
rudimentary behavior	motor asymmetries
crawling	

The Developmental Continuum

Phase	Approximate age	Stage
Reflexive/ Spontaneous	conception	Prenatal
Rudimentary	birth	
	6 mo.	Infancy
	2 years	
Fundamental Movement		Early Childhood
	6	
Sport Skill		Later Childhood
	12	
Growth & Refinement		Adolescence
	18	
Peak Performance		Adulthood
	30	
Regression		Older Adulthood
	70	

THE BEGINNINGS OF HUMAN MOVEMENT are those characteristic behaviors that appear during the prenatal and infancy stages of development. Coinciding with these stages that cover the first two years of life are the reflexive/spontaneous and rudimentary phases of motor behavior. This chapter describes and explains the importance of reflexive and stereotypic (spontaneous) behaviors. It also documents the development of early voluntary movement with regard to postural control, locomotion, and manual control. Evidence of early motor asymmetries and theoretical views on the topic also will be discussed.

■ *Reflexive Behavior*

Objective 8.1

➤ It already has been established that motor development has its origins in the prenatal period. Reflexes can be elicited in the fetus as early as the second or third month after conception, and most are present by the time of birth or before. In fact, many of the superficial, cutaneous reflexes are present by the fifth or sixth fetal month. **Reflexes** are involuntary movement reactions elicited by such forms of sensory stimuli as sound, light, touch, or body position. They are controlled primarily by the subcortical areas (lower brain centers), which are also responsible for numerous involuntary, life-sustaining processes such as breathing and heart rate.

The body's initial movement responses are controlled in the subcortical areas due to the maturational stage of the central nervous system (CNS). As the nervous system matures, reflexes come under the command of the brain stem and midbrain rather than remaining solely under spinal cord control. Finally, as the cerebral cortex (higher brain center) matures, most of these transient reflexes gradually become inhibited and voluntary motor behavior eventually takes over. The motor area of the cerebral cortex generally is considered to be minimally functional in the developing fetus and newborn infant, thus most movement behavior is thought to be primarily involuntary. The human organism in the first six months to one year is essentially a reflex machine that undergoes a continuous process of neuromuscular functional maturation. Of the estimated 27 major infant reflexes (Lorton & Lorton, 1984), most are suppressed (disappear) by 6 months of age in the typical developing child and few are observable after the first year. However, some reflexes, such as coughing, blinking, and sneezing persist throughout life. There are also indications that specific reflexes reemerge due to neurological trauma or insult.

Importance of Reflexes in Infant Development

The importance of reflex behavior primarily is associated with its role in stimulating the CNS and muscles, in infant survival, and in its use as a diagnostic tool for assessing neurological maturity. Until the information-processing mechanisms become mature enough to consciously formulate motor programs and execute movement responses, reflexes are a primary mode of stimulating the CNS and muscles. It is suggested, though somewhat speculatively, that this mode of initial stimulation is vital to optimal growth and development of the mechanisms that will eventually control voluntary motor behavior. This supposition is based partly on the fact that reflexive behaviors stimulate neural pathways, memory trace activity, and muscle tonicity. Several researchers have supported the notion that reflexes play a dominant role in the development of muscle tone that, in time, becomes critical to the performance of future voluntary actions. In an article published in *American Scientist*, Easton comments that "normal motor coordination is based to a huge extent on the reflexes" (1972, 591). Theoretical views on this topic will be discussed later in this chapter.

The presence of some reflexes offers infants certain survival advantages with regard to seeking nourishment and, perhaps to a lesser degree, protection. Two prime examples of these *primitive reflexes* are the rooting reflex and the sucking reflex. The *rooting (search) reflex* is exhibited when newborns automatically turn their mouths toward the mother's nipple (or bottle) when it touches their cheek or lips. In the *sucking reflex*, newborns reflexively suck on anything that touches their lips. Interestingly, the neonate is not born with the voluntary capacity to ingest food. Thus, the sucking reflex enables the newborn to feed by involuntary means.

While perhaps not as critical to survival as the reflexes related to feeding, certain involuntary responses also have been described as *protection mechanisms*. One example of this type of survival response is the *Moro reflex*. When a newborn is startled or begins to fall, the arms and legs fling outward, the hands open, and the fingers spread. As the reflexive action for protection continues, the arms draw close to the body, the fists clench, the eyes open, and the infant lets out a loud wail. Although some primitive reflexes do not readily appear to have any survival value, it has been speculated they once served a protective function. The assumption is that certain primitive protective reflexes evolved from lower primates to human infants, as in the case of the *palmar grasp* (or *grasping reflex*). Upon tactile stimulation of the infant's palm, the hand will close reflexively around an object and grip tightly. Researchers have speculated this reflex evolved among primates so infants could cling to their mothers as they moved about.

Reflexes are not only important to the survival of infants, but also serve as an indicator of general neurological status. The genesis of reflex behavior is well documented with regard to onset, persistence, and disappearance. Since infant reflexes occur within predictable age ranges, pediatricians have used these behaviors extensively as diagnostic tools for assessing neurological maturity. The failure of reflexes to appear, their prolonged continuation, or their uneven strength characteristics may cause the physician to suspect neurological impairment. Two universal assessments of neonatal behavior (described in chapter 12) are the *Apgar scale* and the *Brazelton scale;* both include reflex measures as indicators of neurological adequacy. The Moro, Babinski, and asymmetrical tonic neck reflexes commonly are used with infant assessment scales and during normal physical examinations. These measurements can provide highly critical information. For example, if the asymmetrical tonic neck reflex perseveres past the time it normally disappears (about 6 months), it is an indication that cerebral palsy or other neurological impairment may be present (Lorton & Lorton, 1984).

Although most measures of reflex behavior indicate generalized neurological status, they may be used in a selective way by specialists to determine the presence of localized neurological defects of such areas as the cranial nerves, spinal roots, and spinal cord (e.g., spina bifida).

Types of Reflexes

Objective 8.2 ➤ Although it may not be possible to precisely and systematically classify reflexes into neat categories, they generally may be grouped under the descriptors of primitive, postural, and locomotor.

Primitive reflexes primarily are associated with the infant's instinct for survival and protection. Upon stimulation, the infant reflexively seeks nourishment with the rooting and sucking responses and shows indications of protecting itself with the Moro and grasping reflexes. Though it can be debated whether these primitive reflexes are actually vital to infant survival and safety, indications are that these behaviors aid the fetus in orienting itself in its prebirth environment (Milani-Comparetti, 1981). The term *primitive* may be appropriate in view of the infant's ultimate potential; however, the term also may be associated with the level of neurological control. Because most of these reflexes are mediated by the lower brain centers (e.g., spinal cord and lower brain stem) as opposed to the higher centers of control (e.g., midbrain and cerebral cortex), use of the word *primitive* in this context also seems to be appropriate. Compared with the other types of reflexes, most of the primitive responses are functional prenatally and can be elicited in utero. As the cerebral cortex matures and gains control of lower brain functions (around 3 to 4 postnatal months) many of the primitive reflexes are suppressed.

As the higher brain centers begin to function and suppress the lower control centers, postural reactions enter the infant's repertoire. **Postural reflexes** provide the infant with the ability to react to gravitational forces and changes in equilibrium. These involuntary reactions are the mechanisms by which the infant is able to maintain an appropriate posture with a changing environment. General functions of these reflexes include coordinating movements of the head, trunk, and limbs to keep the head upright; maintaining equilibrium; rolling over; and attaining vertical postures. There is also a protective response with postural control, as evidenced with the parachute reflex. When infants are tilted forward (face down) from an upright position, they reflexively extend their arms as a protective mechanism to brace against the forward displacement.

It is not unusual to find classification methods that use only the primitive and postural categories. However, another group of reflexes has enough common characteristics to justify including a third category. **Locomotor reflexes** are unique in that they resemble later voluntary locomotor movements. Involuntary responses such as the reflexes associated with climbing, walking (stepping), and swimming have been described as precursors of the voluntary movements of the same name.

TABLE 8.1

Approximate Timetable of Selected Reflexes

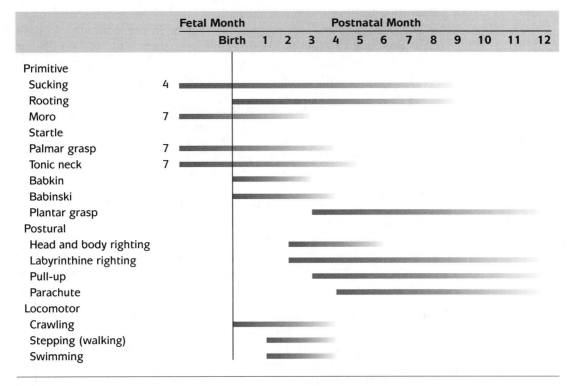

	Fetal Month		Postnatal Month											
	Birth	1	2	3	4	5	6	7	8	9	10	11	12
Primitive													
Sucking	4												
Rooting													
Moro	7												
Startle													
Palmar grasp	7												
Tonic neck	7												
Babkin													
Babinski													
Plantar grasp													
Postural													
Head and body righting													
Labyrinthine righting													
Pull-up													
Parachute													
Locomotor													
Crawling													
Stepping (walking)													
Swimming													

Source: Data from J. O. Forfar and G. C. Arneil, *Textbook of Paediatrics*, 2d ed. Copyright © 1978 Churchill Livingston, New York, NY.

Although these reflexes normally are suppressed by the fifth or sixth month, their voluntary counterparts do not appear until months later. Consequently, there has been much debate concerning their possible linkage. This issue will arise again in the discussion of the various theoretical views concerning the role of reflexes in motor development.

A fourth group of involuntary responses, known as *tendon reflexes*, should be noted with regard to their initial appearance. These reflexes are used throughout the life span to evaluate neuromuscular response (primarily contraction) and are present in standard sites of the jaw, biceps, knee, and ankle by the second day of postnatal life.

The following section does not attempt to describe all infant reflexes. Rather, its purpose is to discuss those involuntary responses considered most appropriate to the study of motor development. For a more detailed description of specific reflexes, refer to the work of Fiorentino (1981) and Forfar and Arneil (1998). Table 8.1 summarizes the approximate timetables for appearance, persistence, and disappearance of selected reflexes.

Primitive Reflexes   One of the earliest involuntary responses to appear is the *sucking reflex*. This response is evident in the 4-month-old fetus as it protrudes its lips in unmistakable preparation for sucking. Some babies have sucking blisters at birth caused by this sucking action during the prenatal state. In newborns, the sucking reflex is elicited by anything that touches its lips.

In conjunction with the sucking response, the tongue and pharynx adequately adapt to swallowing so the newborn can feed. Newborns can suck and inhale simultaneously and swallow between breaths about three times faster than adults. After a couple of weeks, most newborns have mastered the complex function of synchronized sucking, swallowing, and breathing.

The reflexive behavior of sucking for nourishment is joined with the instinctive response to seek food using the *rooting reflex*. This response is activated by a light touch on the cheek, which causes the newborn to turn its head toward the stimulus in search of nourishment. This response also is referred to as the *search reflex*. Although the sucking response appears to be voluntary around the third month of infancy, characteristics of the reflex are still evident until 6 to 9 months of age, when feeding is totally under voluntary control. The rooting reflex follows a similar timetable, it persists until approximately the ninth month.

When the newborn is startled or begins to fall, its arms and legs extend outward, its hands open, and its fingers spread in the instinctive protective response called the *Moro reflex* (figure 8.1). As noted earlier, the Moro reflex commonly is used for assessing generalized neurological status. The response can be elicited in several ways. One way is abruptly to remove support from the newborn's head by allowing it to drop sharply backward a short distance and then catching it with the hand. Another way to produce the reflex is to make a loud noise by clapping or slapping a table. After the arms and legs extend in response to the stimulus, the limbs return to a normal flexed position against the body. The Moro reflex crystallizes in the seventh fetal month and normally disappears by the third month of postnatal life.

Although quite similar to the Moro response, the *startle reflex* may not appear until months after the Moro reflex has disappeared (at about 7 months). When startled the infant initially flexes its arms and legs rather than extending them as in the Moro reflex. The startle response normally is suppressed by the end of the first year; however, less intense indications of it may persist throughout the life span.

Grasping reflex behavior is one of the most well-known and interesting responses in the infant's involuntary movement repertoire. This reflex is evident when a small rod or someone's finger touches the newborn's palm. The fingers (excluding the thumb) fold tightly around the

■ *Figure 8.1*

Moro reflex:
(a) position of rest,
(b) extension of
limbs

a.

b.

■ *Figure 8.2*

The grasping reflex

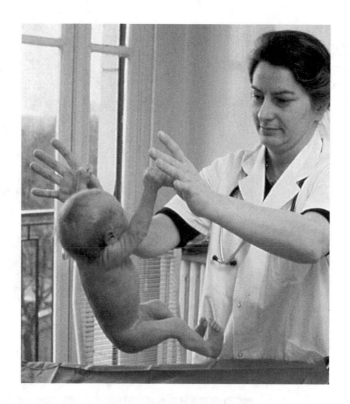

object with a grasping action. The reflex is present by the seventh fetal month, though in a weaker form, and gradually grows stronger for several weeks after birth. The reflex then weakens and is suppressed entirely by the time the infant is about 4 months old. Around this time the involuntary response is replaced by the initial stages of voluntary grasping, or manual control. This association will be described later with regard to the developmental progression of manual control.

Another interesting facet of involuntary grasping behavior is its strength characteristics (figure 8.2). When pulled toward suspension while involuntarily clinging to a rod with both hands, infants typically are able to support more than 70% of their body weight (Eckert, 1987). In a classic study of the grasping reflex, Richter (1934) recorded the suspension time, of 37 newborns 1- to 23-days-old who grasped with both hands. Large individual differences were evident, but only one infant failed to hang for any length of time. The longest suspension of 128 seconds equals that found among the better efforts of adults. It also has been noted that strength of the reflex is greater about two weeks after birth.

Two forms of the *tonic neck reflex* have been identified: asymmetric and symmetric. Both responses appear at about 7 fetal months of age and disappear by approximately 5 months of age. The asymmetric tonic neck reflex can be elicited by placing the infant in a supine position (on

■ *Figure 8.3*

Tonic neck reflexes:
(a) asymmetric,
(b) symmetric
when tipped
backward, and
(c) symmetric
when tipped
forward

a.   b.   c.

its back, face upward) and turning the neck so the head faces either side. In response to the stretch of the neck muscles as the neck turns, an increase of tonus in the limbs is triggered. The infant exhibits a fencer's on guard position (figure 8.3a) as the limbs extend on the side of the body in which the head is facing and flex on the opposite side.

Right-side limbs respond differently than the left-side limbs in the asymmetric pattern. In the symmetric tonic neck reflex the limbs move symmetrically, a response that can be elicited by placing the infant in a supported semistanding position and tipping the neck forward or backward. If tipped backward, which causes the neck to extend, the infant's arms will extend reflexively and the legs will flex (figure 8.3b). If tipped forward, which causes flexion of the neck, the infant's arms also will flex and the legs will extend (figure 8.3c).

One unusual infant reflex is the *Babkin reflex*, also known as the *palmar-mandibular reflex*. This response can be elicited by providing pressure simultaneously to both palm, which causes the infant to exhibit one or all of the following behaviors: mouth opens, eyes close, neck flexes, and head tilts forward. The Babkin reflex can be elicited at birth and normally disappears by the third month.

The *Babinski* and *plantar grasp* reflexes are involuntary responses to stroke stimulation along the sole of the infant's foot. In the Babinski reflex, which is present at birth, pressure applied to the sole of the foot causes the infant to reflexively fan out and extend its toes (figure 8.4 on page 252). This reflex normally is suppressed by the fourth month. Around this same period in the infant's life, stroking the sole will induce the plantar grasp reflex in which the toes contract or flex as if attempting to grasp the object. The plantar grasp reflex may persist through the first year of life.

Postural Reflexes *Head and body righting* are reflex behaviors believed to form the basis for future voluntary rolling movements. Both involuntary responses appear around the second month and persist until about 6 months of age. The head (and neck) righting reflex can be elicited by gently turning the infant's body in either direction while in the supine position (on its back). The infant will respond reflexively by righting, or turning, its head in the same direction. In contrast, the body-righting reflex is elicited by turning the head in one direction while the infant is in a supine position. The body will reflexively right itself by turning in the same direction—first the hips and legs and then the trunk.

The *labyrinthine righting reflex* characteristically involves both righting and gravity reactions. This reflex enables the infant to maintain an upright body posture; it is believed to contribute to the ability to move in a forward direction. The first evidence of this reflex is seen around 2 months when the infant, while lying on its stomach, attempts to orient its head to gravity and look up. It is this upright head position while the infant is on its hands and knees at around 6 months that establishes the posture for forward locomotion.

The labyrinthine righting reflex can be elicited by holding the infant in an upright position and tilting its body forward, backward, or to the side. In response, the infant will reflexively attempt to maintain an upright posture of the head by moving it in the direction opposite that in which the trunk was moved (figure 8.5). The head tends to maintain the original upright posture with relation to gravity. This response also detects functioning of the otolith organs housed in the labyrinth of the inner ear. The labyrinthine righting reflex generally appears around the second month of life, becomes stronger during the middle of the first year, and normally disappears by 12 months.

■ *Figure 8.5*

The labyrinthine
righting reflex

The *pull-up reflex* is an involuntary attempt to maintain an upright position. The response is elicited by placing the infant in an upright sitting position while holding its hands and carefully tipping it backward or forward. In response, the infant will flex or extend its arms in an apparent effort to maintain the upright posture (figure 8.6). This reflex usually appears around the third month and disappears by the end of the first year. It has been suggested this involuntary response is related to the attainment of voluntary upright posture.

Also referred to as propping reflexes, the *parachute reflexes* serve as protective and supportive movements for the infant. Protective responses are evident when the infant is tipped off balance in any direction.

■ *Figure 8.6*

The pull-up reflex

Parachute reflexes:
(a) protective
reaction to sudden
downward
movement,
(b) protective
reaction to being
tilted from a
balanced position,
(c) propping
reaction using one
arm for support in
reaching for a toy

a.   b.

c.

Forward and downward parachute reflexes are present around the fourth
month. The forward response is elicited by holding the infant in an
upright position and tilting it toward the ground. In response, the infant
reflexively extends its arms in a protective movement to break the fall
(figure 8.7a). The downward response is observed when the infant sud-
denly is lowered downward (from an upright position) a distance of
about three feet. The infant's legs will extend and spread, and the feet
will rotate outward.

These reflexes also are seen when the infant is tilted off balance in
either direction from a sitting position (figure 8.7b). The sideward propping movement usually is not observable until around the sixth month.
The backward response usually is not observable until sometime between 10 to 12 months. In response to being tilted backward, the infant
also may rotate the body to avoid falling in that direction. Until these
reflexes are present, infants will make no attempt to brace or catch

themselves when falling. It is not unusual for these protective responses to persist beyond the first year.

Parachute reflexes are supportive as well as protective movements. The supportive response is observable when the infant extends an arm for support while reaching with the other hand (figure 8.7c). It may be assumed this supporting (propping) action enables the infant to attain a better visual perspective of the surroundings and perform other tasks such as reaching, grasping, and crawling.

Locomotor Reflexes   The *crawling reflex* can be observed from birth and, as noted earlier, there is a definite similarity of movements between this response and the voluntary pattern that appears months later. If the infant is placed in a prone position (on the stomach) and pressure is applied to the sole of one foot or both feet alternately, the infant will reflexively crawl using its arms and legs (figure 8.8). There is some speculation that this reflex (and others in this category) is a precursor to the voluntary crawling pattern, even though there is a distinct time lag between the disappearance of this reflex and the appearance of the voluntary pattern. While the crawling reflex normally disappears by the fourth month, voluntary crawling generally is not observed until around the sixth or seventh month. The crawling reflex is important for the development of sufficient muscle tone for voluntary crawling.

The *stepping reflex* is one of the most debated involuntary responses in the infant's repertoire. The primary point of contention is its assumed link with voluntary walking behavior. Normally present by the end of the first week after birth, this reflex can be elicited by holding the infant upright with the feet touching a flat supporting surface. Pressure on the bottom of the infant's feet will cause it to reflexively respond with crude but characteristic walking movements. The reflex will consist of a distinct knee lift but will not involve an arm swing or hip motions. A variation of the stepping response is the *placing reflex*. This reflex is similar in kinetics to the stepping reflex but is elicited by bringing the front of the infant's foot lightly in contact with the edge of a table. The infant

■ *Figure 8.8*

The crawling reflex

■ *Figure 8.9*

The stepping reflex

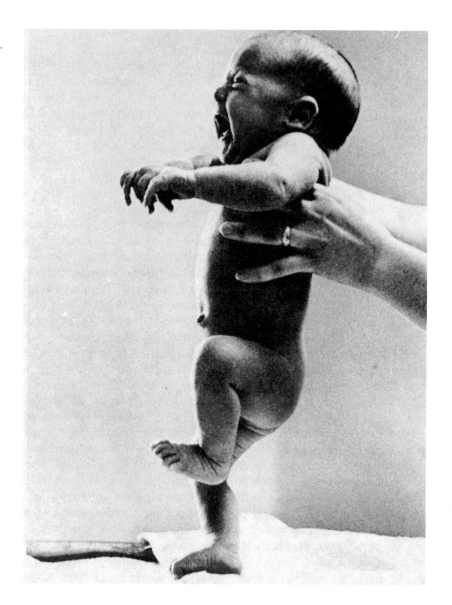

THINK ABOUT IT

Of the types of reflexes, how would you rank their importance?

responds by appearing to place the foot on the table (figure 8.9). It also may appear as though the infant is lifting its foot over an object. The stepping reflex normally persists through the fourth month.

The *swimming reflex* is one of the most interesting involuntary responses seen in infants and can be elicited during the second week after birth by holding the infant horizontally in the water with its head up or over the surface of the water. The infant responds by moving the arms and legs rhythmically in a swimming movement pattern (figure 8.10). Researchers also have noted that a breath-holding reflex is

▪ *Figure 8.10*

The swimming
reflex

elicited in the newborn when its face is placed in the water. However, a
month or so later, an infant may experience severe anxiety when its head
is submerged. This involuntary response usually disappears by about the
fourth month.

Theoretical Views of Reflex Behavior and Voluntary Movement

Objective 8.3   ➤ The developmental evolution of reflexive behavior into voluntary
motor control can be described generally. However, an explanation of
how and why these changes occur has been debated from several dif-
fering viewpoints. The relevance of the survival reflexes has stimulated
some debate, especially with regard to their phylogenetic origin, but the
primary issue from a motor behavior context has been related to the possible connections between involuntary responses and voluntary movement. This has been especially true of the reflexes that resemble
voluntary movements, such as grasping, crawling, stepping (walking),
and swimming.

One prevailing point of debate is whether the link between specific
reflexes and the later voluntary movements they resemble is a direct or
indirect relationship. Most viewpoints support the general notion that
reflex behavior, to some degree, forms the basis for later voluntary movement. In essence, reflexes do not actually disappear but, rather, are suppressed and integrated into the hierarchy of controlled behavior. Other

researchers have proposed that early reflexes are independent of voluntary control and thus actually do disappear.

Tied to the theoretical view of a *direct connection* between the two types of responses is the notion that stimulation of the reflex positively will affect later voluntary control. This point of view has been supported by research on the effects of stimulation on stepping and reaching reflexes. Researches in one well-known series of studies (review by Zelazo et al., 1993) had infants "practice walking" by stimulating their stepping reflex. They then compared the results with various control groups. In general, results indicated that infants whose stepping reflex was stimulated not only exhibited a prolonged phase of persistence and an increased response frequency, but they also began to walk voluntarily at an earlier age than the infants who had not practiced walking. One noted limitation of this research is that it is not known when the infants would have begun walking without stimulation. Bower (1976), who subjected infants to practice reaching movements during the involuntary phase, obtained similar results; the emergence of voluntary reaching was accelerated and, in some cases, children experienced no disappearance phase. Results such as these have led researchers to speculate that not only is there a direct link between specific involuntary reflexes and later voluntary control, but the disappearance phase may be due to simple disuse.

Dynamic systems research (e.g., Thelen, 1995; Thelen & Ulrich, 1991) also supports the general theory of continuity between specific reflexive movements and voluntary control. This view differs somewhat from Zelazo's theory that a reflex is transformed to a voluntary action by practice. Rather, it is suggested that increased stepping frequency and the earlier onset of independent walking may simply be the result of strengthening the infant's musculature. In one set of studies, Thelen and Fisher (1982) found that kicking and stepping reflexes involve the same neuromuscular functioning and suggest the reflex disappears because muscle growth does not keep up with leg growth. That is, the muscle is not strong enough to lift the leg mass in the upright position. In the horizontal position the pull of gravity is less, so kicking can occur. Therefore, the researchers suggest the stepping reflex actually is linked to later walking through spontaneous kicking. Studies involving the analysis of involuntary stepping and the walking patterns of independent walkers also report transition stages can be detected that link the initial coordinative patterns of the newborn with later independent walking (Thelen & Cooke, 1987; Thelen & Ulrich, 1991). In essence, there appears to be an underlying behavioral continuity that is masked by a pattern of presence-absence-presence, rather than a true disappearance.

The more *traditional view* of reflexes is that those resembling later voluntary movements (primarily locomotor reflexes) must disappear before voluntary behavior can occur (Pontius, 1973; Wyke, 1975). Proponents of this view contend there is a certain independence between involuntary responses and the voluntary movements they resemble because of the natural gap of several months between them. This time lag, they suggest, indicates there is no continuity and thus no direct link between reflexive behavior and later voluntary movement.

Milani-Comparetti and Gidoni (1967) and Molnar (1978) suggest a somewhat different but related view. They contend that certain primitive reflexes must disappear and that certain postural and locomotor reactions must appear before specific, voluntary motor skills can be attained. In their view, these postural and locomotor reflexes become supportive elements in the attainment of voluntary movement behavior. For example, Molnar's information suggests that only after the righting reactions appear is voluntary rolling possible. And, in turn, the appearance of the righting reflexes depends on the inhibition of the primitive asymmetric tonic neck reaction (Roberton, 1984). The same research also indicates that the plantar (foot) grasp must be suppressed before voluntary walking can occur. Similar transitions can be found for other voluntary motor behaviors.

Casting some doubt on the idea that a reflex must disappear before its voluntary counterpart can appear is reported evidence that both the reflexive and voluntary patterns coexist in the infant (Touwen, 1988). In a longitudinal study of 50 infants from birth to the time of independent walking, Touwen found no indications of a sequential order of development in which reflexes appear and are suppressed by the developing voluntary activity. The results of his investigation led the researcher to conclude that support is lacking for the contention that reflexes should disappear in normal infants before particular voluntary behavior can develop.

The role of reflexive behavior in the later development of voluntary movement remains unclear, though each view presented raises questions worthy of consideration. Available evidence seems to suggest that *specific reflexes play at least an indirect role in preparing the infant for later voluntary movement.* Partial justification for this assertion is based on the fact that reflexes play a significant role in the regulation, strength, and distribution of infant muscularity. Most developmentalists determine this supportive element to be vital to the attainment of voluntary movements. This same line of reasoning may be used with other readiness elements such as postural control and balance for which specific reflexes can provide practice.

■ *Spontaneous Movements (Stereotypies)*

Objective 8.4 ➤ In contrast to reflex behavior, **spontaneous movements** are stereotypic repetitive motions that appear in the absence of any known stimuli. Compared to rudimentary behaviors, stereotypies cannot be characterized as voluntary, goal-oriented motor behaviors. Thelen

(1996) describes normal infant stereotypies as *transitional behaviors*, because they are performed when some level of control over body parts is involved, but intentional, goal-oriented action is not yet possible. These early patterns of coordinated movement have been observed as early as the 10th fetal week (e.g., alternating legs movements and kicking). They occur with increasing frequency and peak between 6 and 10 months of age. Stereotypic behavior such as persistent rocking, waving, and other nonpurposeful spontaneous movements are considered abnormal in older children and adults.

In her pioneering efforts in this area, Thelen (1979) identified 47 distinct stereotypic movements. Of these, the most common and first noticed is rhythmical leg kicking (single leg, two leg, and alternate leg). These patterns, along with various feet movements, seem to reach their peak between 6 and 8 months of age. Other commonly found stereotypies are arm waving, arm waving with an object, arm banging against a surface (with or without an object), and finger flexion. Noteworthy of these movements is that the peak frequency for hand and arm stereotypies is between 8½ to 10½ months. However, whereas spontaneous arm movements may appear just after birth, hand movements typically are not evident until 3½ to 5½ months. Stereotypic finger movements also appear in the first few months after birth but reach their peak frequency between 6 and 8 months, approximately 2½ months before hand and arm stereotypies do.

In a more recent investigation of spontaneous arm movements in neonates (3 to 5 days old), results suggested "there is clearly more to neonatal (spontaneous) movements than thrashing and swiping or elicited reflexes" (Hofsten & Rönnqvist, 1993, page 1057). The researchers found these early movements are subject to several sets of organizing constraints. That is, though appearing to be random, they actually have an underlying temporal (timing) structure. Once again this adds credence to the underlying dynamic properties of the human body.

Other characteristic stereotypies include arching the back and rocking when on hands and knees, rocking and bouncing when sitting, and bouncing while standing with support. These movements typically reach their peak later than the other stereotypies.

THINK ABOUT IT

How can we be sure stereotypies are not purposeful and goal-oriented?

Although these movements do not appear to be goal-oriented and their purpose is not evident, it is apparent their appearance is predictable and orderly. Thus, it may be suggested they are of developmental significance. This conclusion is based on the observation that stereotypic kicking characteristically precedes and accompanies voluntary control of the legs, spontaneous finger flexion normally precedes voluntary grasping attempts, and rocking on the hands and knees precedes creeping. Thelen suggests this type of predictive behavior reflects a specific stage process of neurological maturation that controls specific motor actions. These stages of normal maturation prepare the infant for more complex use of the neural pathways that complement skilled motor actions.

■ *Figure 8.11*

Common stereo-
typies: (a) alter-
nate leg kicking,
(b) single leg
kicking, (c) kicking
with both legs
together, (d) arm
waving with
object, (e) rocking
on hands and
knees, (f) arm
banging against
a surface, and
(g) finger flex

Although stereotypies have not been determined clearly to be precursors of voluntary motor behavior, the fact that newborn infants can
exhibit this degree of neuromuscular coordination with relatively little
CNS activity has been a revelation. Figure 8.11 shows seven of the more
common stereotypic behaviors. Refer to Sprague and Newell (1996), the
chapter on normal infant stereotypies by Thelen, for an excellent review
of the topic (see Suggested Readings).

■ *Rudimentary Behavior*

Objective 8.5 ➤ **Rudimentary behavior** occurs in that phase of motor development
that spans the period from birth to approximately 2 years of age. As the
infant's nervous system matures, a gradual increase in basic voluntary
motor behavior occurs. During the first 6 to 10 months of the infant's
life, these *initial voluntary movement responses* coexist with various reflexes
and stereotypies. As more voluntary behavior is achieved, the infant
develops a basic level of postural control, locomotion, and manual control. The acquisition of these basic abilities, in turn, provides the foundation for fundamental movement skill abilities.

Rudimentary movements, to a large extent, are based maturationally and appear in a very predictable sequence. However, experience with the environment through various challenges (e.g., gravity) and *affordances* play a significant role in development. The order of motor control generally develops in a cephalocaudal-proximodistal direction. That is, functions appear and develop earliest in the infant's head and neck, then in the shoulders and upper trunk, and later in the lower trunk and legs. The order also proceeds proximodistally from the shoulders, to the elbows, and then to control of the fingers. Progression also is characterized by the performance of gross motor before fine motor acts. This is evident in the development of manual control when, for example, infants initially use their whole arm to corral a toy before they are able to grasp it securely with a hand.

The remainder of this chapter describes the general sequence of early voluntary movement behavior with regard to the achievement of postural control, rudimentary locomotion, and manual control.

Postural Control

Objective 8.6 ➤ The ability to maintain body posture and to move the body voluntarily into a desired position underlies all motor behavior. Postural control requires a dynamic interaction of neural and muscuoskeletal systems. The infant must be able to perceive and assess sensory information, and generate forces to make adjustments in body position. In general, the development of these rudimentary abilities begins with control of the head and neck muscles and proceeds in a cephalocaudal direction until the infant is able to stand alone, a course of rapid development during the first year of postnatal life. However, before the infant can stand without support and progress to the landmark achievement of upright locomotion, a number of developmental milestones must be reached. Figure 8.12 depicts the general sequence of postural control and approximate age at which 50% to 75% of infants achieve these milestones (Bayley Scales, 1993; Denver Developmental Screening Test, 1990).

Head and Upper Trunk Although some involuntary behavior may be evident at birth, the newborn has minimal voluntary control over the head, neck, and upper trunk. At about 1 month the infant gains enough control of its head to hold it erect momentarily when supported at the base of the neck. When prone the infant can hold its head up only for seconds; the movement is unsteady and the angle of vision is quite low.

By the second month, the infant is able to hold its head and chin steadily off a supporting surface while in the prone position. The head can be lifted as much as 30 degrees above the horizontal plane, thus allowing for greater visual field. At 3 months the cephalocaudal progression is even more evident in that the infant is able to hold its head and chest up off the surface using arm support. By the fifth month, the

■ *Figure 8.12*

Sequence of
rudimentary
postural control

Head and upper trunk	Approximate age (mos)
Holds head erect voluntarily	1
Holds head and chin up	2
Holds chest up with arm support (prone)	3
Elevates head when supine	4–5

Rolls (turns)	
Side to back	2
Back to side/stomach to side	3–4
Back to stomach	5–6
Stomach to back	8

Sits	
With support	3–4
Alone	5½–6½
Gets into sitting position	8
Sits down	9

Stands	
Holding on	6–8
Pulls self to stand	7½–9½
Alone	11–13

infant can accomplish the more difficult task of lifting the head off the surface when on its back.

Rolling (Turning) Rolling the body requires a certain level of control over the head, neck, and trunk. The first signs of voluntary rolling appear at about 2 months with the infant turning from its side to its back. By approximately 4 months the infant can roll from a supine position to the side and from the prone position to the side. As the infant matures and gains greater control of the hips and shoulders, more advanced abilities become evident such as rolling from the supine to prone position at around 6 months. The most difficult task, rolling from the prone to the supine position, normally is achieved by 8 months.

Sitting By approximately 3 to 4 months infants, while being supported, can sit with their heads relatively steady. The first attempts at sitting without support (after being placed into position) are characterized by an extreme forward lean, which may be an attempt to gain control of the lumbar region. By 6 months the infant is able to remain in the sitting position for a short time without additional support. However, before the infant can independently position itself into a sitting posture, it must have some basic body rolling ability (indicating some control of the upper body) and possess various support reactions (e.g., parachute reflexes). By 8 months infants generally can position themselves from a prone or supine position into a sitting posture and remain there without support.

A rather important early achievement is the ability to sit down from a crouched or standing position. This task requires additional postural control and flexibility, especially if the infant is attempting to position itself in a chair. The ability to sit down with reasonable control normally is achieved around 9 months of age.

Standing The achievement of upright posture while standing is a major milestone in the infant's first year of development. With the ability to gain control over gravity and remain upright, the infant is ready to proceed with efforts to achieve upright locomotion (walking), perhaps the most monumental landmark in development. The first attempts to stand may occur early when the infant is held under the armpits by a parent and brought into contact with a surface. The ability to remain in the standing position while holding on to something usually occurs by the seventh or eighth month. By about 9 months of age the infant becomes capable of pushing or pulling itself to a standing position. Typically the infant can stand unassisted by the end of the first year. The infant does this by first getting to its knees, pushing itself upward using the power of the legs, and pulling downward with extended arms.

Rudimentary Locomotion

It generally is acknowledged that the two most basic motor skills in the human repertoire are the maintenance of upright posture and bipedal locomotion. Within roughly the first six months of life the infant develops postural control, the ability to detect changes in the body's center of gravity in relation to the base of support.

Before infants will attempt the complex task of forward upright locomotion (walking), they will move about their surroundings in a variety of ways. As early as the third month infants have been observed to *scoot* along in a sitting position, using one leg to push the body along. However, basic forward locomotion normally begins during the second six months after birth. Although virtually all infants will develop through the orderly progression of moving forward in a prone position with crawling and creeping movement patterns, some also will use more unorthodox methods such as edging sideways like a crab and walking on all fours.

After they are able to pull up to an upright standing position around 8 months, some infants may be observed to *cruise* around by moving unsteadily from spot to spot while holding on to furniture or similar supports. This form of walking with support usually is done with sideways motion, which enables the infant to use the arms for support and control. Cruising is an important behavior since it provides opportunities to improve strength and postural control, and learn to adjust with the flow of perceptual information. By the age of 13 months, most infants will have achieved the single most important milestone in motor development: independent walking.

Although walking is considered a fundamental motor skill, which is the topic of the next chapter, much of its development and refinement occur before the rudimentary phase of motor behavior and infancy is over (figure 8.13 on page 266).

Crawling and Creeping Both *crawling* and *creeping* are well-known terms, but they sometimes are used in the developmental literature in ways that cause confusion. Some popular infant assessment batteries describe creeping as a precursor to crawling, whereas others note creeping as the advanced form of prone locomotion. By dictionary definition, crawling is slow movement by dragging the prone body along the ground; creeping is the act of moving the body along slowly and close to the ground on the hands and knees. Though their differences are evident, both are slow, deliberate forms of progress. Many individuals tend to perceive creeping as a slower (thus less mature) form of locomotion. However, most contemporary references to motor development and this text use crawling to designate the movement that precedes creeping.

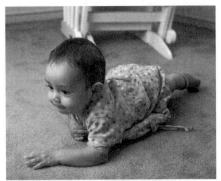

Locomotor ability	Approximate age
Crawling (body drag)	6–8 months

Creeping (abdomen clear)	8–10 months

Walking

With support	9–10 months
Alone (well)	12–14 months
Backward	14–18 months
Stairs (up and down)	2–4 years
Perfected	4–5 years

■ *Figure 8.13*

Sequence of rudimentary locomotor abilities

Crawling represents the infant's first purposeful efforts at prone locomotion, which normally occurs between the ages of 6 to 8 months. Infants crawl using their arms and legs to drag the body along a surface. An important characteristic of this ability is that the abdomen remains in contact with the surface. Infants may use only their arms and legs, or a variety of arm-leg combinations to achieve forward progress. Important prerequisites to crawling are control of the muscles of the head, neck, and upper trunk. It may be speculated that for crawling and creeping, certain reflex movements (e.g., asymmetrical tonic neck, labyrinthine, body righting, and crawling) provide some of the stimulus for neural and muscular development.

Creeping occurs approximately two months (between 8 to 10 months of age) after the appearance of crawling. In contrast to crawling, creeping movements involve moving in a prone position on hands and knees with the abdomen clear of the surface. Initial efforts are characterized by minimal elevation off the supporting surface and a *homolateral pattern* of movement—that is, the leg and arm of one side move together, alternating with the limbs of the opposite side. Shortly after sufficient strength has developed to support the abdomen above the surface, the infant's elevation increases, as does the flexion and extension of the limbs. These factors support the more efficient *contralateral pattern* of movement in which the right leg and left arm are used together, alternating with the left leg and right arm. Creeping appears to be an enjoyable mode of locomotion for the infant. In fact, infants who have become independent walkers at times revert to creeping as the desired form of speedy travel. By the end of the first year, most infants have become very efficient creepers and use this pattern to move up and down stairs. For a excellent review of this behavior from a dynamic systems perspective, refer to Freedland and Bertenthal (1994).

THINK ABOUT IT

If all physical properties were equal in two infants, why is it likely that one will walk before the other?

Walking **Walking** is movement by means of shifting weight from one foot to the other, with at least one foot contacting the surface at all times. Walking is perhaps the single most significant milestone in motor development, and its characteristics have probably been researched more than any other motor skill. Although some infants may be observed taking their first independent steps at 8 or 9 months, most children will not walk independently with any degree of efficiency until approximately 13 months of age. Children usually will not achieve the mature walking pattern until the age of 4 or 5 years. Before these efforts can be attempted, the infant must possess a certain level of upright postural control as evidenced by the ability to pull up to a standing position (achieved around 8 months) or stand without assistance (achieved around 12 months). With at least some control of upright posture, infants will begin walking with the support of a parent holding their hands, or by cruising, usually laterally, from point to point while holding on to furniture or other supports (achieved around 8 to 10 months).

■ *Figure 8.14*

Initial (immature) walking pattern; rear and side views

Source: From Wickstrom *Fundamental Motor Patterns* (3rd ed.). 1983 Lea & Febiger.

Rear

Side

MOVEMENT PATTERN DESCRIPTIONS. Even when the infant walks independently, the movement pattern is usually immature (figure 8.14). Balance is easily lost and falls are frequent in initial walking efforts. To compensate for the general sense of instability, the infant uses a relatively wide base of support and takes short steps. The leg action is inefficient, as demonstrated by the short steps with limited leg and hip extension. Little, if any, trunk rotation is evident. Contact with the ground is flat-footed with one knee locked and the other knee bent (figure 8.14). Out-toeing is also present with minimal ankle movement and a slight pelvic tilt. Arm action is characterized by a high guard position in which the limbs are fixed and do not swing on each stride.

With the mature walking pattern each leg alternates between a supporting phase and a swinging phase. The heel strikes the surface first as the back leg pushes off, which shifts the weight to the front leg. The body leans forward slightly after the lead foot contacts the surface. The weight then is transferred from the heel to the outside of the foot, ball of the foot, and toes. The base of support is approximately shoulder-width, and the feet are parallel to each other with toes pointed forward. The arms swing rhythmically in opposition to the legs; the right arm swings forward with the left leg and the left arm moves forward with the right leg.

Infants also exhibit some characteristic patterns while walking up and down stairs. This skill is sometimes referred to as climbing stairs, although in the truest sense, climbing involves use of the upper body. Initial efforts of walking up stairs are characterized by *marking time*. With this pattern, the infant places one foot forward to the next step, then follows with the other foot to the same step. This pattern is repeated with each succeeding step. Marking time without the support of a handrail or another person's hand generally occurs between the ages of 24 and 28 months.

By the age of about 3 years, the child will progress to the more advanced *alternate stepping* movement pattern (without support). With this pattern, the first foot moves to the first step, the other foot is placed on the second step, and the cycle is repeated. Descending stairs by marking time occurs just a few months after the child learns to walk up the stairs. However, the ability to descend using the alternating step without support does not occur until around 4 or 5 years of age, about a year (12 to 15 months) after the child learns to ascend the stairs without support.

DEVELOPMENTAL CHARACTERISTICS. The walking pattern improves gradually from initial independent walking (around 13 months) to maturity at about 4 or 5 years of age. According to Shumway-Cook and Woollacott (2001), there are three requirements for successful locomotion that apply to walking: a rhythmic step pattern, control of stability, and the ability to modify gait to changes in the environment. The following general developmental trends parallel the transition from initial to mature walking:

1. The *base of support* (dynamic base) narrows to within the approximate lateral dimensions of the trunk (figure 8.15 on page 270). This normally occurs by 4½ months after the onset of independent walking. In general, *maturation of the equilibrium system* is critical to independent walking.
2. *Foot contact* changes from flat-footed to the heel-toe pattern. The appearance of heel-striking commonly is achieved by the age of 19 months. Toe stepping is common in novice walkers who have not yet reached the more advanced pattern.
3. *Foot angle* changes show a decrease in the degree of toeing out. In-toeing is usually rare and considered abnormal.

Change in arm
position as base of
support narrows

4. The single knee-lock pattern is abandoned for the more mature *double knee-lock* variation. This pattern involves heel-strike with knee extension followed by slight knee flexion as the body moves forward over the supporting leg, then extension once again at the push-off phase. This action creates a greater range of leg motion.

5. *Pelvic rotation* increases to allow full leg motion and oppositional movement of the upper and lower body segments. This action normally is observed in infants by 14 months of age.

6. The high-guard *arm position* (elbows flexed and abducted) is gradually lowered and oppositional arm swinging starts. The infant's first efforts at arm swing are frequently not equal and regular; both hands might swing forward in unison. A mature arm action involves movement of the opposite arm and leg together with slight movement at both the shoulder and elbow of each arm. The change in arm position usually parallels a narrowing base of support and is achieved at approximately 18 months (figure 8.15).

7. *Step and stride length* increase, which reflects greater application of force and greater leg extension at push-off. Step and stride length nearly double between 1 and 7 years of age, then increase by approximately 50% by adulthood (see table 8.2). In general, step and stride length increase linearly with increasing leg length. With this, there is a decrease in *double-support*—that is, time when both feet are in contact with the ground.

8. *Walking speed* increases and *step frequency* (steps per minute) decreases during the development of walking (see table 8.2). Sutherland (1984)

TABLE 8.2

Developmental Characteristics of Gait Length and Speed

Age (yr)	Step Length (cm)	Stride Length (cm)	Steps/Minute	Walking Speed (cm/s)
1	21.6	43	175.7	63.7
2	27.5	54.9	155.8	71.8
3	32.9	67.7	153.5	85.5
7	47.9	96.5	143.5	114.3

Source: Data from Sutherland, 1984

notes that younger people normally must take more steps per unit of time to increase walking speed, which is due primarily to lack of neuromuscular control.

DYNAMIC SYSTEMS RESEARCH. Along with basic infant reaching, one of the most active lines of developmental biodynamics research has been conducted on walking using the dynamic systems approach. Numerous studies have been reported in the last decade or so; what follows is a glimpse of selected pioneering achievements.

As noted earlier (review chapters 1 and 7), the dynamic systems approach seeks to identify and explain the *processes* associated with motor control and of change. For example, experiments by Thelen and Ulrich (1991) have noted that some infants as young as 3 months exhibit well-coordinated, alternating stepping movements typically not common until several months later. In the experiment, infants were held by an adult over a motorized treadmill to facilitate the *stepping action* (see figure 8.16 on page 272), not a stepping reflex that can no longer be elicited after about 2 months. By holding the infant upright, balance and leg strength (subsystems), critical *rate controllers* in independent walking, were supported, therefore allowing the apparently more mature neuromuscular component to emerge. This study supports the general dynamic systems hypothesis that the development of motor control is an *emergent* rather than a prescribed (preset) process turned on in the brain. Walking emerges as a consequence of sufficient development and cooperation of contributing subsystems that are quite adaptive for use in other contexts as well. As you may recall, this *functional adaptability* also was noted as a characteristic of neuronal group selection (Edleman, 1987). Other constraints, such as environmental contexts (walking surface, slope, etc.) also contribute to behavior.

Clark and Phillips (1993) added to the dynamic systems literature by studying the dynamic properties of intralimb coordination in infants over the course of their first 12 months of walking. The researchers note

■ *Figure 8.16*

Experimental setup Thelen and her colleagues used to study dynamic components of upright locomotion

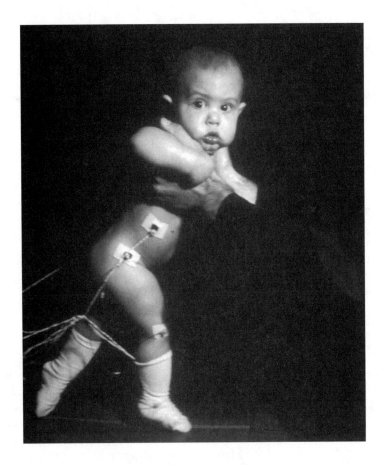

others have suggested that such components as body mass, limb length, and strength contribute to the dynamic system. Clark and Phillips observed that two additional control parameters, force production and balance, also play integral roles in independent walking. It is noted that the propulsive forces needed in coordinated walking are potentially destabilizing, but the infant's *self-organizing* system appears to compensate by spending more time with both feet on the ground than the more forceful adult does. The novice walker begins quite slowly but after a few months produces gait parameters that are much more adultlike. The researchers suggest that perhaps to compensate, the infant's control parameters are being *scaled* to contribute to stability and coordination.

While studying arm posture during early acquisition of walking, from high guard to coordinated alternating arm-swing, Ledebt (2000) concluded (confirmed) that efficient walking is not a prewired synergy or pure reflection of neural maturation. Rather, it is a motor behavior that must be learned. Infants in this study self-organized their movements to adapt the most efficient means to overcome the problem of destabilization while shifting their weight and moving forward. This

THINK ABOUT IT

What are the developmental constraints in learning to walk?

TABLE 8.3

General Sequence of Rudimentary Manual Control

Approximate Age (months)	Characteristics
Newborn	Reflexive and spontaneous reaching and grasping
4	Initial voluntary efforts
	Corralling (both limbs)
	Palmar grasp
5–6	Smooth arm and hand action
	One hand/pseudo thumb opposition
8	Accepts two objects
9–10	Pincer grasp (thumb opposition)
14	Adult-like reaching and grasping
18	Effective release

same example of *self-organization* seems to apply with learning to ski, roller-blade, or walk on ice.

As you will recall from previous discussions, one of the main principles of dynamic systems research is that behaviors emerge from the constraints that surround them such as the organism, environment, and specific task. These findings present us with examples of how the environment influences the developmental dynamics of motor behavior.

Clearly future research of this type will add significantly to our understanding of the mechanisms and processes that govern the development of motor behavior.

Manual Control

Objective 8.7 ➤ In addition to the attainment of basic postural control and upright locomotion, the first two years are characterized by several developmental milestones that involve manual coordination. Three terms commonly are used to describe this area of motor development: prehension, manipulation, and manual control. **Prehension** is the initial voluntary use of the hands as characterized by basic seizing or grasping. In contrast, **manipulation** refers to skillful use of the hands, such as in stringing beads or threading a needle. Skillful manipulative behaviors usually are not observed until the middle childhood years (ages 5 to 8), even though they are a basic part of the early childhood curriculum. The term **manual control** encompasses both descriptors by referring to the developmental characteristics of hand movements. The three basic components of manual control are reaching, grasping, and releasing. Table 8.3 shows the

THINK ABOUT IT

Cite specific examples of affordances that could stimulate the development of early manual control.

general sequence of rudimentary manual control and the approximate age that particular characteristics appear.

Non-Goal-Directed Behavior   The first reaching and grasping movements appear as reflexes and spontaneous movements. Involuntary grasping usually appears in the seventh fetal month and disappears by 4 months of age. Spontaneous arm and hand (flexion and grasping) movements also have been observed prior to and during voluntary manual behavior (e.g., Hofsten & Rönnqvist, 1993; Prechtl & Hopkins, 1986). Spontaneous prereaching (arm) and finger movements may appear as early as newborn to 3 months, whereas stereotypic hand movements are generally observed between 3½ to 5½ months. These seemingly nonpurposeful stereotypic behaviors normally parallel voluntary efforts and reach their peak between 6 and 12 months of age (Thelen, 1979). Figure 8.17 illustrates some commonly found spontaneous (stereotypic) behaviors involving arms, hands, and fingers.

Goal-Directed Behavior   By 4 to 5 months, most infants make their initial *goal-oriented* efforts in reaching and grasping. With regard to the reaching segment, researchers using a dynamic systems perspective report that initial movements (trajectories) are jerky and do not follow a straight-line path (Konczak & Dichgans, 1997; Thelen et al., 1996). However, within a few months of experience, infants make remarkable progress, and their reaches become smoother and much straighter over the first year. By age 7 months, the ability to make corrections based on visual information is quite functional. Interestingly, Konczak and Dichgans also noted that some of the basic patterns of coordination found in these infants were observed in early spontaneous movements, which provide evidence for continuity of developmental behaviors. It also has been suggested that, even though young infants lack the fine motor control of adults, they learn to adjust their trajectories as a consequence of previous *experience* that they match with their current level of control (Berthier, 1996).

Learning to stabilize the body in a reaching posture and control movement speed are important factors in the early development of goal-oriented reaching and subsequent grasping. Recent dynamic systems research with young infants provides convincing data that support the general claim *that virtually every movement is nested into a postural set* (Reed, 1989). This suggests a functional relationship between manipulative behavior and level of postural control. This assumption has some anecdotal support as derived from recent laboratory studies of infants' reaching and grasping behavior. For example, van der Fits et al. (1999), while studying postural adjustments during spontaneous and goal-directed reaching in the first 6 months of postnatal life, observed that even before the onset of successful reaching (around 4 to 5 months), arm movements were accompanied by a high amount of postural activity.

■ *Figure 8.17*

Examples of spontaneous (stereotypic) movements of the arms, hands, and fingers:
(a) arm waving with object,
(b) arm banging against a surface,
(c) banging both arms together with object, (d) arm sway, (e) and
(f) finger flexion,
(g) hand rotation, and (h) hand flexion

More specific, early reaching success required the need for head stabilization, which the authors believed facilitates the processing of visual information. With increasing age and reaching success, the amount of postural activity decreased. The same general conclusion was reached in an earlier review of several contemporary studies by Berthenthal and Von Hofsten (1998). They found that for mastery of reaching to occur, the head must be stabilized for the infant to gaze toward the intended reaching target. The researchers also speculated on a nested hierarchy of postural support involving the eyes, head, and trunk. It also was stressed that trunk control is critical in providing a base of support to allow free movements of the arms and hands. This latter observation was given support by studies showing the quality of reaching movements improved when infants mastered postural skills such as sitting without support (e.g., Rochat & Goubet, 1995).

With regard to grasping, first efforts usually are characterized by a corralling action in which both arms and hands work together to pull in the object. At this point, the infant picks up the object by using the immature palmar grasp. With this form of manual control the infant grasps the object without thumb opposition and instead uses the thumb and fingers as a unit to hold the object against the palm of the hand. Evidence indicates that young infants successfully alter grip size based on orientation and size of the object (Corbetta et al., 2000; Hofsten & Rönnquist, 1988). That is, children learn to integrate (self-organize) perceptual information characteristics of the task and environment with their developing motor system.

During the fifth to sixth month, development normally reaches the level of reaching and grasping with one hand using *pseudo thumb opposition*. Here the thumb opposes the fingers (but not the finger tip as in true opposition) to pick up an object; there is minimal contact of the object with the palm. Infants also may transfer an object from one hand to the other during this period. By 8 months infants normally exhibit the ability to receive two objects (holding one object in the opposite hand).

A major developmental milestone that usually occurs between 9 and 10 months is the ability to grasp small objects using true opposition of the thumb with one finger. Often referred to as the *pincer grasp*, this advanced form of manual control progresses to the level of fine motor coordination using the thumb and forefinger to manipulate objects.

With regard to learning to grasp large objects with two hands, Fagard and Jacquet (1996) note a few interesting observations. First, infants younger than 11 months did not perceive the need to use both hands to grasp a large object as well as older infants (12 to 13 months of age) did. Younger infants tended to activate their second hand only after the first one completed its trajectory, whereas older infants displayed more bimanual flexibility. The researchers concluded that a critical factor in development appears to be visuomanual *experience*.

To summarize, the sequence of manual control moves from no thumb opposition, to pseudo-opposition, to true opposition. This developmental pattern also involves a shift in the positioning of the grasped object from the little finger side (ulnar) to the thumb side (radial). During the course of development, grasped objects are positioned to occupy a more radial and distal position next to the thumb and index forefinger rather than in the palm. Figure 8.18 illustrates the basic grasping techniques and changes in object positioning. By the time the infant is 14 months old, reaching and grasping have evolved into a smooth, coordinated adultlike action.

■ *Figure 8.18*

(a) Basic grasping techniques and (b) changes in object positioning

No opposition   Pseudo-opposition   True opposition

a.

Distal end

b.

As a general (simplified) description of the developmental progression of reaching and grasping, Eckert (1987) provides the following as modified from Landreth (1958).

1. Visual location of an object moves to the attempt to reach for the object.
2. Simple eye-hand coordination moves to progressive independence of visual effort with ultimate expression in activities, such as piano playing and typing.
3. Initial maximal involvement of body musculature moves to a minimum involvement and greater economy of effort.
4. Proximal large muscle activity of the arms and shoulders moves to distal fine muscle activity of the fingers.
5. Early crude raking movements in manipulating objects with the hands move to the pincerlike precision of control with the opposing thumb and forefinger.
6. Initial bilateral reaching and manipulation move to ultimate use of the preferred hand.

Unquestionably, *releasing* is a difficult component of manual control. The ability to control and relax the muscles in the arms and hands to provide a well-coordinated and accurate release is one of the final acquisitions in the development of manual control. Although a crude form of object release may be observed as early as 8 months when the infant opens its hand and simply allows the object to drop, accuracy of release normally is not achieved until 18 months of age.

Related to the ability to grasp and accurately release objects is the infant's perception of object weight and ability to control the amount of applied force. Prior to about 9 months of age, the application of force with the grasp appears to be unrelated to the weight of the object. Regardless of object weight, infants apply a similar force in the arm and grasping movements. By 9 months the infant normally can adjust the force used to grasp objects of varying weights, but only *after* the initial grasp of the object (Palmer, 1989). Not until approximately 18 months of age can the infant *anticipate* the weight of objects (after repeated presentations) and apply the appropriate amount of force. By this age most infants apparently acquire the perception that similar objects weigh more or less based upon their length. Therefore, by approximately 18 months of age, infants have acquired the general ability to reach, grasp, and release objects in a relatively well-coordinated manner.

Use of Visual Information Obviously, the perception and use of visual information are critical to the development of manual control via reaching. To succeed at reaching, infants must integrate visual and kinesthetic input and accommodate their movements to the constraints of the task. Several weeks prior to goal-oriented (voluntary) successful grasping at around 4 months, the infant projects arm and hand movements in the presence of visible objects (e.g., Hofsten, 1991). Figure 8.19 illustrates the general experimental setup used to study reaching in neonates.

With the onset of goal-oriented behavior, the use of visual stimuli in reaching movements can be described as visually guided and visually elicited. The first stage, *visually guided*, describes the infant as learning to grasp by bringing both hand and object into view, thus guiding the hand toward the object (e.g., Bushnell, 1985). Several studies have reported *visually elicited* behavior beginning around 6 to 7 months of age (Clifton et al., 1993; Robin et al., 1996). That is, the infant visually sights the object and follows with a trajectory, without need for sight of the hand. A common experimental setup is to have infants reach for a moving object in the light, then reach for a glowing object in the dark so they cannot see their hands. In essence, infants at this stage of development can grasp a moving object successfully without sight of their reaching hand. Robin and colleagues suggest further that this behavior adds to the weight of evidence that emphasizes the importance of

■ *Figure 8.19*

Example of experimental set-up used to study reaching in neonates

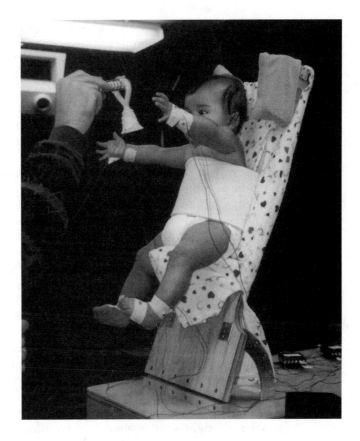

proprioceptive (kinesthetic) control of reaching. However, the use of visual information, whether visually guided or elicited, does play a vital role in reaching behavior. By about 9 months, reaching becomes less dependent on visual feedback and more ballistic, with corrections made toward the end instead of during the movement.

Motor Asymmetries

Objective 8.8 ➤ Some of the most evident behavioral manifestations of brain lateralization are **motor asymmetries.** That is, although the human body (and hemispheres) is symmetrical in general appearance, the paired limbs (hands, feet) and sensory organs (eyes, ears) are used in an asymmetric manner. Complementing this phenomenon is the fact that the cortex of the right hemisphere controls muscular activity in and receives sensory input from the left half of the body; the left hemisphere has a complementary role in conscious movement on the right side of the body (chapter 2). Other terms often used interchangeably with motor (and functional) asymmetries are *lateral preference* and *lateral (hemispheric) dominance*. Lateral dominance generally means that one side of the brain has developed to the point of establishing dominance for motor control; therefore the individual has an internalized lateral preference for use of one side with a specific action or task. Although lateral preference most often is identified as *right-sided* or *left-sided*, there are individuals who do not consistently favor the use of one limb or the other on a specific task; these individuals are identified as *mixed-sided*.

Theoretical Views   Perhaps the most evident and intriguing manifestation of motor behavior is that the vast majority of people are right-sided. Complementing this phenomenon is the much debated issue of whether motor asymmetries stem from innate biological factors inherited from parents or are learned behaviors influenced by environmental contexts. In other words, is handedness (or footedness) learned, or is it primarily genetically based (inherited)? Despite volumes of literature dating back over a century (e.g., Broca, 1865; Brown-Sequard, 1877), no single theory that explains the nature and developmental characteristics of this phenomenon has been widely accepted. However, most reviews on the subject conclude there is an underlying biologically based explanation. For example, Van Strien states in sum, handedness appears to be determined by genetic, intrauterine and perinatal factors, (2000, 58).

One of the most widely accepted theoretical positions is the genetic model proposed by Annett (1985, 1996). According to the general tenets of *Annett's Right-Shift Theory*, while the majority of the population has a strong right-shift genetic factor underlying cerebral asymmetry, the remaining portion of individuals may not express a dominant limb due to a weaker right-shift gene or lack of this inheritance (no right-shift factor). This suggests that environmental factors could influence the distribution of limb preference (right, left, or mixed) in this portion of the population. Arguments by Corballis and Morgan (1978; see also Corballis, 1983) also suggest that limb preference is specified innately, but they contend that in most of the population there is a *left-right maturational gradient* programming the left hemisphere to mature more rapidly than the right hemisphere, thus providing the bias toward right-sidedness in limb preference

In essence, although functional asymmetries may have origins in genetic makeup and possess maturational characteristics, few theorists would deny that specific behaviors may be modified by cultural/environmental factors (i.e., experience). More specifically, while *direction* (right, left, or mixed) of limb preference may be more fixed to biological foundations, the *degree* of preference could vary considerably depending on experience (e.g., McManus et al., 1988). Thus, experience may account for developing a strong or weak phenotype (functional asymmetry).

Although there have been some exceptions, research in general has supported the variant developmental trend for handedness and footedness. This has been evidenced by a general shift toward right-sidedness with increasing age (from early childhood) for hand preference (e.g., Dargent-Paré et al., 1992; McManus et al., 1988; NCHS, 1987) and foot preference behavior (as reported in a review of the literature by Gabbard and Iteya, 1996). A comprehensive review of infant motor asymmetries also suggests there is insufficient behavioral evidence to conclude that motor asymmetries are fixed (invariant) at birth and unchanging thereafter (Provins, 1992).

With regard to gender, an interesting theory proposed by Geschwind and Galaburda (1985) (also see review by Finegan, et al. 1992) suggests that due to potentially higher levels of prenatal testosterone in males, neuronal growth in the left hemisphere slows, hence weakening contralateral control. This suggests less right-sidedness and more left-dominance in males. Support for this, or any theory suggesting gender bias however, has not been widely accepted.

THINK ABOUT IT

Which functional asymmetry, handedness or footedness, do you think is more affected by the environment, and why?

Early Infant Motor Asymmetries Well before children are capable of understanding and responding reliably to conventional preference inventories, evidence of asymmetric bias may be observed. Remarkably, indications of handedness have been observed before birth! Using ultrasound observations of fetuses during the last two trimesters, Hepper and colleagues (1991, 1998) noted a marked bias for arm movements and thumb sucking of the right side. The conclusion of two reviews on early infant asymmetries found the majority of newborns and young infants exhibit reflexes and spontaneous movements that are stronger and more coordinated on the "right side of the body" (Grattan et al., 1992; Provins, 1992). Types of responses favoring the right side include spontaneous head turning, spontaneous fisting, rooting reflex, asymmetric tonic neck response, right foot lead in walking reflex, and the plantar and palmar grasps. Also worthy of note is that the asymmetry described was found only in the motor (efferent) parameters (strength and coordination) and not the sensory (afferent) parameters. This may be indicative of the developmental state of the population observed (primarily neonates). As mentioned earlier, although the relationship appears complementary, the question of whether right-biased involuntary movement behaviors in infants are the basis for right-sided voluntary responses in older persons still is being debated.

Complementing the development of motor control during childhood is the emergence of *functional asymmetries* such as handedness, footedness, and eye preference. The development of these behaviors is most evident during the early childhood years and will be discussed in the next chapter.

Summary

Early movement behavior is categorized by movements associated with reflexes, spontaneous actions, and rudimentary behavior. Reflexes are involuntary movements controlled by the subcortical areas of the brain. They primarily are associated with the stimulation of the CNS and muscles, infant survival, and their usefulness as a diagnostic tool for assessing neurological maturity. The three general categories of reflexes are primitive, postural, and locomotor. Theoretical viewpoints concerning the relationship between reflex behavior and voluntary movement focus on whether the link is direct (continuity view) or more indirect (reflexes must disappear before voluntary actions emerge). Most are suppressed by 6 months of age, and only a few are observable after the first year.

Spontaneous movements are stereotypic, rhythmic patterns of motion that appear in the absence of any known stimuli and do not appear to serve any apparent purpose. Some of the more frequently observed stereotypies include kicking, waving, rocking, and bouncing. Stereotypies are observable early in fetal life and reach a general peak between 6 to 10 months of age. Since their appearance is predictable and orderly, it has been suggested they are of developmental significance.

The first two years of life are characterized by the development of several rudimentary behaviors that follow the general trend of cephalocaudal-proximodistal growth and motor control. In general, the development of postural control begins with control of the head and neck muscles and proceeds in a cephalocaudal direction until the infant is able to stand alone. Forms of early locomotion that precede independent walking are scooting, cruising, crawling, creeping, and walking with support. The theory that walking is an emergent rather than prescribed (preset) process has been confirmed by dynamic systems research. Independent locomotion emerges as a consequence of sufficient development and cooperation of several contributing subsystems.

The first signs of hand use in the form of reaching and grasping appear as reflexes and spontaneous movements during the prenatal stage. Rudimentary (initial) voluntary manual control, referred to as prehension, develops rapidly during the first two years in the form of reaching, grasping, and releasing abilities.

Several motor asymmetries (linked to brain lateralization) are evident during the first two years of life. With regard to its origin, the primary debate focuses on what extent these behaviors stem from biological factors or the environment (learning).

Think about It

1. Of the types of reflexes, how would you rank their importance?
2. How can we be sure stereotypies are not purposeful and goal-oriented?
3. If all physical properties were equal in two infants, why is it likely that one will walk before the other?
4. What are the developmental constraints in learning to walk?
5. Cite specific examples of affordances that could stimulate the development of early manual control.
6. Which functional asymmetry, handedness or footedness, do you think is more affected by the environment, and why?

Suggested Readings

Fiorentino, M. R. (1981). *A basis for sensorimotor development: The influence of the primitive, postural reflexes on the development and distribution of tone.* Springfield, IL: Thomas.

Forfar, J. O., & Arneil, G. C. (1998). *Textbook of paediatrics.* 5th ed. New York: Churchill Livingston. Refer to chapter on reflexes.

Shumway-Cook, A., & Woollacott, M. (2001). *Motor control.* 2nd ed. Baltimore, MD: Williams & Wilkins. Refer to chapter on posture/balance.

Spraque, R. L., & Newell, K. M. (Eds.). (1996). *Stereotyped movements: Brain and behavior relations.* Hyattsville, MD: American Psychological Association.

Thelen, E., & Smith, L. (1994). *A dynamic systems approach to the development of cognition and action.* Cambridge, MA: MIT Press.

WebLinks

Esther Thelen's Infant Motor Development Laboratory at Indiana University
http://php.indiana.edu/~gormleyf

Information on Biomechanics (See the section on Gait and Locomotion)
www.per.ualberta.ca/biomechanics

International Society on Infant Studies
www.isisweb.org

Society for Research in Child Development
www.srcd.org

Motor Behavior during Early Childhood

OBJECTIVES

Upon completion of this chapter, you should be able to

9.1 Provide a brief overview of the fundamental movement phase of motor behavior.

9.2 List and describe basic terminology associated with fundamental movement behavior.

9.3 Discuss the methods used to study motor pattern development and the type of questions that each attempts to answer.

9.4 Compare the composite and component approaches to describing movement pattern characteristics.

9.5 Identify key descriptive and developmental characteristics associated with fundamental locomotor and manipulative motor skills.

9.6 Describe the key developmental characteristics of manual manipulation.

9.7 Identify the basic developmental aspects of functional asymmetries.

KEY TERMS

locomotor skills	standing long jump
nonlocomotor (stability) skills	hopping
manipulative skills	galloping
fundamental movement skill	sliding
movement pattern	skipping
process characteristics	throwing
product values	catching
composite approach	striking
component approach	kicking
prelongitudinal screening	ball bouncing
running	climbing
jumping	manipulation
leap	bimanual control
vertical jump	functional asymmetries

The Developmental Continuum

Phase	Approximate age	Stage
Reflexive/ Spontaneous	conception	Prenatal
Rudimentary	birth	Infancy
	6 mo.	
	2 years	Early Childhood
Fundamental Movement	6	
Sport Skill	12	Later Childhood
Growth & Refinement	18	Adolescence
Peak Performance	30	Adulthood
Regression	70	Older Adulthood

Objective 9.1   AFTER THE ACQUISITION of rudimentary motor abilities, the individual's movement repertoire expands to include fundamental movement behaviors. The period during which these behaviors emerge normally spans the early childhood years (from approximately ages 2 to 6 or 7), a period of landmark significance for motor development. This phase of motor behavior sometimes is referred to as the movement foundation. This is based on the notion that the elements of movement behavior that develop and emerge during this period provide a substantial part of the motor skill foundation upon which more complex motor programs are formed.

Fundamental movement behaviors may be classified into three general motor skill groups: locomotor, nonlocomotor, and manipulative. **Locomotor skills** are movements that transport an individual through space from one place to another; examples are walking, running, and skipping. **Nonlocomotor (stability) skills** involve axial movements and movements of balance executed with minimal or no movement of the base of support; examples are bending, twisting, and swaying. **Manipulative skills** include fine motor manual movements and gross motor skills that involve the control of objects primarily with the hands and feet; examples are throwing, catching, kicking, and striking. From this foundation children begin to perform movement activities that include more advanced combinations of skills and specificity and require greater temporal and spatial accuracy.

This chapter focuses on fundamental motor skill development and places specific emphasis on those skills in which developmental motor patterns have been established.

■ *Fundamental Motor Skill Development*

Basic Terminology

Objective 9.2　➤ The development of fundamental motor skills is perhaps the most extensively researched area of motor development because the study of basic developmental movement patterns is considered by many to form the core of the field. As early as the 1930s, researchers sought to identify the sequence and primary developmental components of basic movement patterns. In recent years, this area of inquiry has continued to be active through the efforts of several established and promising researchers.

The terminology associated with fundamental movement skills is a vocabulary that has developed over the years of research in that field of scientific inquiry. Much of the following discussion was derived from the works of Wickstrom (1983).

Fundamental Movement Skill　Also referred to as a *basic motor skill*, a **fundamental movement skill** is a common motor activity (e.g., walk, run, jump, and throw) with specific movement patterns. It also is believed these basic skills are general, in that they form the foundation for more advanced and specific movement activities.

Movement Patterns　Often used interchangeably with the term *motor pattern*, a **movement pattern** is the basic functional structure of a fundamental motor skill. The primary description involves a series of movements organized in a particular time-space sequence. The term also is used in reference to common elements observable in more than one motor skill. For example, several throwing and striking skills share common movement pattern elements in terms of arm, trunk, and leg action. Another term frequently associated with the identification of movement elements is *movement form*. This term also is used to describe the *process* rather than the *product* (performance) characteristics of movement.

Proficiency in movement pattern execution has been described using terms ranging from *immature* (or initial) to *mature*, and from *minimal* form to *sport skill* form. Each term identifies the developmental movement pattern characteristics of children in the approximate age range of 2 to 7 years. Immature and minimal descriptors generally depict the minimal standard of a movement pattern characteristic of children 2 to 3 years of age.

With practice, by the end of the sixth year most children acquire at least some features of the *mature movement pattern*. This pattern represents the composite of the common elements skilled performers used. Mature pattern performance is skill- rather than age-related. That is, with practice and maturity most children will acquire some, or perhaps all, mature pattern characteristics; however, others may not achieve a mature level until years later, if ever. This appears to be especially true of the overhand throwing pattern and standing long jump (with the two-foot take-off and landing).

Mature fundamental movement patterns that have been adapted to the special requirements of a particular advanced movement activity such as pitching in baseball (from basic throwing) and running hurdles (from basic leaping) are known as *sport skill movement patterns*. These advanced skill movements retain most of the characteristics found in fundamental patterns and generally appear during the sport skill phase of motor behavior (later childhood from 6 to 12 years). Wickstrom describes the general pattern of transition from minimal to mature as a *developmental motor pattern*. More specifically, this pattern meets the minimal requirements but does not equal the features of optimal execution.

Methods for Studying Change

Objective 9.3 ➤ Several perspectives may be taken when observing and analyzing motor pattern development. Tools of assessment range from simple observation using the human eye to sophisticated three-dimensional cinematography using computers to calculate and analyze even slight movement changes. Much of the available literature on movement pattern development is based on descriptive analysis that uses relatively subjective interpretation. Over the years, however, an increasing number of researchers have deemed it more appropriate to use a biomechanical approach in analyzing movement changes.

This trend has become evident in recent research activity that studies coordinative structures (dynamic systems theory). *Biomechanics* is the physics of human motion, a study of the forces produced by and acting on the body. Three associated terms are *kinematics*, *kinetics*, and *kinesiology*. *Kinematics* refers to the temporal and spatial characteristics of motion. *Kinetics* is concerned with the forces that act upon (i.e., cause, modify, facilitate, or inhibit) motion. *Kinesiology* frequently is used synonymously with the terms *biomechanics* or *applied* (functional) *anatomy*. The term *kinesiology* literally means the *science of motion*.

The study of movement pattern change generally includes collection of the following types of specific information: descriptive characteristics of the movements in a pattern; range of motion at each joint; muscle action; angular velocities accompanying segmental movement; timing of the movement sequences; time devoted to each phase of a pattern; and projection angles and velocities. Commonly used tools and techniques of the biomechanical approach include anthropometry (to measure body dimensions); timing devices; optical devices (cameras, stroboscopy, videography, computer-linked cinematography); electrogoniometry (joint action); electromyography (electrical activity of muscle); dynamography (force production characteristics); accelerometry (acceleration); and computer modeling. For a more detailed discussion of the analysis of human movement and the study of developmental biomechanics refer to Adrian and Cooper (1994) and Hall (2003).

Much of the literature related to the development of fundamental movement patterns is based on qualitative descriptions. That is, the focus is on changes in "form" (**process characteristics**) rather than "performance" **product values.** Product values are quantifiable measures of performance such as the number of yards a ball is thrown, running velocity in seconds, and the height of a jump in feet and inches.

Objective 9.4

➤ Researchers have used various approaches to describe and interpret *observable* movement changes using qualitative information. Currently, two practical yet scientific approaches have drawn considerable attention: the composite approach and the component approach. To some degree, both are *stage* oriented and employed primarily to identify movement pattern changes across time and describe developmental trends. The **composite approach** (Painter, 1994) describes motor pattern changes through a series of discrete steps (or stages) in the developmental process. Characteristic of this approach is the attempt to break down movement pattern changes into a *sequence* of stages that covers all parts of the body; hence, it also is known as the *total (whole) body approach* (Seefeldt & Haubenstricker, 1982). Identified for each stage (e.g., Step 1, 2, etc.) are the actions of various primary body parts (e.g., for the skill of throwing, the arm action, trunk action, and leg action). The number of stages inevitably varies from skill to skill.

The **component approach** (e.g., Roberton, 1977, 1978) proposes that movement pattern changes must be divided into substages to gain more accurate developmental information. Under this approach, each body component (rather than the general pattern) is followed through the development process. For example, if the stage theory uses the general description of stages 1, 2, and 3 in the development of the throwing pattern, the component approach might identify five arm action stages but only three marked changes for the legs. Obviously, for research purposes this approach provides more precise scientific information relative to studying changes. On the other hand, the composite approach may be quite useful as a practical assessment for teachers and coaches.

THINK ABOUT IT
What is the role of nature/nurture in the development of fundamental movement patterns during early childhood? Consider information from previous chapters to support biological change.

The desired outcome of any hypothesized developmental sequence is that it is a valid representation of most children. As mentioned in chapter 1, one of the best methods of developmental research is the longitudinal design. Roberton et al., (1980) have developed a **prelongitudinal screening** technique that accommodates such a purpose. The first step is to hypothesize a developmental sequence as a result of numerous observations for children of different ages and experience. Then data would be collected from an appropriate number and age range of subjects. Subjects' performances are evaluated and compared with the hypothesized longitudinal model. The desired outcome is that the youngest (and less-experienced) subjects exhibit the less proficient motor pattern characteristics, while the older subjects perform advanced (mature) patterns. To establish validity over time, subjects are retested periodically (e.g., yearly) to determine whether, for example, a child who originally was identified at Step 1 fits the model for Step 2.

The following section discusses the process characteristics associated with key fundamental movement patterns that emerge during early childhood. In addition to a summary of movement pattern and developmental characteristics for each skill, examples of component and composite sequence models are included. For instructional (teaching) purposes, focus on the mature pattern should be helpful.

■ *Movement Patterns (Process Characteristics)*

Running

Objective 9.5 ➤ **Running** is a natural extension of walking and is characterized by activity in which the body is propelled into flight with no base of support from either leg. This is in contrast to walking, in which one foot is always in contact with the surface. Because it contains a nonsupport phase, running is less stable than walking and therefore demands more bodily control. Most children take their first running steps at about 18 months and exhibit a true flight phase (minimum standard) between 2 and 3 years of age. By the age of 5 most children attain a reasonably skillful running form, and speed becomes a primary stimulus for performance. The general development of a skillful running pattern usually occurs without need for specific help or instruction. However, depending on the nature of the running task (e.g., sprints and long-distance running), education usually is needed to attain mastery.

MOVEMENT PATTERN DESCRIPTIONS. The description of the developmental pattern for running has been established primarily on

■ *Figure 9.1*

Initial running
attempts of a
15-month-old

running performance at maximum velocity (short sprints of 30 to 50 yards). Sprint-action analysis is used because it yields relatively constant performance, and the high degree of effort required produces maximum movement and acceptable reliability. During the initial (immature) stages of running, there is no observation flight phase and the base of support is relatively wide (figure 9.1). The stride is short with the feet rotated outwardly and laterally. The center of gravity is forward and foot-to-surface contact is usually flat-footed with some children exhibiting a tiptoe style. Arm swing is relatively rigid and more lateral and horizontal than vertical.

In the mature stage, the arms are bent at the elbows in approximate right angles and are swung vertically in a large arc in opposition to the legs. The recovery knee is raised high and swung forward quickly, while the support leg bends slightly at contact and then extends completely and quickly through the hip, knee, and ankle. Stride length and duration of the flight phase are at their maximum. There is little rotary movement of the recovery knee or foot as stride length increases. Figure 9.2 shows characteristics of the mature pattern in a young girl. The essential characteristics of the mature running pattern are as follows:

1. The trunk maintains a slight forward lean throughout the stride pattern.
2. Both arms swing through a large arc in a vertical plane and in synchronized opposition to the leg action.
3. The support foot contacts the ground approximately flat and nearly under the center of gravity.

■ *Figure 9.2*

The mature
running pattern

4. The knee of the support leg bends slightly after the foot has made contact with the ground.
5. Extension of the support leg at the hip, knee, and ankle propels the body forward and upward into the nonsupport phase (*flight phase*).
6. The recovery knee swings forward quickly to a high knee raise and there is simultaneous flexion of the lower leg, which brings the heel close to the buttock.

Unfortunately, little developmental information is available on the long-distance running pattern, even though it is considered a fundamental skill. Since almost all national physical fitness assessment batteries have been revised in recent years to include tests of distance running (rather than sprints), it is anticipated that more research in this area will follow. There are postural similarities between sprinting action and long-distance patterns, but many mechanical differences are evident. Proper mechanics and speed are primary factors in sprinting, but efficiency, pace, and endurance are paramount to the distance runner. Due to the sprinter's need for maximum forward propulsion, knee lift and rear kickup of the recovery leg are higher and the sprinter's arms move more vigorously. In contrast, the distance runner normally displays less knee flexion, uses less arm motion, contacts the ground with more of a heel-to-toe action, and displays more vertical movement. The sprinter normally relies on a combination of long stride and high frequency, whereas the distance runner exhibits a relatively short stride with low frequency and pace to conserve energy. Although the concept of pace is generally difficult for young children, the long-distance running pattern is acquired by 5 years of age.

DEVELOPMENTAL CHARACTERISTICS. Among the numerous developmental studies of the running (for speed) movement pattern, the following major trends are frequently noted:

1. Length of stride increases. This developmental trend coincides with the age-related increase in running speed.
2. Base of support narrows.
3. Relative amount of vertical movement decreases so there is greater horizontal displacement of the center of gravity.
4. Relative distance of the support foot from the center of gravity at contact decreases.
5. Hip, knee, and ankle extension during the takeoff increases.
6. Duration of the nonsupport (flight) phase increases.
7. Support knee flexion on contact increases.
8. Knee flexion in the recovery leg increases, as exhibited by the closeness of the heel to the buttock on the forward swing.
9. Height of the swing of the forward knee (recovery leg thigh) increases.
10. Lateral leg movements and out-toeing are eliminated.

11. Arm action evolves from the immature high and middle guard positions (rigid and held laterally) to elbows flexed at approximate right angles that move in opposition to the legs.

Table 9.1 presents Roberton and Halverson's (1984) component view of the running pattern.

TABLE 9.1

Developmental Sequence (Components) for Running

LEG ACTION COMPONENT

Step 1   The run is flat-footed with minimal flight. The swing leg is slightly abducted as it comes forward. When seen from overhead, the path of the swing leg curves out to the side during its movement forward. Foot eversion gives a toeing-out appearance to the swinging leg. The angle of the knee of the swing leg is greater than 90° during forward motion.

Step 2   The swing thigh moves forward with greater acceleration, which causes 90° of maximal flexion in the knee. From the rear, the foot is no longer toed-out and the thigh is not abducted. The sideward swing of the thigh continues, however, which causes the foot to cross the body midline when viewed from the rear. Flight time increases. After contact, which may still be flat-footed, the support knee flexes more as the child's weight rides over the foot.

Step 3   Foot contact is with the heel or the ball of the foot. The forward movement of the swing leg is primarily in the sagittal plane. Flexion of the thigh at the hip carries the knee higher at the end of the forward swing. The support leg moves from flexion to complete extension by takeoff.

ARM ACTION COMPONENT

Step 1   The arms do not participate in the running action. They sometimes are held in high guard or, more frequently, middle guard position. In high guard, the hands are held about shoulder high. Sometimes they ride even higher if the laterally rotated arms are abducted at the shoulder and the elbows flexed. In middle guard, the lateral rotation decreases, which allows the hands to be held waist high. They remain motionless, except in reaction to shifts in equilibrium.

Step 2   Spinal rotation swings the arms bilaterally to counterbalance rotation of the pelvis and swing leg. The frequently oblique plane of motion plus continual balancing adjustments give a flailing appearance to the arm action.

Step 3   Spinal rotation continues to be the prime mover of the arms. Now the elbow of the arm swinging forward begins to flex, then extend during the backward swing. The combination of rotation and elbow flexion causes the arm rotating forward to cross the body midline and the arm rotating back to abduct and swing obliquely outward from the body.

Step 4   The humerus (upper arm) begins to drive forward and back in the sagittal plane independent of spinal rotation. The movement is in opposition to the other arm and to the leg on the same side. Elbow flexion is maintained; the elbow oscillates about a 90° angle during the forward and backward arm swings.

Source: Data from Roberton & Halverson (1984)

Jumping

Jumping is a motor skill in which the body is projected into the air by a force generated by one or both legs and then lands on one or both feet. One of the most diverse and fundamental of all motor skills, jumping patterns range from simple leaping (a one-foot takeoff and opposite-foot landing) to hopping (jumping from one foot to the same foot rhythmically).

For the young child the primary challenges of jumping are sufficient leg strength to propel the body off the ground (for a longer period than required in running) and the ability to maintain postural control in the air and upon landing. For these reasons, most jumping patterns are considered more difficult than walking or normal running.

Some sources document the first stage of jumping as an exaggerated step down from a higher level (stairs or box) at about 18 months. But it is generally agreed that the first true jumping movements do not occur until the child is able to project the body off the ground into flight. This form of jumping, described as a **leap,** is normally evident by approximately 2 years, when the child propels himself or herself forward and upward into flight with one foot and lands on the other foot. Though simple leaping is achieved by the age of 2, maximum height and distance (flight) are not accomplished until approximately age 4 or 5.

Table 9.2 shows the sequence of general jumping patterns and approximate age of skillful achievement. It should be emphasized that achievement levels are for the basic patterns of jumping, and that these movements provide the elements for more advanced jumping variations (sport skills) commonly displayed by older children (e.g., running long jump, triple jump, and high jump).

Of the several jumping variations, the patterns that have received the most attention in the developmental literature are the vertical jump, the standing long jump, and the hop.

TABLE 9.2

General Sequence Jumping Patterns

Movement	Approximate Age of Skillful Achievement (Yr)
One-foot takeoff and opposite-foot landing (simple leap)	2–2½
One-foot takeoff and two-foot landing	
Two-foot takeoff and one-foot landing	5
Two-foot takeoff and landing (vertical jump; standing long jump)	5–6
One-foot takeoff and same-foot landing (hop)	5–6

Both the vertical jump (for height) and the standing long jump (for distance) involve a two-foot takeoff and landing, as well as distinctive preparatory, takeoff, flight, and landing phases. In the mature form of both skills, the jumper must (a) initiate a preparatory crouch, (b) vigorously swing the arms forward and upward to initiate the action, (c) extend the legs rapidly to propel the body from the ground, (d) extend the entire body during flight, and (e) flex the hips, knees, and ankles to absorb shock upon landing.

The standing long jump pattern is slightly more difficult than the vertical style, due primarily to the angle of projection and the coordination of arm action with the leg movements required. The long jump requires the body to be propelled forward and upward. This necessitates the center of gravity to be slightly ahead of the base of support at takeoff, which may create difficulty in maintaining forward balance; there is a strong tendency for the novice to step out with one foot to avoid falling. At this angle (about 45 degrees) the jumper also must swing the legs forward under the trunk in preparation for landing, whereas in the vertical jump the legs and trunk remain relatively vertical throughout execution.

Although rhythmical hopping (one foot to the same foot repeatedly) does not require maximum effort, it is the more difficult and complex of the three forms noted. The difficulty lies primarily in the requirement of greater leg strength and better balance, as well as the ability to perform controlled, rhythmical movement. All three of the jumping patterns, however, exhibit common developmental changes in relation to increased depth of preparatory crouch and increased use and effectiveness of arm action. With few exceptions, initial jumping patterns lack effective arm action. As a general rule, leg action is considerably more advanced than arm movements in the early stages of jumping. With maturity, arm movements are used effectively to aid in takeoff propulsion and in maintaining stability through flight and upon landing.

Vertical Jump   The **vertical jump** movement pattern involves a two-foot takeoff and landing with the primary purpose of achieving maximum height. Assessment of pattern characteristics usually is conducted by observing the skill while the individual reaches for an overhead target that elicits maximum reach. This form of vertical jumping often is described as the jump-and-reach version. If the jumping task does not include purposeful reaching (to a target) by the arms, less mature pattern characteristics usually are displayed. Although mature process characteristics of the vertical jump have been observed in children as young as 2 years, most children do not achieve mastery until approximately age 5.

MOVEMENT PATTERN DESCRIPTIONS.   In the performance of skillful vertical jumping, the knees are bent in a preparatory crouch and the arms are lowered with the elbows slightly flexed. As the knees

■ *Figure 9.3*

Arm positions in novice jumpers

The arm position of the child on the left is the most effective of the three for attaining maximum reach

straighten the arms swing upward. The body stretches and extends as far as possible into vertical flight. The landing should be on the balls of the feet, with knees flexed to absorb the force of impact. However, the novice jumper frequently displays the following immature characteristics: (a) minimal preliminary crouch, (b) arms fixed at the middle or high guard position, (c) slight forward lean at takeoff, and (d) quick flexion at hips and knees following takeoff. An important factor in accomplishing maximum reach is the position of the shoulders and nonreaching arm at peak height. Figure 9.3 illustrates three arm positions commonly observed in novice jumpers when reaching for an overhead target.

In the mature vertical jump pattern, the preparatory phase is characterized by flexion at the hips, knees, and ankles. A vigorous forward and upward lift by the arms initiates the jump, and thrust is continued by forceful extension at the hips, knees, and ankles. Just prior to the peak of the jump, the nonreaching arm is pushed downward. This movement tilts the shoulder girdle laterally and raises the hand of the reaching arm higher. Upon landing, the ankles, knees, and hips flex to absorb the shock (figure 9.4 on page 296).

DEVELOPMENTAL CHARACTERISTICS. The following general developmental trends have been noted in the vertical jump pattern:

1. A gradual increase in preparatory crouch.
2. Increased effectiveness of arm opposition.
3. Improved extension at takeoff and in flight.
4. Change from a forward flexion of the head throughout the jump to deep dorsiflexion (backward) during the entire sequence.
5. Greater extension of the trunk at the crest of the reach.

■ *Figure 9.4*

Mature vertical
jumping pattern

Standing Long Jump   The **standing long jump** (two-foot takeoff and landing) for maximum horizontal distance may be considered the standard fundamental jumping skill. This form of jumping has been included in numerous motor and physical fitness assessment batteries over the years to determine jumping ability in relation to maximum distance (product). Research on the early childhood years, however, has brought focus to the development of process characteristics. These components form the basis for several advanced jumping variations older children use in a sports setting. As noted earlier, the standing long jump pattern is slightly more difficult than the jump-and-reach due primarily to the angle at which the body is projected. Although most children achieve a relatively high degree of vertical jump proficiency by age 5, mastery of the standing long jump usually is not observed until age 6.

MOVEMENT PATTERN DESCRIPTIONS. Skillful execution of the standing long jump requires, in general, a deep preparatory crouch and forward lean of the body that is counterbalanced by swinging the arms backward and then forcefully forward. Both feet leave the ground together with the angle of takeoff at approximately 45 degrees. The body achieves extension during flight, and the landing is on both feet. However, arm, leg, and trunk action in the initial (immature) stages of jumping are quite limited. The jumping action is not initiated effectively by the arms because of their limited swing. Several ineffective arm positions may be observed in the novice jumper. Two of the most common are arms held rigidly at the side with elbows flexed and a winging position. At takeoff, which is usually at an angle of less than 30 degrees from vertical, the trunk is propelled in more of a vertical direction with little emphasis on the length of the jump. The preparatory crouch is limited and generally inconsistent with regard to the degree of leg flexion. Extension of the hips, legs, and ankles is incomplete at takeoff, and one leg frequently precedes the other upon takeoff and upon landing. Figure 9.5 shows two immature movement patterns for the standing long jump. In figure 9.5b the child displays the characteristic winging arm position.

■ *Figure 9.5*

Initial patterns of the two-foot take-off. (a) Arms are held rigid at the sides with elbows flexed; (b) Arms are held in a winging position.

With maturity and practice, greater coordination of arm and leg movements is achieved to result in a mature movement pattern. The mature pattern is characterized by a relatively deep preparatory crouch, while the arms swing backward and upward (figure 9.6). At takeoff, both feet leave the ground together, with the thrust initiated in a horizontal direction at an angle of approximately 45 degrees. As the body moves forward, the hips, legs, and ankles extend in succession. During flight, the hips flex, which brings the thighs to a position nearly horizontal to the surface. The lower legs extend prior to landing. When the body lands on both feet, the knees bend and the body weight continues forward and downward. The arms reach forward to keep the center of gravity moving in the direction of the flight.

DEVELOPMENTAL CHARACTERISTICS. General developmental trends in the standing long jump movement pattern are similar to the developmental characteristics described for the vertical jump-and-reach:

1. An increase in the preparatory crouch.
2. Greater efficiency in use of the arms as displayed by an increase in the forward swing in the anteroposterior plane.

■ *Figure 9.6*

Mature stages of the horizontal jumping pattern

3. A decrease in the takeoff angle; theoretically, a projectile angle of 45 degrees is ideal.
4. An increase in total body extension at takeoff.
5. Greater thigh flexion during flight.
6. A decrease in the angle of the leg at the instant of landing.

Hopping

Hopping is a coordinated one-foot takeoff and landing on the same foot repeatedly. It is considered the most difficult form of basic jumping because hopping requires greater leg strength and better balance, as well as the ability to perform controlled, rhythmical movement compared to other jumping patterns. Prerequisite to hopping is the ability to balance on one foot momentarily (static balance), a skill not acquired until approximately 2½ years of age.

Since hopping is a dynamic (moving) skill, repeated steps generally are not observed until after the age of 3 years. By 3½ years of age most children can hop one to three steps; by the age of 5, the ability to hop 10 consecutive times is commonly seen. However, in a study of the process components of children ages 3, 4, and 5, Halverson and Williams (1985) found few children who displayed advanced levels of hopping and therefore concluded the development of this skill may not reach the mature stage until the age of 6 years or older. The researchers also concluded that females are developmentally more advanced than the males. This finding appears consistently in the literature.

MOVEMENT PATTERN DESCRIPTIONS. The early attempts at hopping are performed primarily in place with little forward movement. The general pattern is usually jerky with little extension and flexion of the support leg. As a result, the hop has minimal elevation and landings are flat-footed. As one would expect, arm opposition is ineffective (held in the high guard position and to the side for balance) and the nonsupport (swing) leg often is lifted high and held awkwardly to the side or in front of the body.

As the child's balance, leg strength, and coordination improve, arm and leg actions gradually transform into a smooth rhythmical mature movement pattern. Mature hopping is characterized by arm opposition that moves forward and upward in synchrony with the swing leg. The other arm moves in direct opposition to the action of the swing leg.

Longitudinal data reported by Roberton (1990) suggest that advanced, smoothly timed arm opposition is the last component of hopping to develop and sometimes takes more than 10 years to achieve. Prior to takeoff, the weight of the child is transferred along the foot to the ball before the knee and ankle extend to takeoff. The support leg reaches maximum extension on takeoff, while the swing leg leads the upward-forward thrust with a pumping action. During this action, the swing leg

Figure 9.7

Mature hopping pattern

passes behind the support leg (when viewed from the side). Upon landing, the hip, knee, and ankle joints flex to absorb the shock (figure 9.7).

DEVELOPMENTAL CHARACTERISTICS. The following major developmental trends have been observed in hopping behavior:

1. A decrease in the amount of forward body lean.
2. An increase in arm action effectiveness from stabilization to efficient arm opposition.
3. A change from leg clearance by flexion to clearance as a result of leg thrust.
4. Improvement in the use of the nonsupportive (swing) leg, from an inactive forward position to a forward-upward swing connected with takeoff.
5. An increase in range and speed of movement at the hip, knee, and ankle of the support leg.
6. Change in landing from immediate extension that follows knee and ankle flexion to a delay in extension while the body pivots over the foot.

Galloping, Sliding, and Skipping

Galloping, sliding, and skipping are locomotor skills that consist of a combination of basic movements. Due to their increased complexity, they normally are not mastered until the end of the early childhood years. The relatively late appearance of these skills (around age 4) may be expected because they require a certain level of dynamic balancing ability. As children master the ability to propel their body weight onto the forward foot, these patterns begin to appear.

Galloping, which is usually the first of these three skills to emerge, combines the basic patterns of a walking step and the leap; it is an uneven rhythmical pattern. The mature movement pattern is characterized by a slight forward lean and a thrusting forward of the lead leg. The lead foot supports the body weight, while the rear foot quickly closes behind the lead foot and takes the weight. During this cycle there is extension and flexion of both legs with a momentary suspension of both feet in the air. In a series of gallops, the same foot takes the lead and contacts the ground with a heel-toe action. The arms swing freely from the shoulders during execution. In comparison to sliding and skipping, opportunities for galloping and the motivation to gallop as a mature physical activity appear limited.

Sliding is similar to galloping except the direction of movement is sideways. When sliding to the right, the right foot moves sideward and takes the weight, and the left foot follows quickly. As with galloping, the same foot always takes the lead. The first step is usually a slow gliding movement, and the second is a quick closing step. Foot contact is normally on the balls of the feet, with the weight shifted from the lead to the follow-up foot. After the follow-up foot catches the lead foot, a slight jump (momentary suspension) is displayed. At this time the body is ready for a quick change of direction or continuation in the same pathway. Arms are held in a relaxed position at approximately waist level and to the side. (See figure 9.8.)

Of the three locomotor skills noted, **skipping** is typically the last to be mastered (between the sixth and seventh year). The general pattern involves stepping forward on one foot, quickly hopping on the same foot, duplicating the process on the opposite foot, and so on. Complexity lies in the fact that it consists of a *step-hop pattern* performed in an uneven rhythm. To perform a step-hop on one foot requires additional skill in timing of sequential movements as well as a substantial degree of balance. Another aspect of its complexity is that the step-hop is performed on one foot before the weight is transferred to the other foot.

Characteristic of mature skipping is a well-coordinated and continuous cycle of weight transfer to the opposite foot and the subsequent step-hop. The trunk is held erect with the head focused in a forward direction. The arms swing freely and in opposition to leg action. The

■ *Figure 9.8*

Sliding

■ *Figure 9.9*

Skipping

support knee and ankle extend for takeoff (which creates momentary suspension) and flex upon landing. The nonsupport leg flexes to aid elevation of the hop. The balls of the feet receive the weight of the body. Figure 9.9 shows the movement pattern in skipping.

Since young females tend to be superior at hopping, it is not surprising the literature shows them to be better skippers also. For example, Haubenstricker and colleagues (1990) found females 2 to 9 years of age were consistently more advanced at skipping than males at all ages were. Males appear to be about six months to one year behind in the qualitative aspects of skipping in comparison to females. Although it is speculative, this difference could be a result of females' greater interest in and subsequent practice of the skill, as well as the fact that females have a slight edge in biological maturity for chronological age.

Throwing

Throwing is a complex manipulative skill in which one or both arms thrust an object away from the body and into space. During the early childhood years, children display many different throwing patterns. There does not appear to be any definite or precise developmental order for the onset of the variations. The pattern a child uses depends on several factors, including size of the child, size of the object, and age. Of the three most common variations (overarm, sidearm, and underhand), the unilateral overarm style is used most commonly and has been studied the most thoroughly.

The first signs of the overarm pattern appear around the age of 6 months when the child executes a crude throw that involves limited use of the arm while he or she is in a sitting position. Though a wide variation in skill level may be observed at all ages, the majority of children are skillful throwers by age 6. As noted, some individuals may never acquire the mature stage of a specific motor skill. The mature overarm throwing pattern is a motor skill that has a relatively high incidence of individuals (especially females) who do not reach mastery.

Data from a longitudinal study that documented pattern changes of kindergarten children to the seventh grade support this finding (Halverson et al., 1982). By the seventh grade, 80% of the males achieved the mature level in upper arm action compared to only 29% of the females. This trend was also evident for actions of the forearm and trunk. The presence of immature throwing patterns among adult females also is not uncommon, which demonstrates not all movement patterns reach the mature level during childhood or even adolescence.

As one might expect, instruction and adequate opportunity for practice are significant factors in the development of throwing technique among children; however, these factors do not appear to affect ball-throwing velocity (Halverson et al., 1977).

MOVEMENT PATTERN DESCRIPTIONS. Although conducted over 65 years ago, Wild (1938) is recognized as having directed one of the most definitive studies of developmental form in overarm throwing. Through cinematographic analysis of throwing form in children from ages 2 to 7 years, the researcher identified four developmental stages (see table 9.3). Subsequent observations have confirmed much of the characteristics described; as a composite model, they present a good example.

Stage I is characterized by minimal trunk rotation and projection of the ball primarily by elbow extension. Virtually all movement is in the anterior-posterior plane. During the entire series of movements, both feet remain stationary and the body faces toward the direction of the throw.

Stage II is distinguished primarily by movements that occur in the horizontal plane. The feet remain stationary but rotation of the pelvis and spine are evident. Greater projection force also is attained from the forward and downward follow-through.

The most noticeable occurrence at Stage III is the appearance of a step forward with the delivery. In the preparatory phase, the weight is shifted onto the left (or rear) foot while the body is rotated to the right. The arm is moved obliquely upward and behind (over) the shoulder and set in a flexed position. During delivery, the weight is transferred onto the foot on the same side as the throwing arm (ipsilateral), as the body rotates to the left and the arm projects forward. Upon completion of the follow-through, the body faces partially to the left (for a right-hander), in contrast to facing forward that took place in the preceding stages.

In Stage IV (mature pattern), the thrower displays proper opposition by transferring weight to the foot opposite the throwing arm (contralateral). This action facilitates greater trunk rotation and, along with the horizontal adduction of the arm during the forward swing, enables the thrower to achieve maximum body leverage. Wickstrom (1983) provides additional clarification (composite) of the mature throwing pattern.

TABLE 9.3

A Summary of Wild's Four Developmental Stages (Composite) of Throwing

Stage I (2–3 yrs)	Stage II (3½–5 yrs)	Stage III (5–6 yrs)	Stage IV 6½ yrs and older)
Throw is arm-dominated Preparatory arm movements involve bringing the arm sideways-upward or forward-upward. Thrower faces the direction of intended throw at all times. No rotation of trunk and hips is evident. Feet remain stationary during the entire throwing act.	Body moves in horizontal plane instead of anterior-posterior plane. Throwing arm moves in a high oblique plane or horizontal plane above the shoulder. Throwing is initiated predominately by arm and elbow extension. Feet remain stationary, but rotary movement of the trunk is observable.	Forward step is unilateral to the throwing arm Arm is prepared by swinging it obliquely upward over the shoulder with a large degree of elbow flexion. Arm follows through forward and down-ward and is accompanied by forward flexion of the trunk.	Forward step is taken with the contra-lateral leg. Trunk rotation is clearly evident. Arm is horizontally adducted in the forward swing.

Source: Data from Payne & Isaacs (1987), as interpreted from Wild (1938)

Preparatory Phase
1. The body pivots to the right with the weight on the right foot; the throwing arm swings backward and upward.

Execution Phase
2. The left foot strides forward in the intended direction of the throw.
3. The hips, then the spine and shoulders, rotate counterclockwise as the throwing arm is retracted to the final point of its reversal.
4. The upper arm is rotated medially, and the forearm is extended with a whipping action.
5. The ball is released at a point just forward of the head with the arm extended at the elbow.

Follow-Through
6. The movement is continued until the momentum generated in the throwing action is dissipated. Figure 9.10 on page 304 depicts the mature overarm throwing pattern.

Roberton and Halverson (1984) (table 9.4 on pages 305 and 306) offer a more precise developmental (component) analysis of the overarm

■ *Figure 9.10*

Mature overarm throwing pattern

THINK ABOUT IT

How do table 9.3 (composite of throwing) and 9.4 (components for throwing) compare?

throwing pattern. Although some of the component sequences have been hypothesized from other studies and have not been validated, this model adds significantly to our understanding of the specific developmental changes that occur. Research based on this model has verified that development within component parts may proceed at different rates in the same individual or at different rates in different individuals.

DEVELOPMENTAL CHARACTERISTICS. These developmental trends have been noted in relation to the overarm throwing pattern:

1. A gradual shift of movement from a predominantly anterior-posterior plane to a horizontal plane.
2. Transition from the use of a stationary base of support to weight transfer on the same side as the throwing arm, followed by functional arm-foot opposition.
3. An increase with each successive throwing pattern in effective mechanical projection as evidenced by throwing velocity.

For an excellent description of critical features that can be used to qualitatively analyze and improve performance of the overarm throw, refer to Knudson and Morrison (2002) in the Suggested Readings.

Catching

Catching is a fundamental, gross motor, manipulative skill that involves visually tracking an incoming object, stopping its momentum, and gaining control of it with the hands. Receiving objects with the hands is a complex movement pattern for children. This is due primarily to the fact that catching requires coincident timing ability. Recall that coincident timing is a form of temporal accuracy that involves timing self-movements with an object. This action includes a series of complicated perceptual judgments that can vary considerably, depending on catching conditions. In addition, David and colleagues (2000) point out from a

TABLE 9.4
_____

Developmental Sequence (Components) for Overarm Throwing

TRUNK ACTION COMPONENT

Step 1   *No trunk action or forward-backward movements.* Only the arm is active in force production. Sometimes, the forward thrust of the arm pulls the trunk into a passive left rotation
(assuming a right-handed throw), but no twist-up precedes that action. If trunk action
occurs, it accompanies the forward thrust of the arm by flexing forward at the hips.
Preparatory extension sometimes precedes forward hip flexion.

Step 2   *Upper trunk rotation or total trunk block rotation.* The spine and pelvis both rotate away
from the intended line of flight and then simultaneously begin forward rotation, thus acting as a unit or block. Occasionally, only the upper spine twists away, then toward the
direction of force. The pelvis then remains fixed, faces the line of flight, or joins the rotary
movement after forward spinal rotation has begun.

Step 3   *Differentiated rotation.* The pelvis precedes the upper spine in initiating forward rotation.
The child twists away from the intended line of ball flight and then begins forward rotation with the pelvis while the upper spine still twists away.

PREPARATORY ARM BACKSWING COMPONENT

Step 1   *No backswing.* The ball in the hand moves directly forward to release from the arm's original position when the hand first grasped the ball.

Step 2   *Elbow and humeral flexion.* The ball moves away from the intended line of flight to a position behind or alongside the head by upward flexion of the humerus and concomitant
elbow flexion.

Step 3   *Circular, upward backswing.* The ball moves away from the intended line of flight to a position behind the head via a circular overhead movement with elbow extended, an oblique
swing back, or a vertical lift from the hip.

Step 4   *Circular, downward backswing.* The ball moves away from the intended line of flight to a
position behind the head via a circular, down, and back motion, which carries the hand
below the waist.

HUMERUS (UPPER ARM) ACTION COMPONENT DURING FORWARD SWING

Step 1   *Humerus oblique.* The humerus moves forward to ball release in a plane that intersects the
trunk obliquely above or below the horizontal line of the shoulders. Occasionally, during
the backswing, the humerus is placed at a right angle to the trunk, and the elbow points
toward the target. It maintains this fixed position during the throw.

Step 2   *Humerus aligned but independent.* The humerus moves forward to ball release in a plane
horizon-tally aligned with the shoulder, which forms a right angle between humerus and
trunk. By the time the shoulders (upper spine) reach front facing, the humerus (elbow) has
moved independently ahead of the outline of the body (as seen from the side) via horizontal adduction at the shoulder.

Step 3   *Humerus lags.* The humerus moves forward to ball release horizontally aligned, but at the
moment the shoulders (upper spine) reach front facing, the humerus remains within the
outline of the body (as seen from the side). No horizontal adduction of the humerus
occurs before front facing.

(continued)

Table 9.4 *continued*

FOREARM ACTION COMPONENT DURING FORWARD SWING

Step 1   *No forearm lag.* The forearm and ball move steadily forward to ball release throughout the throwing action.

Step 2   *Forearm lag.* The forearm and ball appear to lag, i.e., to remain stationary behind the child or to move down or back in relation to the child. The lagging forearm reaches its farthest point back, deepest point down, or last stationary point *before* the shoulders (upper spine) reach front facing.

Step 3   *Delayed forearm lag.* The lagging forearm delays reaching its final point of lag until the moment of front facing.

ACTION OF THE FEET

Step 1   *No step.* The child throws from the initial foot position.

Step 2   *Homolateral step.* The child steps with the foot on the same side as the throwing hand.

Step 3   *Contralateral, short step.* The child steps with the foot on the opposite side from the throwing hand.

Step 4   *Contralateral, long step.* The child steps with the opposite foot a distance of over half the child's standing height.

Source: Data from Roberton & Halverson (1984)

dynamic systems perspective that postural control may be a significant constraint on successful catching performance. Unfortunately, evidence concerning the emergence of catching skills is insufficient to provide a precise developmental description. Part of the difficulty in studying catching behavior is due to the numerous variables that influence the measurement of performance (e.g., ball size, ball speed and distance traveled, method of ball projection, and angle and level of the receiver). Because of these and other conditions under which catching has been researched, it is difficult to compare and contrast various studies.

Although throwing and catching have a close functional relationship, catching proficiency normally follows throwing proficiency. A primitive form of catching that involves trapping can be observed in 2- and 3-year-olds, but the reports of children who achieve proficiency at this skill indicate they typically range in age from 6 to 8 years. However, these figures are based on two-handed catching in relatively stable conditions; the ability to catch a ball under more complex conditions continues to develop well into the upper elementary years (from age 10 to 12).

MOVEMENT PATTERN DESCRIPTIONS. The first attempts to stop and control a moving object occur when a ball is rolled toward a child seated on the floor with legs apart. Initially, the child will stop the ball by corralling and trapping it against the legs. With adequate practice, the child will develop the ability to coordinate arm movements with the velocity of the ball and thus trap it with the hands. As the child rises from the relatively stationary sitting position, he or she develops the ability to chase, stop, and gain control of a moving or bouncing ball. This series of achievements is important in the progression leading to comprehensive catching ability.

The first attempts to catch an aerial ball with two hands are relatively passive. That is, the child simply holds its arms out stiffly in front of the body, regardless of the angle and height of the incoming object. Little or no effort is made to move the body to adjust to the ball's flight. At the point of contact with the ball, the hands exhibit very little give; the momentum is not attenuated. In addition, there is little, if any, flexion at the knees to help absorb the shock of the ball's velocity.

A common observation in novice catchers is a negative reaction and fear of the ball. These characteristics include turning the head to the side, a slight backward bending of the trunk away from the incoming ball, and closing the eyes. These characteristics are more common in 4-, 5-, and 6-year-olds but apparently are rare in younger children. Seefeldt (1972) speculated that fear of an aerial ball is not a natural phenomenon but may be a conditioned response from earlier failures at the task. In this stage of development, success in catching is as much (or more) dependent on the accuracy of the throw as it is on the ability of the catcher. Figure 9.11 on page 308 shows two variations of the immature two-handed catching pattern.

As development approaches mastery, the child displays greater coordination by adjusting the body and the hand and arm positions to accommodate the ball's flight. In addition, the catcher learns to give with the object, thus allowing the body to absorb the momentum of the projectile. The following general characteristics summarize the movements associated with the mature two-handed catching pattern:

1. Body is in alignment with incoming object.
2. Feet are slightly apart and parallel or in forward stride position.
3. Arms are held relaxed at sides (or in front of the body), and elbows are flexed.
4. Hands and fingers are relaxed and slightly cupped (pointing to object).
5. Eyes follow the flight of the object.
6. Hands move forward to meet approaching object.
7. Arms give upon contact to absorb the force, and fingers close around the object. Contact and closure are simultaneous with both hands.
8. Body weight is transferred from front to back.

DEVELOPMENTAL CHARACTERISTICS. Since the qualitative evidence concerning the emergence of catching skills is insufficient for a precise developmental description, only generalized observations about developmental trends and characteristics can be made:

1. Catching ability, in general, progresses from trapping (using the arms, body, and hands) to catching an object using the hands exclusively.

Two variations of immature catching pattern

In the upper sequence the child displays a fear reaction. The child in the lower sequence exhibits urgent actions. He responds to the ball only after it has touched his hands, then traps it against his chest.

2. Movement pattern action improves from a relatively passive reception (e.g., simply holding the arms out and trapping after contact) to adjusting the body to the flight of the object.

3. Positioning of the body improves to be in line with the oncoming object.

4. Arm action improves from a stiff outstretched position to a position in which the elbows are flexed and give occurs upon contact to absorb the object's momentum.

5. With practice and a subsequent increase in confidence, fear reactions to catching an aerial ball decrease in most individuals.

Figure 9.12 illustrates the mature two-hand catching pattern (with a small ball). Although no developmental sequence model for two-hand catching has been validated for all components, table 9.5 presents an update of that endeavor (Strohmeyer et al., 1991). Table 9.6 (on page 310) is an example of a process-oriented rating scale for catching.

Figure 9.12

Mature two-hand catching pattern

TABLE 9.5

Developmental Sequence (Components) for Catching

PREPARATION: ARM COMPONENT

Step 1   The arms are outstretched with elbows extended, awaiting the tossed ball.

Step 2   The arms await the ball toss with some shoulder flexion still apparent, but flexion now appears in the elbows.

Step 3   The arms await the ball in a relaxed posture at the sides of the body or slightly ahead of the body. The elbows may be flexed.

RECEPTION: ARM COMPONENT

Step 1   The arms remain outstretched and the elbows rigid. There is little to no give, so the ball bounces off the arms.

Step 2   The elbows flex to carry the hands upward toward the face. Initially, ball contact is primarily with the arms, and the object is trapped against the body.

Step 3   Initial contact is with the hands. If unsuccessful in using the fingers, the child may still trap the ball against the chest. The hands still move upward toward the face.

Step 4   Ball contact is made with the hands. The elbows still flex but the shoulders extend, which brings the ball down and toward the body rather than up toward the face.

HAND COMPONENT

Step 1   The palms of the hands face upward. (Rolling balls elicit a palms-down, trapping action.)

Step 2   The palms of the hands face each other.

Step 3   The palms of the hands are adjusted to the flight and size of the oncoming object. Thumbs or little fingers are placed close together, depending on the height of the flight path.

BODY COMPONENT

Step 1   No adjustment of the body occurs in response to the flight path of the ball.

Step 2   The arms and trunk begin to move in relation to the ball's flight path, but the head remains erect, which creates an awkward movement to the ball. The catcher seems to be fighting to remain balanced.

Step 3   The feet, trunk, and arms all move to adjust to the path of the oncoming ball.

Source: These sequences were hypothesized by Harper (1979), cited in Roberton & Halverson (1984), and updated by Strohmeyer, Williams, & Schaub-George (1991).

TABLE 9.6

Example of a Process-Oriented Rating Scale for Catching

0 = Initial body contact: subject makes no attempt to contact the ball.

1 = Arm and/or body contact, miss: initial attempt to contact is made on the arms and/or body, and the ball is missed.

2 = Arm and/or body contact, save: initial contact is on the arms and/or body, and the ball is retained.

3 = Hand contact, miss: initial contact is made by the hands, but ball is then dropped immediately or dropped following arm or body contact.

4 = Hand contact, assisted catch: hands make initial contact. The ball is juggled but retained by using arms and/or body for assistance.

5 = Hand contact, clean catch: the ball is contacted and retained by the hands only. The ball may be brought into the body on the follow-through after hands gain control.

Source: Data from Payne & Isaacs (1987), as derived from Hellweg (1972), & Isaacs (1980)

As noted earlier, the conditions under which catching behavior has been measured vary considerably. Obviously, catching a large ball tossed slowly in front of the body at chest level while stationary is the easier form of catching. Several factors may influence catching performance (e.g., ball velocity, trajectory angle, and ball color), but one of the most consistently noted in the literature is ball size.

As may be expected, catching performance is achieved at a certain level of performance with a large ball before the same level is attained with a smaller ball. Mature catching, using the hands only, seems to appear earlier if the child also practices with a small ball. This practice seems to induce the child to think of using only the hands when catching a small ball, rather than using an arm/chest trap. When a larger ball is introduced to children after they have attained some proficiency using a small ball, they seem more likely to resort to the immature pattern (Payne, 1985). The best catching performance seems to be elicited using a ball that can be cupped in the hands (e.g., tennis ball size) but one that is not so small it requires extraordinary visual-motor control.

Striking

With **striking,** a part of the body or an implement is used to give impetus to an object. Depending on the striking situation, the skill can be executed using a variety of body parts (most commonly a hand, a foot, or the head) and a variety of implements (e.g., paddle, racquet, or bat). Striking skills also can be performed using various movement patterns; the most common the overhand, sidearm, and underhand patterns.

Kicking, also considered a striking skill, is discussed separately because of its unique pattern characteristics.

Unfortunately, relatively little information is available on the developmental sequence of striking ability. As in the case of catching, a number of factors may affect striking performance, including the size, weight, and length of the implement used, the physical characteristics of the object to be struck, and the speed of the incoming object (whether stationary or moving).

Young children frequently display skillful striking patterns before they gain the ability to contact a moving ball with enough frequency to provide reasonable quantitative measurement. Of the various striking skills, the ones most commonly used are the one- and two-handed sidearm striking pattern in the horizontal plane. A well-defined sidearm pattern may be evident in some children at approximately 3 years of age, but the mature pattern generally is not achieved until age 4 or 5. The ability to consistently intercept a moving object is more difficult and continues to improve through the late elementary years (from ages 10 to 12).

MOVEMENT PATTERN DESCRIPTIONS. Striking appears to develop in much the same sequential order as throwing in terms of general age level of performance. In the initial stage, the child uses an overarm chopping action (with or without an implement) in a vertical plane. From that initial stage the child seems to progress slowly through a downward series of planes that are more horizontal (sidearm) or even underarm.

The position of the object, however, influences the angle of the arm's approach. Most striking skills are performed with a sidearm pattern. One of the techniques most used for eliciting and assessing developmental sidearm striking characteristics is to require the individual to forcefully strike (with a racquet or bat) a stationary ball suspended at approximately waist level.

Initial efforts at sidearm striking are similar to immature pattern attempts at overarm throwing. That is, the individual chops at the ball by using an overarm pattern that consists of bending forward slightly, extending at the elbow, and using minimal trunk and leg action. The general striking action is predominantly flexion and extension of the forearm. In addition, the individual usually directly faces the object (instead of standing sideways to it). If a step forward is taken (though none may be evident), it is taken with the foot on the same side as the striking arm (homolateral) (figure 9.13 on page 312). Therefore, as with immature throwing, arm motion occurs primarily in the anterioposterior plane.

With maturity and practice, the individual gradually lowers the striking plane to the horizontal and abandons the arm-dominated movement pattern. Although the one-arm and two-arm variations of the striking skill have their own unique characteristics, each involves the same basic sequence of three movements: the step, the turn, and the swing. Basic actions within this sequence are as follows:

1. In the preparatory phase, the feet are positioned approximately shoulder-width apart.
2. Body weight is shifted initially away from the intended hit, and then in the direction of the strike (sideways to the target), while the shoulders and arms are coiled in the opposite direction. That is, for right-handers, the weight is shifted onto the right (rear) foot. The individual steps with the opposite foot into the hit to apply a straight-line direction of force. The length of the step is slightly greater than one-half of the individual's height.
3. Hips and spine are rotated in rapid succession in the same direction as the weight shift.
4. The arm (or arms) swings around and forward (horizontally) in close succession with the other rotary movements. The swing is performed through a full range of motion to apply adequate force.
5. The wrist (or wrists) is cocked in preparation for the strike and uncocked just prior to contact with the object.
6. Eyes follow the flight of the ball until just before contact is made.
7. Follow-through after contact.

Figure 9.14 describes the mature one-arm striking pattern. The only additional basic characteristic unique to the two-arm striking pattern

■ *Figure 9.15*

■ *Figure 9.15*

Mature two-arm
striking pattern

(batting) is the position of the elbow. That is, in the preparatory phase, the lead elbow is held up and out from the body with the bat held off the shoulder (figure 9.15).

DEVELOPMENTAL CHARACTERISTICS. The following developmental trends and characteristics have been noted for the sidearm striking pattern:

1. Increased use of a forward step or a forward weight shift to initiate the pattern.
2. Increased range of motion in the various joints during the swing.
3. Increased hip and trunk rotation preceding the action of the arm(s) in the swing.
4. Change of wrist action from a relatively stiff position to a more distinct cock and uncock action during the swing.

Table 9.7 on page 314 describes a developmental sequence (composite) for striking with a bat.

Kicking

Kicking is a fundamental manipulative skill in which the foot strikes an object. Unfortunately, information on developmental kicking behavior has not been extensive. Although the characteristics of mature pattern variations and general trends have been reported, qualitative changes made within the various components are not well documented. Another limitation has been that kicking performance (distance and accuracy) of

TABLE 9.7

Developmental Sequence (Composite) for Striking with a Bat

Stage 1   The motion is primarily posterior-anterior in direction. The movement begins with hip extension and slight spinal extension and retraction of the shoulder on the striking side of the body. The elbows flex fully. The feet remain stationary throughout the movement, with the primary force coming from extension of the flexed joints.

Stage 2   The feet remain stationary, or the right or left foot may receive the weight as the body moves toward the approaching ball. The primary pattern is the unitary rotation of the hip-spinal linkage about an imaginary vertical axis. The forward movement of the bat is in a transverse plane.

Stage 3   The shift of weight to the front-supporting foot occurs in an ipsilateral pattern. The trunk rotation-derotation is decreased markedly in comparison to stage 2, and the movement of the bat is in an oblique vertical plane instead of in the transverse path as seen in stage 2.

Stage 4   The transfer of weight in rotation-derotation is in a contralateral pattern. The shift of weight to the forward foot occurs while the bat still is moving backward as the hips, spine, and shoulder girdle assume their force-producing positions. At the initiation of the forward movement the bat is kept near the body. Elbow extension and the supination-pronation of the hands do not occur until the arms and hands are well forward and ready to extend the lever in preparation to meet the ball. At contact the weight is on the forward foot.

Source: From V. Seefeldt and J. Haubenstricker, 1974, Developmental Sequence for Striking with a Bat. Unpublished material, Michigan State University, East Lansing, MI. Reprinted by permission of John L. Haubenstricker.

children younger than 4 or 5 years is difficult to measure in quantitative terms. Most research data on the development of fundamental kicking behavior have been collected on pattern characteristics using the placekick with a stationary ball. The placekick is considered the basic foundation upon which other skills such as kicking a moving ball, dribbling, and punting are developed. These forms of advanced kicking usually are not achieved until some degree of placekicking skill has been acquired and additional perceptual abilities developed. As with catching and striking, variations in speed and position of the ball in space significantly can alter the level of difficulty.

The ability to kick a stationary ball (with minimal form) appears around the age of 2. But the mature pattern is not achieved by most children until 5 or 6 years. It should be noted that proficient kicking, like proficient throwing, may not be achieved through the natural course of childhood development.

MOVEMENT PATTERN DESCRIPTIONS. Before an individual can execute a true kicking action, the kicker must be able to maintain an upright posture while balancing momentarily on one foot and imparting force to an object with the other foot. This ability, which is normally present by 2 years, provides the basis for initial kicking behavior.

The immature stage of kicking is characterized by a limited range of action in the propelling leg and minimal backswing and follow-through. There is little movement of the upper body, and the arms are held out from the sides for balance. The kicking leg frequently is deeply flexed while it contacts the ball. General leg movements are described as a "pushing" action and may be displayed with either leg. During the early stages of this skill, the child also may respond to a ball placed in front of the body by running into it.

As the child attempts to kick more forcefully, range of leg motion increases (more backswing and follow-through), forward lean of the trunk increases, and the arms elevate to aid in maintaining balance. Opposition of the arm and foot also begins to develop. The following actions are fundamental to the mature pattern of all basic kicking variations:

1. Preparatory forward step on the support leg to rotate the pelvis backward on the opposite side and to extend the thigh of the kicking leg.
2. The support foot is placed to the side and slightly behind the ball.
3. Forward pelvic rotation and swing of the kicking leg with simultaneous flexion at the hip and at the knees.
4. Vigorous extension (whipping) of the lower part of the kicking leg.
5. Momentary slowdown or cessation of thigh flexion as the lower leg whips into extension just before the foot makes contact with the ball.
6. Forward swing of the opposite arm in reaction to the vigorous action of the kicking leg (arm/leg opposition).
7. Follow-through is forward and toward the midline.

Figure 9.16 (see page 316) illustrates four typical stages of kicking behavior as described by Deach (1950).

DEVELOPMENTAL CHARACTERISTICS. The following developmental trends and characteristics have been noted for the placekicking movement pattern:

1. An increase in the range of preparatory movement at the hip and the knee of the kicking leg.
2. An increase in the range of motion in the kicking leg.

■ *Figure 9.16*

Deach's four stages of kicking behavior (a) The girl keeps her kicking leg nearly straight and exhibits minimal coordination of rest of her body; (b) increased flexion of the kicking leg (precontact) and some arm opposition; (c) increased preliminary hip extension, greater range of leg motion, and additional body adjustments; and (d) the mature form of kicking behavior.

a.

b.

c.

d.

3. A tendency to start farther behind the ball and move the total body forward into the kick.
4. An increase in compensatory trunk lean and arm opposition.

Ball Bouncing and Dribbling

Ball bouncing and dribbling propel a ball in a downward direction. It has been speculated that the development of bouncing originates as the child drops a ball, causes it to bounce, and attempts to strike the object repeatedly. As the child's control of the ball progresses, the term *dribbling* is used to describe the action; minimal form commonly is determined by the ability to bounce a ball three or four consecutive times.

Although some 2-year-olds may exhibit a minimal degree of skill in two-handed bouncing, the mature pattern of one-handed dribbling in a relatively stationary position is not mastered until approximately 5 or 6 years of age. Dribbling proficiency while moving is much more complex than dribbling in a stationary position and is considered a sport skill. The difficulty of this skill is attributed, in part, to the fact that the ball loses forward speed after each bounce and a special push is necessary to maintain the desired forward speed.

MOVEMENT PATTERN DESCRIPTIONS. Although a specific developmental sequence has not been validated, the following general progression has been noted:

1. Bouncing and catching.
2. Bouncing and slapping on the rebound.
3. Dribbling with the ball in control.
4. Dribbling with the individual in control.
5. Dribbling as a sport skill such as that used in basketball activities.

Young children at the lowest skill level typically hold the fingers of the striking hand close together (often hyperextended) and display a distinct slapping motion. Minimal elbow extension follows a quick retraction of the hand after contact (figure 9.17). Because of their limited eye-hand coordination, inexperienced dribblers often strike the ball inconsistently. In essence, the ball controls the dribbler.

■ *Figure 9.17*

Immature and mature dribbling

The upper series demonstrates the slapping motion characteristic of immature dribbling. The lower series shows a mature dribbling action.

DEVELOPMENTAL CHARACTERISTICS. The transition from immature to mature dribbling action is characterized primarily by a progression that moves from slapping to pushing the ball. To achieve the mature form of multiple controlled bounces requires greater consistency in hand position at contact and more continuous contact from the upper part of the rebound through the downward pushing action. Maximum control also necessitates that the proportionate size of the hand and ball allow the dribbler to control the direction of the ball by placing the hands at the center of the ball's mass.

In contrast to the inexperienced dribbler, a pushing action is used to propel the ball with the elbow nearly fully extended. The dribbling arm stays extended with fingers pointed toward the ball and recontacts it after it bounces approximately two-thirds of the way up from the rebound. Upon contact, the forearm flexes and moves up with the ball; the hand remains in contact with the ball until after the downward push for the subsequent bounce. The fingers stay spread out to conform to the shape of the ball and the height of the bounce is maintained at approximately waist level (figure 9.17).

Climbing

Climbing is a fundamental locomotor skill that involves ascending and descending movement using the hands and feet. The upper limbs usually initiate primary control. Climbing, an outgrowth of creeping, often is performed before walking, especially if the opportunity to practice is made available. Unfortunately, little information is available concerning the developmental process components used in climbing. Depending on the conditions under which climbing takes place (ladders, frames, nets, ropes, or stairs), a number of movement pattern variations may be used. Most information available on climbing patterns (as defined in the context of upper body involvement) has been derived from ladder and stair climbing observations.

MOVEMENT PATTERN DESCRIPTIONS. Two basic movement patterns appear to predominate during ladder and stair climbing: the immature pattern of marking time and the advanced cross-lateral pattern. During the initial stages of climbing, movement is characterized by *marking time*. That is, the child steps up or down to the appropriate level with the same foot each time. This is followed by movement of the trailing foot to the same level (figure 9.18). The dominant arm initiates and guides the action, which is followed by leg movement on the same side. As with the foot action, both arms are placed on the same level before the next cycle begins.

With increased maturity and practice, the child progresses to the alternate-foot ascent and descent described as the *cross-lateral pattern*. That is, rather than placing both feet on the same level, the child

■ *Figure 9.18*

Marking time
pattern: (a) start
and (b) completion

a. b.

THINK ABOUT IT

Of the fundamental
skills described in
the Movements
Patterns section,
which ones are
culturally gender-
biased in children's
play and youth
sport activities?

alternates sides and places only one foot on each level (figure 9.19). Hand placement may vary from positioning both hands on the same level before following with leg action to the more advanced alternating pattern (matching the leg movements). With practice and confidence, the child prefers to reach for the next highest level, therefore displaying the alternating cross-lateral pattern with the arms as well.

DEVELOPMENTAL CHARACTERISTICS. Though there are wide differences in climbing ability at every age level, children as young as 2 years have been observed to display initial climbing patterns. By 6 years the majority of children are reasonably proficient climbers and

■ *Figure 9.19*

Cross-lateral
pattern: (a) start
and (b) completion

a. b.

exhibit the mature pattern characteristics. The skill of ascending an apparatus usually is achieved before an individual attempts to descend. Children are usually capable of skillfully descending ladders or stairs by 5 years of age. As one might expect, the physical characteristics of the climbing apparatus markedly may affect climbing performance (e.g., the angle, height, and distance between ladder rungs or step risers). It is not uncommon for children who normally use advanced climbing techniques when operating at low heights to revert to immature and cautious marking time movements when attempting to climb at a significantly greater height.

▦ *Fine Motor Manipulative Behavior*

Objective 9.6 ➤ In the discussion of early motor behavior (chapter 8) several developmental milestones were noted in relation to manual control. The primitive and rudimentary behaviors of reaching, grasping, and releasing that flourish during the prenatal stage and the first two years of life represent three developmental categories: reflexes, rhythmic stereotypies, and prehensile behaviors. The grasping (palmar) reflex appears prenatally and is suppressed by the fourth postnatal month. Rhythmic stereotypies appear in the arms, hands, and fingers shortly after birth and reach their peak during the second half of the first year. The peak of proficient prehensile behavior normally is displayed by 18 months of age. During this period most children are reasonably proficient in coordinating basic reaching and grasping skills, as evidenced by their ability to use a precision pincer grip and to effectively release objects.

The final stage of manual control (that is, before regression) is **manipulation.** Manipulation refers to skillful and refined use of the hands, such as in stringing beads, drawing, and writing. The development of several aspects of manipulation occurs during the early childhood period and shortly after (up to around 8 years of age). With an understanding of the development of manipulation skills and early motor behavior characteristics, a relatively complete picture of manual development is created.

Finger Differentiation

Although most children are capable of displaying a pincer (thumb and forefinger) grip around 9 to 10 months, it is several years before they are able to perform precision movements with individual fingers. One task commonly used to evaluate finger differentiation is the test of finger opposition. This task requires the individual to touch each finger, in their order on the hand, to the thumb. Generally the task is scored under speed stress (e.g., the number of cycles of finger opposition are counted within a given time). This finger opposition test frequently is used by

■ *Figure 9.20*

Manual control and speed (moving pegs)

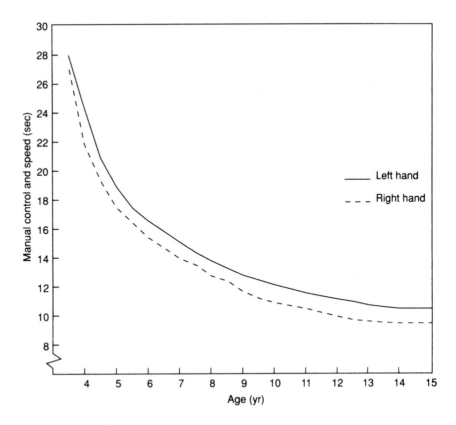

pediatric neurologists to identify possible impairment and by researchers to investigate the developmental characteristics of the hands.

Early signs of individual finger control (differentiation) appear within the first year of life, as evidenced by the appearance of stereotypic finger flexion, pseudo thumb opposition and, as noted earlier, true thumb-to-forefinger opposition by 10 months of age. However, the ability to oppose more than one finger to the thumb does not reveal its beginnings until around age 3. Initial efforts at this age usually require the tester to provide a slow visual demonstration. Regular improvement continues in finger differentiation until about age 8 when performance approximates that of adults.

Other tasks such as stringing beads, moving pegs, and picking up pennies or matchsticks and placing them in a container also are used commonly to determine level of manipulative ability. In general, studies involving these types of tasks have reported similar basic patterns of change. That is, improvement is greater during the early developmental years, with relatively small changes occurring after 8 to 10 years. Figure 9.20 illustrates this trend among individuals from 3 to 15 years of age with the results of a popular test reported by Annett (1970) that measures the speed of moving pegs.

TABLE 9.8

Selected Construction and Self-Help Achievements (Ages 1–4)

Achievement	Approximate Age (Mo)
Drinks from cup	13
Builds tower of two cubes	14
Use spoon	15
Builds tower of four cubes	18
Builds tower of eight cubes	24
Puts on shoes	36
Cuts paper	
Buttons up (clothes)	
Feeds self (spills very little)	
Pours well from pitcher	
Laces shoes	48
Brushes teeth	
Cuts paper following line	

Source: Data from *Denver II* (1990) and *Bayley II* (1993)

Construction and Self-Help Skills

Developmental scales such as the Denver Developmental Screening Test (1990) and Bayley II (1993) typically include several manual construction and self-help tasks. Along with assessing the fine motor abilities used in such tasks as building a block tower, these tasks highlight the importance of manual skills in everyday personal, or self-help, tasks. The attainment of such skills as tying one's shoes, buttoning a coat, holding and drinking from a cup, and feeding oneself with a spoon are considered major developmental achievements. Table 9.8 lists selected construction and self-help achievements attained during the early childhood period and commonly included in developmental assessment scales.

Drawing and Writing

Some of the most investigated aspects of fine motor manual control are the techniques and processes involved in writing and drawing. These skills progress from primitive scribbling and coloring to the highly coordinated and dynamic fine motor movements used to draw figures and write in cursive. In general, the development of drawing and writing follows the *proximodistal* trend, with males lagging behind females at virtually all ages; this is due in large part to females' advanced neurological maturity (e.g., Blote & Haastern, 1989).

◼ *Figure 9.21*

Basic holding grips: (a) the immature power grip and (b) the more advanced tripod

a.

b.

Around the age of 18 months, children can hold a writing or coloring implement (e.g., pencil or crayon) and by 4½ to 6 years have acquired an array of holding grips. Although a number of grips are applicable depending on the implement (e.g., pencil or paintbrush) and the condition (e.g., on a desk or at an upright easel), two basic developmental styles appear to be most prominent: the power grip and the tripod (figure 9.21). From these two basic styles, several variations exist.

The palmar grasp, also referred to as the *power grip*, is usually the initial technique used among children below the age of 3 years. With this style, all four fingers and the thumb are wrapped around the implement and most movement is initiated and guided by the shoulder and arm. The more advanced holding style is the tripod in which the implement is held by the thumb, index finger, and middle finger. During initial use of this style, the child will hold the implement with the proper tripod grip, but movement will still be controlled by the arm rather than hand.

The mature version of the basic tripod is the *dynamic tripod*. At this stage, development has reached the level of using the proper grip and skillfully manipulating the implement with the wrist, fingers, and thumb. The beginnings of dynamic manual control in this context are usually evident by age 4 and progress to a relatively mature level by 7 years, with refinement continuing through early adolescence (Ziviani, 1983).

The development of writing ability also progresses in a proximodistal order. That is, initial movements are through use of the shoulder and arm and then through the elbow. Finally the wrist, fingers, and thumb are used to execute dynamic manipulation. From the ages of 2 to 6 years, children's writing ability increases dramatically as the hand moves closer to the tip of the implement. See the Suggested Readings (Erhardt, 1994) for a detailed description and assessment techniques for the development of prehension skills, including writing and drawing grips.

The child's first attempts at drawing usually occur by accident around the age of 15 months while spontaneously scribbling. *Scribbling* is described as a type of kinesthetic, or motor, babbling similar to primitive vocalizations. This form of early drawing appears to be nonpurposeful and unrelated to any visual model. Depending on experience, by the approximate age of 3 or 4, development has progressed to the level that a definite organization in drawing and copying is evident.

Kellogg (1969), who collected and analyzed more than 1 million drawings done by children, describes the development of drawing abilities as a four-step process made up of the scribbling stage, the combine stage, the aggregate stage, and the pictorial stage.

The *scribbling stage* is characterized by random and repetitive actions that primarily produce circular shapes, then alternating (repetitive) lines. These movements soon become less spontaneous as the child slows down in attempting to control hand movements with visual attention. Less frequently observed lines at this stage are vertical (up-and-down), horizontal (back-and-forth), and diagonal.

The *combine stage* provides evidence the child is beginning to slow down and guide hand movements with the eyes. Characteristic of this stage is the child's effort to enclose space, as in completing a crude circle or square. This is also the period when basic geometric diagrams and combinations of diagrams are created. Common drawings at this stage include spirals, simple crosses, circles, squares, rectangles, triangles, and combinations of these shapes.

In the *aggregate stage*, the child not only combines figures but does so in multiples of three or more. This stage of development represents the ability to create more complex drawings. The final stage of basic drawing development, the *pictorial stage*, designates the child's ability to draw with more precision and complexity. As this ability develops the child begins to draw items from within his or her world with more detail and precision. Frequently chosen items include people (and faces), animals, transportation, and houses.

Most children appear to follow the progression suggested by Kellogg. However, the determination of age-related norms is difficult because this type of skill may be influenced greatly by environmental factors such as opportunities for practice, the particular drawing conditions, and availability of materials.

Most research in the area of drawing ability has been conducted in relation to copying figures. Copying tasks are standard items on most developmental assessment scales under the category of visual-motor coordination. The following discussion describes selected age-related drawing characteristics noted in the literature.

By the age of 2, children can crudely draw circular, vertical, and horizontal lines that follow the appropriate direction. However, the quality of performance among children may vary considerably. Knobloch and Pasamanick (1974) suggest the following general progression and approximate age expectancies for common figure copying: circle (36 months), cross (48 months), square (54 months), triangle (60 months), and the more difficult diamond (72 months). Tracing abilities for all forms are generally mature by 6 years.

The task of forming letters and numbers as required in handwriting tasks presents the child with additional manual challenges. By the age of 4 years, most children are capable of printing at least a few recognizable letters but frequently position them in a disorganized manner on the page. With adequate practice, many 5-year-olds are capable of printing their first names. By 6 years, most children can print the alphabet and the numbers up to 10. Lowercase letters seem to be more difficult to copy than uppercase letters. Younger children (ages 4 and 5) typically write in large letters and numbers that are commonly ½ to 2 inches high. By age 7, the height of the letter decreases to approximately ¼ inch. The ability to space letters remains a difficult task for many children until around 9 years of age.

Bimanual Control

Several manipulative activities require the controlled use of the two hands, or **bimanual control,** in a symmetrical or asymmetrical function. In *symmetrical function*, the two hands perform similar and simultaneous movements, such as those used in clapping and performing selected calisthenic exercises. The other form of bimanual control is more common to general manipulative behavior and is referred to as *asymmetrical function*. This term describes the function in which the two hands make different movements in a coordinated and complementary manner. This ability is evident in the performance of such tasks as cutting paper with scissors, tying shoelaces, and dealing cards. In each of these conditions, one hand is the primary manipulator, while the other functions in a complementary manner to position and stabilize the object.

Although they are not intentional (i.e., voluntary), symmetrical bilateral arm movements can be observed at birth in the form of primitive reflexes (e.g., the Moro reflex) and in the spontaneous behavior of newborns during the first month of life. The earliest patterns of bimanual activity (e.g., hand interplay and clasping) are primarily nonvisual and occur after 3 months of age. By 4 to 4½ months, when crude attempts at voluntary reaching are displayed, arm actions are still basically bilateral and symmetrical, even though one hand contacts the object first. Although some form of asymmetrical behavior also has been noted around this age, it is generally not before the end of the first year that the complementary characteristics of bimanual asymmetrical coordination are unquestionably present. The variety and complexity of tasks that can be performed using bimanual control increase enormously during childhood, though they may be unrefined.

Closely associated with proficiency of asymmetrical bimanual control is hemispheric lateralization and the establishment of a consistent hand preference. Although specific age-related changes are difficult to establish, children display basic mastery of asymmetrical and symmetrical bimanual control by 6 years just after hand preference has been established. From this basic foundation develops the motor control that ultimately manifests itself in the ability to perform complex bimanual skills.

Although age-related characteristics and the nature of developmental change have not been clearly established, a general trend has been noted. Apparently children progress from an early stage of crude bimanual movements that tend to be symmetrical to the development of unilateral behavior, or establishment of a preferred limb. With the development of a preferred and nonpreferred hand evolves more refined bimanual control that culminates in the role differentiation of the hands that is observed in most forms of asymmetrical manipulative behavior. Refer to Fagard (1990) in the Suggested Readings for a more comprehensive review of the development of bimanual coordination in children.

▪ *Functional (Motor) Asymmetries*

Objective 9.7 ➤ Complementing the development of motor control, especially during early childhood, is establishment of limb (hand and foot) and eye preference. As noted in previous chapters (brain lateralization), although the human body (and hemispheres) is symmetrical in general appearance, the paired limbs (hands and feet) and sensory organs (eyes and ears) are used in an asymmetric manner. The behavioral manifestations of this phenomenon are referred to as **functional asymmetries.** For example, in tasks where only one limb can be used, such as throwing or kicking a ball, most individuals exhibit a consistent preference for the use of one limb over the other (also known as handedness and footedness).

Although lateral preference most often is identified as *right-sided* or *left-sided*, some individuals do not consistently favor the use of one limb or the other on a specific task; these individuals are identified as *mixed-sided*. *Ambidexterity* is a somewhat confusing term in a neurological context and one that has received little attention in the developmental psychology literature. This term describes the use of either limb with somewhat equal proficiency on the same task. This characteristic does not necessarily indicate dual dominance of hemispheric control. It generally is believed that individuals possessing this ability with a specific task have adapted or trained their nonpreferred side to be as, or perhaps more, skillful than their dominant side for a specific skill(s). This type of behavior is evident in skilled (practiced) activities such as soccer, handball, and boxing that require proficiency in both limbs.

Following are brief discussions of the developmental characteristics associated with handedness, footedness, and eye preference behavior, which as noted earlier, are closely linked with the development of motor control during early childhood.

Handedness

Of the motor asymmetries, handedness has been investigated more than all the others combined. Hand preference on tasks such as writing, throwing a ball, hammering, stacking cubes, and cutting with scissors is currently the most widely used method of determining *degree* of handedness. It is generally acknowledged that handedness (and footedness) is a trichotomous continuum ranging from left to mixed to right, rather than a dichotomy (right or left only). With a series of tasks, many individuals will not exhibit a totally consistent right or left hand preference.

As noted in chapter 8, individuals generally become more right-handed with increasing age; in addition, approximately 90% of the population establish this preference (e.g., Gilbert & Wysocki, 1992; Hellige, 1993). By the middle of the first year, handedness becomes more evident, with most infants exhibiting a preference for the right hand for visually directed reaching. By 3 to 4 years of age children generally show differential hand preference (about 75% prefer the right limb at this time) and hand skill of a kind comparable to adult characteristics. At about 6 years, handedness (i.e., direction) is stable in most children, with about 90% preferring the right hand.

Is there a disadvantage to being left-handed? For many years, left-handedness was associated with cognitive and language dysfunctions and general motor clumsiness because left-handed individuals more often were found to have such deficits. However, these findings and assumptions were based more on clinical samples and have not been supported by more recent investigations of normal individuals.

Another interesting argument has been the suggestion that children who exhibit consistent (left or right) hand preferences are better

THINK ABOUT IT

Recent theory suggests that even though we have a hand preference, environmental (attentional) stimuli tied to task demands can modify limb selection. Can you think of an example?

coordinated than their inconsistent (mixed) counterparts (Gottfried & Bathurst, 1983; Tan, 1985). The implied underlying premise is that children who are more strongly lateralized (right or left) would exhibit more pronounced functional asymmetries in comparison to inconsistent peers. Although this hypothesis has found some support in general field tests of motor performance, it has not been verified through more rigorous experimental studies. However, the general notion that right-handers are more consistent and more lateralized than left-handers has gained considerable support in recent years (e.g., Hellige, 1993). Evidence has been associated primarily with information-processing (perceptual) abilities.

Footedness

A myriad of data are available on hand preference, but research on foot laterality is relatively limited. Compared to most handedness inventories, which consist of unimanual (e.g., writing, drawing and throwing) and bimanual (e.g., threading bolts, cutting paper and unscrewing lid) motor tasks, recommended foot preference tasks contain both stabilizing and manipulative characteristics. By operational definition, the *preferred* foot is the one used to manipulate an object or to lead out, as in kicking or jumping, while the nonpreferred limb is used as the primary stabilizer (Peters, 1988). Recommended tasks to measure footedness include kicking a ball, figure tracing with toes while standing, and foot stamping a target.

As noted earlier, the developmental course of foot preference behavior follows a similar general developmental trend as handedness; that is, there is a significant shift toward greater right-sidedness with increasing age. In comparison to the development of handedness, however, the genesis of foot preference exhibits a few unique characteristics. During early childhood about twice as many individuals are mixed-footed, compared to persons who do not exhibit a preferred hand. During late childhood a significant shift toward greater right-footedness with a corresponding decrease in mixed-footedness occurs, after which preferences remain relatively stable into adulthood with approximately 80% of adults favoring the right side. The incidence of left-footedness appears relatively consistent across the life span (Gabbard & Iteya, 1996).

What accounts for the mixed-footed phenomenon? One possible explanation is linked in part to Annett's Right-Shift hypothesis. It proposes that in individuals who lack a strong right-shift factor, limb preference may be determined at random. This suggests that environmental factors such as culture (the right-sided world phenomenon) and experience may influence *direction* and/or *degree* of preference. Considerations are that (1) footedness is a more unbiased index of lateral specialization because it is less subject to dextral social pressures than handedness, and (2) activities that require use of the feet (relative to those of the hands) are usually less complex and practiced. From these observations it seems likely the environmental factor that may affect (e.g., strengthen) degree of hand preference during childhood may be less of an influence on foot laterality. This would suggest that in those individuals who do not possess a strong biological propensity for right-side control, the probability of mixed-sidedness would seem greater for the feet than for the hands.

An interesting issue has emerged in contemporary literature associated with footedness: Which is the dominant limb, the one used to stabilize the body or the foot that is mobilized to lead out or manipulate (Gabbard & Hart, 1996)? Indeed, the consensus of research suggests that most humans are right-footed for actions of mobilization (operationally defined as the dominant limb) and left-sided for postural stabilization (Peters, 1988). Two theoretical positions support this general observation. Previc's (1991) neurodevelopmental explanation and MacNeilage's (1991) postural origins perspective both contend that humans are innately predisposed to stabilize on the left side. Although both theories refer to the notion of complementary role function of the limbs (one foot is used for postural support, the other for mobilizing action), tenets from each theory predict that most individuals, when placed in a bilateral or unilateral (stabilizing only) context, would favor the left side for postural control. However, there is evidence that when individuals are placed in a unilateral condition (e.g., one-leg static balance), they also prefer the right limb or have no preference (e.g., Armitage & Larkin, 1993; Hart & Gabbard, 1997; Katsarka et al., 1994). That is, while most individuals stabilize on the left side in the bilateral condition, they switch to the right in the unilateral context of balance. Left-footers also prefer the right or have no preference (mixed-footed) in this context. Similar findings have been noted in bilateral conditions that augment complexity of the stabilizing and mobilizing limbs; for example, when the setup makes stabilizing more difficult than the manipulative action (Hart & Gabbard, 1996). Interestingly, with virtually all foot tasks used in behavioral inventories (since most are bilateral actions), stabilizing requirements such as postural support while kicking a ball and foot tracing letters are relatively simple, compared to the demands of focused mobilization. What does this research suggest? Although these findings are not conclusive, they hint that in foot dominance, the preferred limb is reserved for the more difficult aspect of a behavioral activity. And, foot dominance should be defined operationally, in light of behavioral context (unilateral or bilateral) and demands (level of complexity) of the particular task performed.

Eye Preference

Eye preference can be observed when sighting a telescope or aiming a gunlike instrument. A review of research on eyedness suggests that, as with the other asymmetries described, most individuals prefer the right side, and degrees of right-eyedness increase between childhood and maturity. The levels of right-sidedness in adults, however, are not as high as with hand and foot preference. Approximately 70% of adults prefer the right eye (Bourass et al., 1996; Coren, 1993), whereas values for the same preference in children range between 55% to 60% (Nachshon et al., 1983; Porac et al., 1980). These data also suggest that the major shift over time, which complements the increase in right-sidedness, is a decrease in the incidence of left-eyedness. As with most functional asymmetries, there do not appear to be any differences due to gender.

Summary

Early childhood is characterized by fundamental movement actions that can be categorized into locomotor, nonlocomotor, and manipulative (gross and manual) behaviors. The developmental characteristics of locomotor and gross motor manipulative skills are described according to process-related movement pattern changes. Movement pattern status frequently is identified using terms that represent proficiency ranging from immature to mature, or minimal to sport skill form. The minimal characteristics normally are observed in children at ages 2 and 3. With adequate practice, most children acquire at least some features of the mature movement pattern by the end of the sixth year. However, some individuals may not achieve the mature stage until years later, if ever.

Two general approaches associated with describing and interpreting qualitative movement changes across time are the composite approach and component method. The composite approach describes the sequence of movement pattern changes through a series of total body (general pattern) stages. The component approach divides pattern changes into substages that depict specific body component changes.

A scientific and applied (e.g., teaching) body of information is available concerning the sequential progression and developmental characteristics of most fundamental locomotor and gross motor manipulative skills.

The final stage of manual control appears during early childhood in the form of manipulative behavior. Manipulation refers to the skillful and refined use of the hands, such as that displayed in tasks of finger differentiation, construction and self-help skills, and drawing and writing. As one would expect, the development of manual control abilities generally proceeds in a proximodistal direction.

Bimanual control involves the use of two hands in a symmetrical or asymmetrical function. Bimanual coordination clearly improves during childhood, with the initial actions being more symmetrical before complete role differentiation of the hands can be observed. Mastery of asymmetrical bimanual control seems to be associated with the development of hand preference. With the establishment of a preferred and nonpreferred hand, more highly refined bimanual control develops.

Closely linked to the development of manual and overall motor control during early childhood is establishment of limb and eye preference (functional asymmetries). A general developmental trend for all asymmetries is a shift toward greater right-sidedness with increasing age. Whereas adult right-sided values for handedness and footedness are close, during early childhood a significantly greater number of children express a consistent preference for right-handedness, compared to the lower limbs; thus, handedness appears to mature earlier. Right-eyedness is not as high as with hand and foot preference values at any period.

Think about It

1. Describe what a comprehensive study of walking skills could involve.
2. What is the role of nature/nurture in the development of fundamental movement patterns during early childhood? Consider information from previous chapters to support biological change.
3. How do table 9.3 (composite of throwing) and 9.4 (components for throwing) compare?
4. Of the fundamental skills described in the Movement Patterns section, which ones are culturally gender-biased in children's play and youth sport activities?
5. Recent theory suggests that even though we have a hand preference, environmental (attentional) stimuli tied to task demands can modify limb selection. Can you think of an example?

Suggested Readings

Adrian, M. J., & Cooper, J. M. (1994). *Biomechanics of human movement.* 2nd ed. Madison, New York: McGraw-Hill.

Erhardt, R. P. (1994). *Developmental hand dysfunction.* 2nd ed. San Antonio, TX: The Psychological Corporation.

Fagard, J. (1990). The development of bimanual coordination. In C. Bard, M. Fleury, & L. Hay (Eds.), *Development of eye-hand coordination.* Columbia, SC: University of South Carolina Press.

Hall, S. (2003). *Basic biomechanics.* 4th ed. New York: McGraw-Hill.

Knudson, D., & Morrison, C. (2002). *Qualitative analysis of human movement.* 2nd ed. Champaign, IL: Human Kinetics.

WebLinks

Information on Biomechanics (see the section on Gait and Locomotion)
www.per.ualberta.ca/biomechanics/

Michigan State University Department of Kinesiology Longitudinal Motor Performance Study
http://ed-web3.educ.msu.edu/KIN/Activities/mps.htm

10 *Motor Behavior during Later Childhood and Adolescence*

OBJECTIVES

Upon completion of this chapter, you should be able to

10.1 Provide an overview of the developmental milestones that occur during later childhood and adolescence.

10.2 Discuss the bases for age-related and gender-related quantitative (product) motor performance changes during later childhood and adolescence.

10.3 List and briefly describe the quantitative changes that occur in motor performance.

10.4 Discuss the influence of physical activity and sport participation on motor skill refinement.

KEY TERMS

product performance
gender-related differences
youth sports

physical education
developmentally
 appropriate

The Developmental Continuum

Phase	Approximate age	Stage
Reflexive/ Spontaneous	conception	Prenatal
Rudimentary	birth	Infancy
	6 mo.	
	2 years	
Fundamental Movement	6	Early Childhood
Sport Skill	12	Later Childhood
Growth & Refinement	18	Adolescence
Peak Performance	30	Adulthood
Regression	70	Older Adulthood

Objective 10.1

THINK ABOUT IT

Gender differences are a good example of biological/ environmental interaction. Explain this with regard to sports performance.

The PERIOD FROM LATER CHILDHOOD through adolescence (approximately 7 to 17 years of age) is characterized by several growth and development milestones, many of which are manifested in significant improvements in motor skill performance. Around the beginning of later childhood, individuals begin to use with increasing frequency the fundamental movement abilities acquired during early childhood. At the same time, changes in physical growth, body structure, and physiological development combine to produce greater **product performance**—that is, performance (outcome) values, as opposed to "process" form characteristics (chapter 9). This period also is distinguished by the emergence of sport skill behaviors. In essence, these behaviors are advanced versions of basic skills that are the primary vehicle by which the individual's increased level of motor behavior is displayed. Along with age-related improvements in motor performance that appear in both sexes during this period, **gender-related differences** may also come increasingly into play. This trend is especially apparent during the adolescent growth spurt.

This chapter will focus on the description and bases for quantitative changes in motor performance exhibited during preadolescence and the adolescent years. It also addresses the related issues of gender differences in motor performance and the refinement of fundamental skills as displayed by sport skill behavior.

Bases for Age- and Gender-Related Quantitative (Product) Motor Performance Changes

Objective 10.2 ➤ Quantitative changes in motor performance tend to parallel increasing levels of experience and changes in physical growth, physiological development, and neurological functioning. Previous chapters that described these changes have established that with advancing age, most individuals (both genders) experience increases in such characteristics as body size, muscle mass, strength, cardiorespiratory capacity, and perceptual-motor ability. As a result of these and other developmental changes, virtually all aspects of product-oriented motor performance show an upward trend beginning at the preschool level.

Differences between genders before puberty are minimal but they do exist. As early as 3 years of age, reports suggest that males tend to outperform females on selected tasks of running, throwing, and jumping. Females, on the other hand, appear to excel in hopping, skipping, and tasks requiring fine-motor control, balance, and flexibility (Broadhead & Church, 1985; Morris et al., 1982). Some performance differences have been attributed to biological factors such as body fat, which favor males, and advanced neurological development, which favor females. But it also seems quite likely that at this age level, environmental agents are a primary determinant. Several studies confirm that, beginning at the preschool level, males are generally more active than females (e.g., Baranowski et al., 1993, Branta et al., 1987; Centers for Disease Control and Prevention [CDC], 2000). Complementing this is the fact that parents and teachers usually express specific sex role expectations, which dictate that males and females should behave differently at play and sport. Thomas et al. (1991) note that from a physiological perspective, young females' overall motor performance should be better due to the faster maturation rate prior to puberty. The fact that their overall motor performance generally is not better argues for a sociocultural explanation.

With the onset of the adolescent growth spurt (from age 10 to 12), differences in motor performance product characteristics between the sexes become increasingly evident and generally favor the male. The literature reveals a consistent trend that shows males continue to improve in motor performance on a variety of skills through adolescence, but females have a tendency to peak around the age of 14 and then level off (plateau) or decrease in performance (e.g., Malina & Bouchard, 1991; Thomas et al., 1991). From another perspective, females mature earlier in motor performance, as evidenced by their achievement of adult performance levels at earlier ages than males achieve them (Haubenstricker et al., 1997). Remarkably, Haubenstricker and colleagues at Michigan State University are conducting a longitudinal study that has measured a large group of males and females for over 30 years, beginning at age 5. Their findings complement the aforementioned conclusions; however, their work shows that females' performance on a number of motor tasks continues to improve between 14 and 18 years of age.

THINK ABOUT IT

From your experience, describe cultural gender bias in sports and physical activity.

Although cultural practices and participation levels may significantly influence the range of individual differences within and between genders during this period, numerous biological factors may provide an advantage to males in several motor skill activities. Earlier discussions have highlighted that the primary factors that provide males with a biological advantage over females in motor performance are sex chromosomes and hormones. Most of these factors become increasingly apparent after the age of 10 years. Table 10.1 on page 336 presents a list of selected biological differences between genders. The earlier chapters on physical growth (chapter 3) and physiological changes (chapter 4) are useful for reviewing their discussion of the biological differences between genders.

In general, males tend to be larger and have more muscle mass, less body fat, and a greater oxygen transport capacity than their female counterparts. These characteristics give males the biological advantage in performing activities that require strength, power, and endurance. Because females possess more body fat and less muscle mass, they are at a distinct disadvantage in performing motor tasks that require lifting the body (e.g., jumping) or moving their mass against gravity (e.g., running).

As noted earlier, several research studies that involve children and adults confirm a negative relationship between body fatness and performance on tasks that require the vertical and horizontal movement of the body weight (e.g., Smoll & Schutz, 1990; Thomas et al., 1991). In essence, body fat adds to the mass of the body without contributing to force-producing capacity. Swimming is one activity for which a higher body fat value may be an advantage. Higher values of body fat have been shown to allow individuals to swim higher in the water with less body drag. Though this factor may decrease the difference between the sexes, males still tend to outperform females in swimming events simply because they are stronger.

Structural factors that provide a mechanical advantage also may favor males in sprinting, jumping, and throwing skills. Males have longer arms and wider shoulders, which produce the leverage and rotation

TABLE 10.1

Selected Biological Differences between Genders

Male	Female
Tissue	
Lower percent body fat	
Greater muscle mass (stronger)	
Heavier (greater body density)	
Anatomical structure	Greater angle of insertion of femur (more oblique) to the hip
Taller	
Wider shoulders (more rotation torque)	Lower center of gravity
Longer legs (relative to total height)	Wider hips (relative to shoulder width)
Longer forearms (more lever torque)	Shorter legs
Narrower hips relative to shoulder width	
Larger thoracic cavity (chest girth)	
Physiological functioning	Tends to exhibit better balance and flexibility
Larger heart (greater basal stroke volume and cardiac output)	
Greater maximal oxygen uptake (consumption)	
Faster heart rate recovery	
Greater physical working capacity	
More blood volume	
Greater number of red blood cells	
Higher mean hemoglobin values	
Greater vital capacity	
Greater ventilation volume	
Greater basal metabolic rate (active tissue)	

Source: Data from Brooks & Fahey (1985) and Eckert (1987)

torque needed to forcefully propel objects in throwing or striking activities. Longer legs and narrower hips also may tend to be advantageous in sprinting and jumping tasks. Greater proportionate hip width and angle of insertion of the femur in females has been suggested as a mechanical disadvantage in achieving maximal running speed for sprinting. On the other hand, because females generally have a lower center of gravity and wider hips, they may have the advantage in motor skills that require a high degree of balance. Although females tend to outperform males at virtually all ages on tests of flexibility, current evidence does not suggest that biological factors account for the difference.

Although biological factors such as neurological maturity, body size, anatomical structure, and physiological functioning can influence performance differences, social and cultural agents also may offer the explanation for some of the variation. This may be the case particularly when the motor task involves a high degree of skill (e.g., skipping and throwing) rather than higher levels of basic strength and cardiorespiratory endurance.

Performance of tasks that require a higher degree of skill (i.e., coordination and refinement) can be influenced significantly by practice. Although the trend certainly is changing, males and females in the United States tend to practice only those physical activities traditionally regarded as male-oriented or female-oriented, respectively. That is, young females tend to participate more often in activities that involve skipping, hopping, and perhaps flexibility and fine motor control. Young males of virtually all ages traditionally spend more time in physical activities that practice running, throwing, jumping, and striking skills. Though females today participate in many more traditionally male-oriented activities (e.g., females play baseball, softball, soccer, and football) and vice versa (e.g., males dance and play volleyball), some segments of society still adhere to the more traditional gender roles. It can be speculated this practice may discourage individuals from attaining their potential in specific motor skills.

Assuming the presence of a cultural stymie that, at least to some degree, hinders the level of practice and optimal motor skill potential among females, it is predictable that females will experience an early plateauing effect in their performance compared to males. Interestingly, in describing data collected during the 1950s, Eckert (1987) notes European females continue to improve their running, throwing, and jumping skills up to 16 to 18 years of age. Their American counterparts, in contrast, displayed a leveling off between age 13 and 15. It may be assumed from this data that cultural values have an effect on motor skill performance.

Similar findings of a plateauing effect or decline among females after the age of 12 also have been reported for tests of physical fitness (Thomas et al. 1991). In this instance, it has been speculated that females in our society are less likely than males to be encouraged and motivated to improve their fitness levels through vigorous training. Part of the problem appears to be the perpetuation of the myth that physical activity in females leads to greater masculinization and increases the risk of injury.

Although differences that favor males still exist for most tests of motor performance (especially on strength-related tasks), in recent years females appear to be narrowing that differential. This trend seems to be related to increased participation in physical fitness and sports programs, effective school and university programs, an increase in athletic scholarships and participation opportunities (through Title IX), and a gradual change in society's view of female participation in sports.

THINK ABOUT IT

What is your community's view of female participation in all types of sport?

A word of caution should be given regarding the general interpretation of gender differences. Though clear-cut differences that generally favor males are evident sometimes very early in their development, comparisons normally are based on average performance data by group (males and females). In nearly all motor performance studies large individual differences exist within the sexes at each age level. For example, even though the mean performance of males may be significantly greater on a specific motor skill, the performance of some females certainly may equal or exceed that of some males. Therefore, mean data may be useful from a developmental perspective, but the true developmentalist is also sensitive to individual progress.

Quantitative (Product) Changes in Motor Performance

Objective 10.3 ➤ Running performance commonly is measured by requiring the individual to run as fast as possible (sprint) over a distance of 30 to 50 yards. Performance times usually are reported in tenths of a second and then, for comparative purposes, are converted to feet or yards covered per second. The speed with which an individual can run depends significantly on the length of the stride as well as the stride rate. Stride and leg *length* generally increase with age, whereas stride *rate* remains relatively constant. Thus, an increase in running velocity may not be due to an ability to move the legs more frequently but to propel the body farther with each stride.

Running Speed

Age-related improvements in running speed can be explained in large part by the increase in body size and muscular strength. Figure 10.1 shows performance curves for males and females originally composed by Espenschade (1960) after a review of the literature up to that period. Espenschade reported that velocity in both sexes increases for an average rate of just under 4 yards per second at age 4, to slightly over 6 yards per second at age 12. Males continue to increase in velocity up to age 17 (about 7 yards per second), but females begin to level off or regress slightly beginning around age 13. A review of studies since 1960 confirms this trend for males but reports slightly higher scores for females (Haubenstricker et al., 1997). The review did not find a regression of performance in females after age 13 or 14 but identified a plateauing trend up to age 17. Similar performance patterns have been reported for a test of *agility*, the ability to change the direction of the body rapidly. A popular test is the 30-foot shuttle run. Improvement occurs through childhood with males displaying an edge that increases after 13 years and females plateauing around age 15 (figure 10.2).

▦ *Figure 10.1*

Running speed
curves

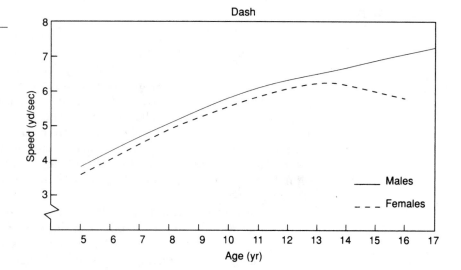

▦ *Figure 10.2*

Agility run scores
(30-foot shuttle)

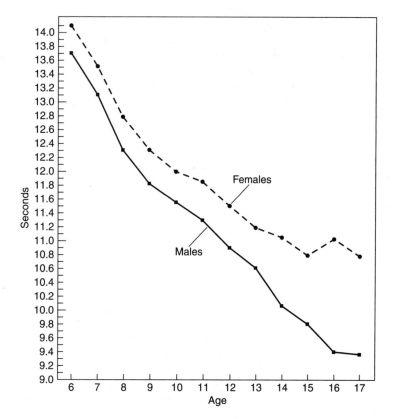

Throwing

The quantitative characteristics of throwing most often are determined by measuring the maximum distance thrown, throwing velocity, and accuracy. Both sexes improve dramatically from childhood to adolescence on all three abilities, but gender differences (that favor males) appear quite early and are relatively large in comparison to other fundamental skills. As noted earlier, it may be speculated that much of the difference that favors males is due to their greater strength, biomechanical characteristics, and the fact that females generally exhibit less mature throwing patterns. Another consideration is the possibility that cultural and social factors provide a positive influence for the development of throwing among males.

Regardless of throwing task, balls projected by the overhand throw have been measured more frequently than those of any other movement pattern. The distance an individual can throw has received the most attention in the developmental literature. Although gender differences are more obvious at the younger ages and become greater over time, throwing distance performance curves show trends similar to those found with running speed performance (figure 10.3). That is, both genders improve up to puberty (12 to 14 years). After this, males continue to improve performance, and females begin to level off and then decline in performance. Unlike running speed performance, however, recent studies do not indicate that female performances in throwing plateau rather than decline after puberty (Haubenstricker & Seefeldt, 1986). Espenschade (1960) reported from a review on the topic that throwing distances for males increased from approximately 24 feet at age 5 to about 153 feet at age 17. In contrast, females threw 14.5 feet at age 5,

■ *Figure 10.3*

Throwing distance curves

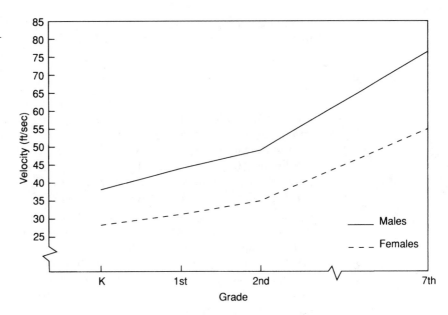

▪ *Figure 10.4*

Longitudinal changes in ball throwing velocities

75.7 feet at age 15, and then declined to 74 feet at age 16. From this data and that reported by Keogh and Sugden (1985), it is clear that both sexes display dramatic improvements in distance thrown during the preadolescent period when scores more than triple. Furthermore, male performance by age 17 more than doubles that of female performance. Females and males apparently increase relatively more in the ability to throw for distance than they do in other fundamental skills.

Although the number of developmental studies has been somewhat limited, changes in horizontal ball velocities (speed) at various ages have been reported. Figure 10.4 shows the results of a longitudinal study of throwing velocity changes from kindergarten through the seventh grade (Halverson et al., 1982). In this study, females improved from an average of 29 feet per second while in kindergarten, to an average of 56 feet per second by the seventh grade. As one would expect, the scores of males also improved over the study period and were significantly greater than those of the females—39 feet per second in kindergarten, to 78 feet per second in the seventh grade. Like distance thrown performance, both males and females improve in throwing velocity dramatically through childhood, and gender differences appear early and are relatively large.

Because testing procedures associated with throwing accuracy have varied considerably, an acceptable developmental description of throwing cannot be given. However, the general statement that individuals improve with age through childhood and that males are usually more accurate than females is well supported. Since distance and the target area usually are confined, and the production of force is not as critical (that is, throwing for maximum distance and velocity), gender differences in throwing accuracy are not as marked.

Jumping

A considerable amount of developmental information has been gathered on jumping ability as measured by the standing (horizontal) long jump and vertical jump. Although data have been amassed from a multitude of studies, the general patterns of change are quite similar.

Figure 10.5 shows general performance curves for the standing long jump. Both sexes improve approximately 3 to 5 inches per year to around age 11; males jump 3 to 5 inches farther than females at each age (Keogh & Sugden, 1985). After that period, males continue to improve to at least age 17, whereas the female scores begin to level off and reach a peak at around age 14. In her review of the literature, Espenschade (1960) determined that at age 17, males achieve an average long jump of approximately 90 inches, whereas females reach a peak of about 64 inches at 14 years of age. Haubenstricker and associates' (1997) more recent report confirms the general trend across time, but it reports somewhat higher scores for females.

Data for the vertical jump (jump-and-reach task) provide similar performance curves to those for horizontal jumping (figure 10.6). Males improve from approximately 2 inches at age 5 to about 17 inches at age 17. Females also show significant improvement by starting out just below the males at age 5 and reaching a peak of approximately 12 inches by

■ *Figure 10.5*

Standing long jump performance curves

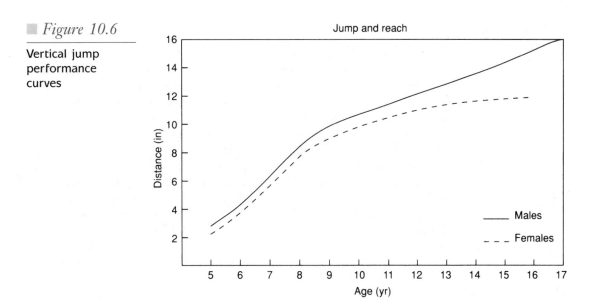

■ *Figure 10.6*

Vertical jump
performance
curves

age 16. As noted in figure 10.6, a plateauing of female performance begins around the age of 11.

Kicking

Perhaps no other fundamental or sport skill has received the attention that has been given to kicking over the last 15 years or so, due to the increasing popularity of soccer in the United States. Unfortunately, even with such focus on this sport, little product data on kicking are available.

The kicking performance of individuals is difficult to measure in quantitative terms prior to the age of 5 years. This is due primarily to lack of experience and lack of ability to judge ball speed and coordinate the movement pattern. After this period, however, the ability to kick a ball with force and accuracy becomes consistent enough to allow a fairly reliable measurement and assessment of ability. The quantitative characteristics of kicking most often are determined by measuring the distance a ball is kicked, velocity, and kicking accuracy. In keeping with the previous general developmental trend noted with running, throwing, and jumping, available data suggest that kicking performance improves with increasing age (for both genders) through childhood regardless of the test; males generally perform better than females. In addition, the differences between male and female kicking performance tend to increase as children get older (DeOreo & Keogh, 1980). However, as noted earlier, much of the available data predate 1970. As of this writing, little has been reported for ages beyond 12 years.

Catching

Catching is a coincident timing task that involves the complex interplay of coordinating visual information and motor behavior to a single point of interception (refer to chapter 6). The information-processing literature suggests the ability of individuals to accurately time their movements to an interception point with a moving object improves through childhood before it reaches a relatively mature level in the early teens. In the review by Williams (1983), it was noted that several developmental trends in the ability to judge the speed, direction, and interception point of a moving object can be observed between the ages of 6 and 11 years. Older children (from ages 9 to 11) are generally much more accurate in judging the flight of a moving object than younger children are. Though these data provide useful information with which to understand the perceptual and motor mechanisms prerequisite to the successful interception of objects, they do not provide specific product performance information. One should also keep in mind that experience has been shown to be a better indicator of coincident timing ability than age is (Kuhlman & Beitel, 1997).

Unfortunately, much of the literature concerning the quantitative characteristics of young children's catching ability is unclear, because many research studies have used scoring systems that reflect the process by which the object is intercepted as well as the actual success of the catch. It also should be noted that although much of the literature describes 6- to 8-year-olds as relatively proficient catchers, much of this information was collected when a large ball was used and the thrower was positioned directly in front of a ball tossed slowly from about 6 feet away.

Studies that have focused primarily on the end product characteristics of catching (i.e., interception and control of the ball), under simple and complex conditions, suggest that males and females display yearly increases in performance through the elementary years and, in some cases, beyond (e.g., Fischman, et al., 1992; Williams & Breihan, 1979). These data appear to parallel the information related to the development of perceptual-motor and coincident timing abilities. In the Fischman et al. investigation, one-hand catching was studied among a sample of 5- to 12-year-olds. Subjects were tossed tennis balls at four different locations (waist height, shoulder height, above the head, and out to the side) from 9 feet away and scored by the number caught. Results indicated that catching performance improved with age, with males outperforming females. One of the noted conclusions is that even 5-year-olds were able to integrate, to some degree, perception and motor response. The literature is mixed with regard to gender differences; therefore, a clearcut statement cannot be made. Along with the general age-related trend of increased catching ability, the literature also suggests that improvement is characterized by the ability to catch increasingly smaller balls and display more sophisticated hand-catching techniques.

Striking with an Implement

Striking is a coincident timing skill that presents difficulty for those who would attempt to establish a precise developmental picture of product performance. This inherent problem is that striking skills are performed in a variety of planes (overhand, sidearm, and underhand) and under widely varying conditions. Along with a wide assortment of striking motions, other variables include the size and type of ball, and the striking implement. The diversity of popular sports that use striking skills includes softball, tennis, hockey, golf, and volleyball. Although a limited number of studies have assessed product characteristics across the broad spectrum of striking, a clear and persistent trend of yearly increases through childhood (and perhaps beyond) has been identified. In contrast to the interception skill of catching, however, most data indicate that males are better strikers than females.

Much of the data on the product characteristics of striking have been collected by measuring striking velocity, distance the ball travels, and number of hits (out of a set number of trials). Williams (1983) reported that velocity with the one-arm and two-arm sidearm motion (using a racquetball racquet) improved substantially for both sexes from 4 to 8 years. Interestingly, one-arm striking performances were slightly better than two-arm striking performances. It has been speculated this is due to a young child's difficulty in effectively timing the motion with two hands. Unfortunately, little information is available in relation to the distance a ball travels after being struck. One generally would expect distance (force) performance trends to parallel those found in velocity scores (as in throwing and kicking); however, there has not been enough evidence gathered to make such a statement.

Perhaps the most commonly used measure of striking performance has been number of hits. Two studies cited most often were conducted by Seils (1951) and Johnson (1962). In both investigations, children were positioned with a bat in a typical batter's stance and asked to strike a ball attached at the end of a rope and swung over the plate. Similar results were found; both sexes increased in their striking ability at successive grade levels; at each grade, males performed better than females.

Although there appears to be a general trend toward improvement through the childhood years, the characteristics associated with change in general striking ability have not been identified clearly.

Hopping

We learned in chapter 9 that hopping is the most difficult form of basic jumping and is an integral part of several advanced movement skills used in games, dance, and gymnastic activities. The movement presents difficulty because it requires leg strength, balance, and controlled rhythmical movement. During the childhood years, hopping is one of the fundamental skills in which gender differences favor the female. In terms of quantitative characteristics, hopping usually is measured by determining (a) the number of consecutive hops completed before balance is lost, (b) the ability to complete a specified distance (usually 25 or 50 feet) while in balance, and (c) the time required to hop a specified distance. Available data suggest that hopping abilities, regardless of the particular type of task, generally improve with age through childhood and females perform better than males. Unfortunately, minimal data are available for individuals beyond the elementary years; thus, the developmental perspective is limited.

By 3½ years of age, most children have the ability to hop repeatedly for three steps (the definition of a true hop); by age 5 the ability to hop 10 consecutive times is normal. Keogh (1965) investigated the ability of children from ages 5 to 9 to hop 50 feet without stopping or exchanging hopping legs. In his findings he reported that with advancing age, an increasing percentage of children completed the distance and females were approximately one year ahead of the males in acquiring the ability. Hopping speed over a specified distance also improves with age during childhood. Cratty (1986) suggests that by age 5, most children can hop a distance of 50 feet in about 10 seconds and females are approximately 3.5 seconds faster than males.

On tests of rhythmical hopping ability, both genders improve with age during childhood. However, as with other tests of hopping ability, females tend to be as much as a year in advance of males. In a rhythmical test consisting of two hops on one foot followed in rhythm by two hops on the other foot, a significantly greater percentage of females than males passed at each age of 5 through 9 years (Keogh, 1968). This type of hopping task seemed particularly difficult for young males; only 3% of 5-year-old males performed acceptably compared to 23% of the females. By age 9 both sexes displayed significant improvement in rhythmical hopping (67% of males passed compared to 87% of females).

Ball Bouncing and Dribbling

Although ball bouncing and dribbling (i.e., three or four consecutive bounces) are two of the most widely practiced fundamental and sport skills, little product data are available. Early research by Wellman (1937) established that an important developmental consideration in ball handling ability is the size of the ball in relation to the size of the hand. According to Wellman's research, 2-year-olds using one hand generally are able to bounce a ball 9½ inches in circumference for a distance of 1 to 3 feet. By the age of 40 months, the distance improves to approximately 4 to 5 feet. By 46 months, a child using both hands can bounce a 16¼-inch ball a distance of 4 to 5 feet, and around the age of 6, the same distance can be achieved using only one hand.

In an unpublished study by Williams and Breihan (1979) as reported by Williams (1983), males and females aged 4, 6, and 8 were asked to use one hand to bounce an 8-inch ball repeatedly within a 12-inch square. Results indicated that performances for both genders improved with advancing age. Whereas males performed better than the females at ages 4 and 6, females were substantially better at 8 years. As a group, the 4-year-olds averaged less than two successful bounces within the square before they lost control. In contrast, 6-year-olds averaged four controlled bounces and the 8-year-olds slightly more than five good bounces.

This topic should be studied more extensively to develop a more complete picture of dribbling as a sport skill. Currently no information is available that assesses dribbling performance in which the child uses the right and left hands while moving.

Balance

As noted in chapter 6 under the discussion of vestibular awareness, the successful performance of virtually all motor skills depends on the individual's ability to establish and maintain equilibrium, or balance. Refer to that chapter for a review of the development of balancing abilities through adolescence.

Motor Skill Refinement

Objective 10.4 ➤ Sports and physical education are two of the most influential developmental factors in motor skill development and refinement during childhood and adolescence. Sport and other physical activity participation normally occur through school programs, spontaneous play activities, and organized youth sport programs. The dramatic increase in nonschool youth sport programs has received considerable attention from developmentalists in recent years.

Youth Sport Participation

Estimates suggest that more than 26 million American children, ages 6 to 17 years, are engaged in an organized program of **youth sports** (Sporting Goods Manufacturers Association, [SGMA] 2002). This figure is 54% of the estimated 48.5 million individuals aged 6 to 17. Females account for about 44% of the total, which represents an increasing trend over the last decade. The term *youth sports* has been applied to any athletic program that provides a systematic sequence of practices and contests for children and youth. Approximately 50 different individual and team sport activities, ranging from baseball to long-distance running, have been identified.

■ *Figure 10.7*

Soccer accounts for a large portion of youth sport participation

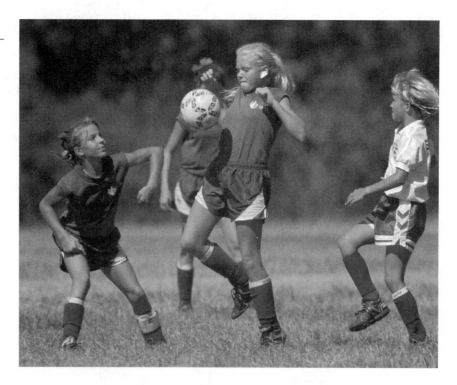

Seefeldt and Branta (1984) suggest six explanations for the increased participation of children in youth sport programs:

1. Passage of Title IX, which mandates equal opportunities in sport at all levels for females. This has had a great impact on overall participation. For example, over the period 1999 to 2000, there was an increase of +41% in the number of females playing on high school varsity teams (SGMA, 2002).

2. Greater accessibility to programs due to the gradual movement of the population from rural to urban residences.

3. Changing lifestyles of adults, including greater concern for health and physical fitness, may be influencing the decisions parents make about children's participation in physical activities that include sports.

4. An increase in the number of women in the workforce. It may be speculated that this has led to an increase in the enrollment of children in activity programs as a caretaking function. It also may be that some single-parent mothers view the coach as an additional role model for their child and want to encourage that interaction. Of course, this could be true for single-parent fathers as well.

5. Glorification of sport. The media's constant focus on the glory of sport undoubtedly leads some parents to involve their child in sport at an early age. Some parents perceive sport involvement as an

avenue through which to increase their child's opportunities for social and financial success.

6. Declining role of public schools in providing sport programs below the high school level. This has stimulated increased involvement by municipal recreation and community agencies in providing activity programs.

Other explanations for the increase in youth sport participation include the fact that children are getting involved at an earlier age; programs for 4- and 5-year-olds are commonplace today. Modifications of popular sports, such as T-baseball and small fry soccer, make such programs more enticing to parents. Increased participation in what is considered nontraditional sport activities (e.g., roller hockey, in-line skating, and snowboarding) and the dramatic increase in the number of programs and events organized for handicapped individuals (e.g., wheelchair bowling, tennis, softball; and Special Olympics) are two other areas of increased involvement in sport activity.

With regard to the increasing trend among 6- to 17-year-olds of selecting nontraditional sport activities, some interesting figures have been reported (SGMA, 2002). In-line skating participation, for example, increased over 600% from 1990 to 2000. Over the same period, gains of 180% were made in snowboarding, 110% in roller hockey, 92% in mountain biking. Perhaps it is no surprise that the popularity of soccer has increased by 76% over the last decade, due in some part, to the success of the U.S. men's and women's team in recent World Cup competition.

The SGMA report also indicated that organized basketball attracted the most members (slightly more than 10 million). The figure was followed by the increasingly popular soccer participation at 9.6 million members. Following these sports were baseball at 7.5 million, slow-pitch softball at 3.6 million, and tackle football at 2.9 million. Once again, females represented about 44% of total participation. It also should be noted that about 10 additional children reported playing at least one team sport, but they were not a formal member of a team. It is estimated that about 40 million formal team members and pick-up players participate in some form of youth sports (figure 10.7).

Interscholastic Sports With regard to participation in interscholastic sports in high school, table 10.2 on page 350 shows figures from 1993 regarding the 10 most popular activities. The report noted that participation among females had increased significantly over the years, especially in soccer, volleyball, and softball. It can be speculated that much of this interest is due to the growing popularity of female sport in general, as evidenced by the increase in programs (and scholarship opportunities) at the college and university levels.

Although involvement in youth sport programs has been found to contribute significantly to the participant's physical, psychomotor, social,

TABLE 10.2

Ten Most Popular Interscholastic Sports

Boys	Rank	Girls
Football	1	Basketball
Basketball	2	Outdoor track and field
Baseball	3	Volleyball
Outdoor track and field	4	Fast-pitch softball
Soccer	5	Soccer
Wrestling	6	Tennis
Cross country	7	Cross country
Tennis	8	Swimming and diving
Golf	9	Field hockey
Swimming and diving	10	Slow pitch softball

Source: National Federation News (1993).

and emotional development, several issues have been raised in relation to potential psychological and physical harm. Frequently addressed issues include the related competitive stress and anxiety, drop-out rate, the physical risks, especially in contact and collision sports, and the effects of intense early participation.

Are youth sports harmful? In chapter 5 we addressed this question with regard to sport training effects and childhood growth—namely, pubertal growth. In general, the evidence suggests that growth is not affected adversely by typical sports training of less than 18 hours per week. Of course, both physical and psychological intensity with fewer or more hours could produce a different conclusion. The importance of this issue prompted the American Academy of Pediatrics to form a statement regarding "intensive training and sports specialization in young athletes" (2000). The primary concern is young athletes who specialize in just one sport may be denied the benefits of varied activity while they face additional physical and psychological demands from intense training and competition. While supporting selected psychological (self-esteem) and physical benefits (cardiac and musculoskeletal growth) of sports training, the report states that little information is available on the possible short-term and long-term health consequences of intensive training in young athletes. One of the difficulties is lack of a clear definition of *specialized* and *intensively trained*. In addition, as a general human development principle, there is a wide variation in individual tolerance to specific conditions. The reports confirms that only a small minority of young athletes experience adverse effects. It appears, however, that those who participate in a variety of sports and specialize only after reaching

■ *Figure 10.8*

In-line skating became a popular activity in the 1990s

puberty tend to be more consistent performers, have fewer injuries, and adhere to sports play longer than those who specialize early. In conclusion the report recommended the following:

1. Children should be encouraged to participate in sports at a level consistent with their abilities and interests. Pushing children beyond these limits is discouraged as is specialization in a single sport before adolescence.
2. The child athlete should be coached by persons knowledgeable about proper training techniques, equipment, and the unique physical, physiologic, and emotional characteristics of young competitors.
3. In the absence of prospective markers of excessive physical stress, physicians and coaches should strive for early recognition, prevention, and treatment of overuse injuries (tendinitis, apophysitis, stress fractures, and shin splints).
4. A pediatrician should regularly monitor the conditions of child athletes involved in intense training.

5. The intensely trained, specialized child athlete needs ongoing assessment of nutritional intake, with particular attention to total calories, a balanced diet, and intake of iron and calcium.

6. A pediatrician should educate the child athlete, family, and coach about the risks of heat injury and strategies for prevention.

Refer to the Suggested Readings for additional information on this topic. Chapter 13 will discuss selected psychological considerations (self-esteem and gender roles).

Ironically, even with the large number of youth participating in sports and other community activities, nearly half of all American youth 12 to 21 years of age are not active on a regular basis. In fact, physical activity declines dramatically with age for both genders during adolescence (CDC, 2002).

School Physical Education

Another potentially powerful source for motor skill and physical fitness development is the school **physical education** program. As noted in chapter 5, the problem of national health among children and adults is clear. For example, more than half of the adults in the U.S. are overweight or obese, and 60% of adults are not active enough physically to reap any significant health benefits. A sedentary lifestyle almost doubles one's risk for coronary heart disease, a condition that can begin to develop in childhood. With regard to children and youth, almost one-quarter of children are now overweight; overall the percentage has doubled in the last 30 years. With this has emerged Type 2 diabetes, which is strongly linked to obesity in adults.

Many children watch too much television and are not active physically, and the overall trend appears to be increasing, especially among young females. Participation in all types of physical activity declines dramatically as age and grade in school increase. For example, nearly 50% of young people age 12 to 21 are not active on a regular basis. This trend results in about 60% of adults who do not achieve the recommended amount of physical activity. Today, only about 25% of children participate in any type of daily physical education. Daily participation in physical education by adolescents has declined dramatically, from 42% to 27% in 1997. See chapter 5 for references and Suggested Readings on this subject.

Most researchers and educators agree that one of the solutions to the problem is *quality school physical education,* more specifically, school programs that are **developmentally appropriate.** This means a program of activities that meets the individual's level of physical and psychological development (e.g., National Association for Sport and Physical Education [NASPE], 1992). Activities may be age-related, but not age-determined, which thus supports the principle of individual differences.

THINK ABOUT IT

Reflect on your physical education experience in schools. Did it promote health-related activity?

NASPE provides a variety of resources (e.g., national standards, appropriate practices, outcomes, and guidelines) to help parents, schools, and communities develop quality sport and physical education programs. Their position is that children and youth should learn how to be active physically in ways that increase physical competence, self-esteem, and enjoyment through physical activity. An example of a quality physical education program would include the following characteristics:

- Instruction by physical education specialists who have baccalaureate degrees;
- Required physical education all grade levels, preferably 30 minutes daily, for at least 150 minutes a week;
- Instruction in a variety of developmentally appropriate physical activities;
- Use of fitness assessment and education to help children understand, enjoy, improve, and/or maintain their physical health and well-being;
- Opportunities through physical activity participation to develop social and cooperative skills and to gain a multicultural perspective;
- Classes designed for ALL children to be involved in activities that provide maximum opportunity to be active continuously;
- Instruction in healthy eating habits and good nutrition.

Summary

The period from later childhood through adolescence encompasses the sports skill and growth and refinement phases of motor behavior and is marked by rapid biological change, increases in product performance, gender-related differences, and the emergence of sport skill behavior. Many of the quantitative (product) changes in motor performance are based on increasing levels of experience and a variety of characteristics associated with the adolescent growth spurt (e.g., increased body size, muscle mass, strength, and cardiorespiratory capacity). Several biological factors may provide an advantage to the male in some motor skill activities, but cultural practices and participation levels significantly can influence wide individual differences within and between the genders. In general, females appear to be closing the gender gap that was quite wide in earlier years. This trend seems to be related to increased participation and a change in society's view of females in sporting activities. However, a general and rather consistent trend in product performance (e.g., run, jump, and throw) change is that both genders improve significantly from childhood to adolescence and that males continue to improve on a variety of skills through adolescence (to at least age 17), whereas females have a tendency to peak around the age of 14.

Organized youth sport programs and school physical education programs are two of the most influential factors in motor skill development and refinement. In recent years there has been a dramatic increase in youth sport participation with a wide variety of activities offered for both genders. Although numerous developmental contributions have been linked to participation in organized youth sport programs, several issues have been raised in relation to their potential to result in psychological and physical harm.

School physical education, if presented in a developmentally appropriate manner, can do much to improve the state of physical fitness in the United States.

Think about It

1. Gender differences are a good example of biological/environmental interaction. Explain this with regard to sports performance.
2. From your experience, describe cultural gender bias in sports and physical activity.
3. What is your community's view of female participation in all types of sport?
4. From your experience, what are the positives and negatives in youth sport?
5. Reflect on your physical education experience in schools. Did it promote health-related activity?

Suggested Readings

American Academy of Pediatrics (2000). *Intensive training and sports participation in young athletes. Pediatrics* 106:154–157.
American Sport Education Program (2002). Champaign, IL: Human Kinetics.
NASPE Coaching Education & Sport publications. See publications under American Alliance for Health, Physical Education, Recreation, and Dance website.

WebLinks

American Academy of Pediatrics (Policy statement on medical concerns in the female child and adolescent athlete)
www.aap.org/policy/RE0003.html

American Academy of Pediatrics (Puberty information for boys and girls)
www.aap.org/family/puberty.htm

American Alliance for Health, Physical Education, Recreation, and Dance (Youth sport skill development resources)
www.aahperd.org

American College of Sports Medicine
    www.acsm.org

American Sport Education Program
    www.asep.com

Centers for Disease Control and Prevention (guidelines for school and community programs, various reports on obesity, physical activity, and health)
    www.cdc.gov

Healthy People 2010
    www.health.gov/healthypeople

National Strength & Conditioning Association
    www.nsca-lift.org/menu.asp

The Institute for the Study of Youth Sports
    http://ed-web3.educ.msu.edu/ysi

The National Alliance for Youth Sports
    www.nays.org

11 *Motor Behavior in the Adult Years*

OBJECTIVES

Upon completion of this chapter, you should be able to

11.1 Provide a brief overview of motor behavior in the adult years.

11.2 Describe the growth and physiological characteristics associated with peak maturity.

11.3 Identify the motor performance characteristics that parallel peak biological maturity.

11.4 Describe the various biological theories of advanced aging.

11.5 Explain the term *regression* and distinguish between chronological and physiological age.

11.6 Briefly introduce and outline the characteristics associated with biological regression and motor performance.

11.7 Describe the changes in movement patterns that occur with advancing age.

11.8 Discuss the relationship between physical activity and longevity.

KEY TERMS

peak motor performance

aging

gerontology

chronological age

physiological age

regression

psychomotor slowing

longevity

The Developmental Continuum

Phase	Approximate age	Stage

Reflexive/
Spontaneous

conception — Prenatal

Rudimentary — birth

Infancy

6 mo.

2 years

Fundamental
Movement — Early Childhood

6

Sport
Skill — Later Childhood

12

Growth &
Refinement — Adolescence

18

Peak
Performance — Adulthood

30

Regression — Older Adulthood

70

Objective 11.1 MUCH OF THE INFORMATION to this point in the text has provided the basis for understanding lifelong motor development by describing the biological and information-processing characteristics associated with motor behavior across the life span. Part Four began with an introduction to the developmental approach to motor performance and identified each of the contributing phases of motor behavior. In keeping with this approach, chapter 8 presented the initial phase of motor behavior by describing actions exhibited prior to birth. Subsequent chapters have traced the evolution of movement abilities and the acquisition of fundamental and basic sport skills through childhood and adolescence.

This chapter describes the final phases and associated behaviors in the lifelong process of motor development. Motor behavior during the adult years is characterized by two distinguishing milestones—peak performance, which is associated with biological maturity during early adulthood, and the emergence of performance regression, which is linked with the latter stages of aging.

The information presented in this chapter constitutes a brief review of those biological distinctions and motor performance characteristics that distinguish adulthood from the other periods of the total life span. A timely discussion of the possible effects of physical activity on longevity also is presented.

Peak Motor Performance

Objective 11.2 ➤Although adolescence generally is accepted as the most distinctive period of biological growth and motor skill development, most individuals reach their peak of physical performance, health, and sexual maturity in early adulthood. It is also during the early adult years that gender differences in motor performance are maximized. Wide variation among young adults is common. But it is during this period in the life span that individuals attain **peak motor performance,** partly because the different physiological systems have become capable of working together so efficiently.

Growth and Physiological Function

Skeletal maturity is one example of continued growth into the adult years. Although most epiphyseal growth is completed in late adolescence (16 to 18 years), the long bones may continue to grow until approximately age 25, and the vertebral column until about age 30. This continued growth in the long bones may add up to one-fourth inch to an individual's height. In addition, certain areas of the braincase do not reach maturity until well into adulthood. This continued growth is evident when men (and women) who wear hats notice they have to purchase larger sizes as they age.

According to most sources, peak physiological function generally occurs between the approximate ages of 25 to 30 years of age (Brooks & Fahey, 1985; McArdle et al., 2001; Smith & Serfass, 1981). As a general rule, females tend to mature at the lower end (22 to 25 years) and males at the upper end (28 to 30 years) of the range. This is especially evident in three of the most influencing factors in motor performance: muscular strength, cardiorespiratory efficiency, and processing speed (reaction/movement time).

Maximum strength for both genders generally is achieved at a time when the muscular cross-sectional area is the largest, which is between the approximate ages of 20 and 30 years. Maximal strength for most muscle groups takes place between the ages of 25 and 29 years. Support for this assertion is shown in figure 11.1, which illustrates that male grip strength values peak in the late 20s and early 30s, and then decline steadily. These

■ *Figure 11.1*

Changes in grip
strength with age

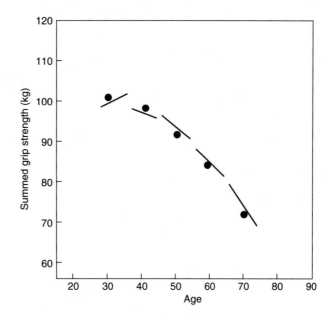

data represent both cross-sectional and a 9-year longitudinal study (Kall-man et al., 1990); note the striking agreement between the two data sets.

Peak physiological function in maximum oxygen consumption and cardiorespiratory work for both genders typically occurs during the third decade. Several reviews and studies report peak values within the range of 25 to 29 years (e.g., Astrand & Rodahl, 1986; deVries & Housh, 1994; Quirion et al., 1987). Figure 11.2 represents a composite of

■ *Figure 11.2*

Changes in maxi-
mum oxygen
consumption
with age

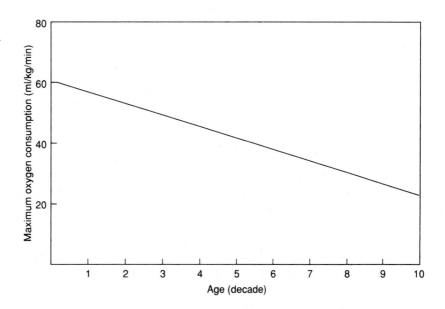

■ *Figure 11.3*

Relationship of age to exercise tolerance (in foot-pounds of work per minute)

Source: Data from Master, *American Heart Journal,* 10:495–510, 1935. C. V. Mosby, St. Louis, MO.

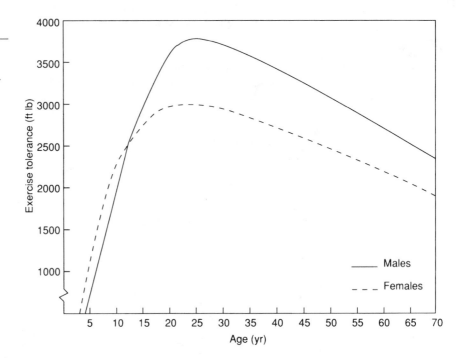

data from 17 published studies (normalized for body weight) and shows the approximate peaking of maximum oxygen consumption around the age of 30 and the steady decline thereafter. Figure 11.3 is a frequently cited illustration that depicts maximum work at various ages based on a two-step climbing test. Based on this information, peak work performance for females is said to occur around the age of 25 years, and for males, approximately three years later. In the early 1960s, Shock and colleagues conducted what is now referred to as a classic aging and physical performance study (Shock, 1962). Included in that series of experiments was a test to determine the amount of work that males could do using a crank ergometer. Among the physiological variables measured were oxygen consumption and cardiac output. The researchers found work rate peaked around the age of 28 years.

The importance of neurophysiological function and processing speed in the performance of a motor act is obvious. Assessments of successful motor performance frequently are based on the combination of perceptual recognition (attention), speed of memory, and neuromuscular response time (reaction/movement time). Processing speed, as determined by reaction time, improves with age up to the early adult years; peak performance occurring in the twenties (Hodgkins, 1962; Wilkinson & Allison, 1989) (figure 11.4).

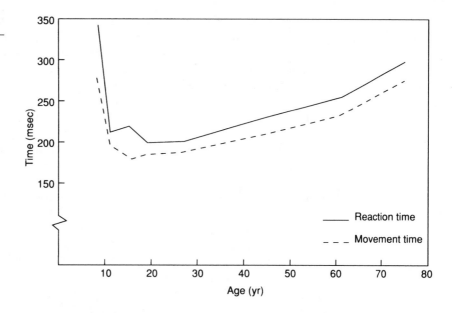

Reaction time and movement time as a function of age

Motor Performance Characteristics

Objective 11.3 ➤ Peak physiological function, which occurs in the approximate range of 25 to 30 years, closely parallels maximal motor performance. A general observation of the sporting world quickly leads to the speculation that college athletes are better than those of high school age, and few professional or Olympic-caliber athletes participate at these levels beyond their early thirties.

Since the majority of physical growth and development occurs during adolescence, the increases in motor performance during the adult years are due primarily to training, practice, experience, and motivation. Peak proficiency may be studied from the perspective of a highly trained population (i.e., athletes) that seeks maximum motor performance, or from the perspective of a population of average or normal ability. Although considerable diversity and variability exist within these groups, and normal is difficult to define, certain trends can be identified.

With the intent of determining age at peak athletic performance, Schultz and Curnow (1988) analyzed records and national ranking from track and field, swimming, baseball, tennis, and golf. In track and field, for example, they examined Olympic results from 1896 through 1980. Overall, the mean age of winners in seven events was about 25. Comparing running events, the average age at peak performance increased with the length of the race: from 22 years in the sprints, 24 years for middle distances, and 27 years for distances of 5,000 meters and greater. For professional baseball players, the mean age of peak performance was consistently around 27 years, based on pitching performances, batting averages, home runs, and runs batted in for nonpitchers (also see Schultz, Musa, Staszewski, & Siegler, 1994). Swimming performance appeared to peak between 18 to 20 years, and record performances in golf were achieved between the ages of 30 to 31 years. An examination of world professional tennis rankings suggested that 24 to 25 years of age was best for optimal performance. Females generally achieved peak performance about one to two years before males. A review of 1993 world record holders at the times the records were broken for open-class track and field, and swimming, reveals similar findings (Stone & Kozman, 1996). Track and field records (male and female ages combined) were broken at 24 to 29 years, while most swimming achievements were attained at ages 17 to 19; the backstroke was the exception at age 24.

Similar findings were reported by Hirata (1979) in the researcher's examination of past records of Olympic medalists (1964–1976). This study included a larger variety of events (than Schultz et al.), including boxing, canoeing, cycling, gymnastics, wrestling, and weight lifting. Although the range of winners' ages was expectedly wide, the average male was approximately 26 years, and the average female was about 23 years of age. Table 11.1 presents a composite of selected events for age at peak performance, based on the findings of Schultz et al. and Hirata.

The conclusion drawn from reviews of the data on this topic has been that younger athletes generally challenge performance records that require greater levels of strength, speed, and endurance. Further, older athletes frequently obtain peak proficiency in activities that require a high skill level and experience but less vigorous physical demands. Although research in this area is limited, it suggests that maximum proficiency in relatively less physically demanding motor skills such as shooting, bowling, golf, and billiards generally occurs after the age of 30.

Another perspective of maximum physical and motor proficiency during adulthood may be formed by observing a more normalized (i.e., not highly trained) segment of the population. Unfortunately, there is a dearth of information concerning the physical and motor proficiency of nonathletic adults. However, available information does allow a comparison of fitness levels between high school students (17-year-olds) and college students (21-year-olds). As table 11.2 shows, the average health-related (i.e., based more on physiological efficiency than skill) fitness performance scores of the 21-year-olds are greater than or equal to those of the younger age group. Superiority is especially evident in the two test items associated with aerobic performance.

Although the information presented is limited and represents a specific segment of the population (one that is relatively active but not highly trained), it does suggest that peak motor performance, in general, is reached after adolescence (17 to 18 years). Unfortunately, data are unavailable on these fitness and motor skill characteristics among relatively inactive segments of the population to use in comparison. One may speculate that due to the influencing effects of a physically active

THINK ABOUT IT

Speculate on a secular trend for peak physiological function and performance 50 years from now. Relate your projections to specific types of activities.

TABLE 11.1

Age at Peak Performance for Selected Events

Age	Male	Female
17		Gymnastics
18		Swimming
19		
20	Swimming	
21		Diving
22	Wrestling, Diving	Running short distance
23	Running short distance, Cycling	
24	Jumping, Boxing, Running medium distance, Tennis	Running medium distance Tennis, Rowing
25	Gymnastics, Rowing	
26		Shot put
27	Running long distance	Running long distance
28	Baseball, Weight lifting	
29	Shot put	
30		Golf
31	Golf	
32		

Source: Data from Schultz & Curnow (1988) and Hirata (1979)

TABLE 11.2

A Comparison of Average Fitness Performance Scores

| Test Item | Gender | AGE | |
		17 Years	21 Years
One-mile run (min:sec)	male	8:20	7:05
	female	10:34	9:23
9-minute run (yd)	male	2,169	2,225
	female	1,729	1,761
Sit-ups	male	44	44
	female	35	37
Sit and reach (cm)	male	31	33
	female	36	36

Sources: Data from The National Children and Youth Fitness Study, *Journal of Physical Education, Recreation and Dance, 56,* (1), 47, 1985; and Norms for College Students Health-Related Physical Fitness Test, American Alliance for Health, Physical Education, Recreation and Dance, 1985.

lifestyle and practice on motor performance after adolescence, performance values for nonactive young adults are not likely to be as high as
those for moderately active individuals.

Considerations of Race

Race implies a biologically distinct group of humans. In considering race
as a factor in development and motor performance, caution in drawing
any final conclusions is warranted. First, race is pure in very few
instances. For example, an African-American is likely to have ancestors
(thus some genetic endowment) of African, West-Indian, Caucasian, and
Spanish descent. Therefore, any practical comparisons between general
categories of race are usually quite generalized. Second, there is considerable variation within racial groups and much overlap among groups
being compared. Any valid observations should view race in a broader
biocultural framework (Malina & Bouchard, 1991). As emphasized
throughout this text, development and motor performance depend on
several factors, of which heredity and the environment are primary
agents. Chapter 13 will provide additional insight with regard to race
and various environmental contexts. This section briefly describes some
biological factors associated with race as reflected in peak motor performance of running and jumping events. The vast majority of research
in this area has been conducted on the comparison between Caucasians
and African-Americans, and will be the focus of this discussion. Given
the increasing proportion in the United States of other racial groups,
such as Hispanics and Asian-Americans, future reports including these
groups should be forthcoming.

Observations and Biological Considerations In a leading running
magazine feature titled "White Men Can't Run," the author notes that
on the all-time list for 100 meters, 44 of the top 50 performers are
sprinters of African origin (Burfoot, 1992). A strong African presence in
other running and jumping events also exists, including the showing of
Kenyans in distance running. The question is, aside from the cultural
bias for such events, are specific athletes of African descent genetically
gifted to perform these activities, compared to Caucasians? As noted in
the general comparison of the sexes (chapter 10), certain anatomical and
physiological characteristics are conducive to specific running and tasks.
Over the years, several research studies have compared Africans and
African-Americans with Caucasians, which has produced some consistent findings (table 11.3).

In general, runners and jumpers of African descent in comparison
to Caucasians appear to have a physiological and biomechanical advantage in such events by possessing less body fat, narrower hips, thicker
thighs, longer legs, lighter calves, a greater proportion of type II (fast-
twitch) muscle fibers (for sprints), and greater VO_2max efficiency (for

TABLE 11.3

Selected Characteristics of the African American Athlete

ANATOMICAL
Greater: lower leg length/thigh length
  biacromial/biiliac breadth ratios (narrower hips relative to shoulders)
  arm length relative to sitting height and stature

PHYSIOLOGICAL
Greater: lean body mass
  density of bone
  proportion of type II (fast-twitch) muscle fibers
  use of VO_2max (uses higher percentage)

Sources: Data from Himes (1988), Ama (1986), Schutte (1984), and Bosch (1990)

THINK ABOUT IT

What does the environment have to do with the discussion on race?

distance runs). Though most attention seems to be on sprinters, Bosch et al. (1990) noted one indication of excellence in distance running when a group of South Africans was able to use a higher percentage of VO_2max than elite Caucasian marathoners did while running a marathon on a treadmill.

In summary, these data provide some biological (genetic) insight into an explanation for excellence in specific running and jumping events by athletes of African origin. Keep in mind there is considerable variation within racial groups and much overlap among groups being compared. In addition, numerous sporting events have not been mentioned, many of which depend on uniquely different sets of skills and physical attributes.

Regression

Biological Theories of Advanced Aging

Objective 11.4 ➤ As noted earlier, (advanced) **aging** is the diminished capacity to regulate the internal environment (e.g., cellular and organismic structures), which results in a reduced probability of survival. Biological aging commonly is equated with biological decline (regression)—such as losses in muscle and bone mass, and cardiorespiratory and neural function—and a general psychomotor slowing of the body. Although the body is aging continuously from conception to death, after about age 30, regression in some form typically develops. There are numerous theories, subtheories, and lines of research on aging; no single hypothesis answers all of the questions proposed. The study of older people and the aging process is known as **gerontology.** The following discussion briefly describes some of the general explanations of biological aging. For a more detailed discussion, refer to Birren and Schaie (1996) and Shephard (1997) in the Suggested Readings. As pointed out in previous chapters and noted in this unit, although advanced aging typically complements a decline in function, physical activity and health habits are significant factors in the rate of degradation. According to McArdle et al., "sedentary living produces losses in functional capacity at least as great as the effects of aging" (2001, 883). The following summary was adapted from a publication of the National Institute on Aging (1993).

Genetic theories. Also referred to as *cellular clock* and *programmed* theories, these views suggest aging is under the direction of the DNA in human genes. Evidently there are proliferative and antiproliferative genes that, in theory, provide checks and balances of biological systems. Antiproliferative genes result in decreased cell division, which represents a weakening agent to the body. Once these genes become more active, regression develops. It seems clear, based on several lines of supportive research, that some sort of genetic program determines the aging process, but our understanding of the specifics remains unclear.

Wear-and-tear theories. The relatively simple premise of this theory is that aging is a result of long-term, accumulated damage to various vital bodily systems. In the course of daily living, the body suffers some damage but repairs itself under relatively normal conditions. With advancing aging, this ability gradually becomes less effective. Although some aspects of this notion appear reasonable, such as wear due to prolonged exposure to sunlight and other damaging elements, there is no evidence that hard work causes early death. To the contrary, vigorous exercise is a factor in predicting longer, not shorter life. Similarly, in some aspects, the brain functions better with use.

Cellular garbage/mutation theories. These theories suggest that with advancing age, the body accumulates cellular garbage (waste products) due to destructive mutation, which results in a decline in functioning. Two of the most noted views on this approach are the *free-radical* and *cross-linkage* theories. Free radicals are highly unstable molecules that react with other molecules in a way that may damage cells and diminish bodily functions. The normal process of cellular metabolism produces some free radicals; others are derived from the environment. Although the body can protect itself against some free radicals, with time the number builds up and results in signs of aging. Related to this view is the cross-linking theory, which focuses on the processes by which different types of molecules are joined together permanently (cross-linked). This results in deterioration such as wrinkling and atherosclerosis. Another substance connected with the wear-and-tear of the body over time is *lipofuscin.* As the body ages, this inert granulated pigment, which accumulates in nerve, cardiac, and skeletal cells, fills spaces and interferes with function. It has been suggested that lipofuscin may be created during metabolism, and it is probably an effect rather than a cause of aging.

Immune system theories. With aging, the immune system's response declines, thus the body's ability to fight many infections diminishes. It is suggested that many symptoms of aging are a result of the accumulated effect of past and present disease the system was or is unable to control. From another perspective, some researchers suggest that with aging, the body loses its ability to distinguish between its own specific materials and threatening foreign organisms (e.g., bacteria, viruses, and fungi). Thus it attacks and annihilates its own tissues at a gradually progressing rate. Although these theories do not address aging of the immune system itself, it stands to reason that life expectancy would increase if the power of the system were sustained.

Hormonal theories. One possible cause for decline in the immune system's effectiveness and the subsequent aging effects has been atrophy of the thymus gland, which influences immune functioning via thymic hormone. Its progressive, age-related loss has been linked with declines in functioning of certain immune cells. Other examples of hormonal influence on characteristics associated with advanced aging are estrogen decline and bone loss in women, and loss of growth hormone, which is related to a decline in muscle mass, bone density, and body fat and the occurrence of thin, wrinkled skin. Individuals who have been treated with growth hormone (discussed in chapter 5) have shown improvements in these areas.

Objective 11.5 ➤ The differences between **chronological age** and **physiological age** become increasingly evident with advancing age. In general physiological function, active individuals appear to be physiologically superior to their counterparts of the same chronological age (see figure 11.5 on page 368). From a general observation of human performance and attitude, this phenomenon is also apparent. Whereas some people consider themselves old by the age of 30, others continue to pursue a highly active lifestyle through old age. Several major championships and records in such sports as track and field, tennis, baseball pitching, and golf have been held by individuals in their forties. One of the truly remarkable athletic feats by an older individual in recent years was accomplished by John Kelley. In the 1992 Boston Marathon at the age of 84 years he completed the course (26 miles, 365 yards) in close to 5 hours. It was the 61st time he had run this race, which he won in 1935 and 1945.

However, though there are numerous benefits from a healthy and active lifestyle during adulthood, it appears that no matter how well people take care of themselves, the effects of advancing age will result in **regression** of physiological processes and motor performance.

■ *Figure 11.5*

General physiological function across the life span for active and sedentary persons

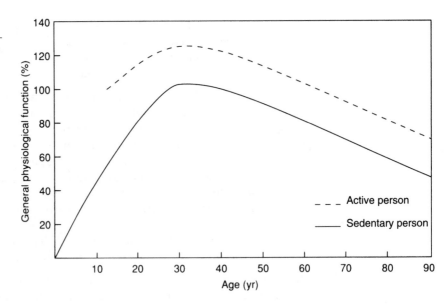

Biological Regression and Motor Performance

Objective 11.6

THINK ABOUT IT

How much do genetics influence the regression of motor behavior?

➤ After an individual reaches peak maturity at approximately 30 years of age, most physiological factors begin to show decrements at a rate of about 0.75% to 1% a year (McArdle et al., 2001; Wilmore & Costill, 1999). This is a general trend of decline, however; differences between individuals and the function of specific organs can vary considerably. There is some suggestion from the research community that up to 50% of the loss usually attributed to physiological aging may be due to inactivity and other poor health habits. The decline in biological capacity and associated motor performance generally is characterized by decrements in cardiorespiratory function, muscular strength, neural function, balance, and flexibility. Additional age-related factors that may affect one's motor performance are changes in the skeletal system (bone tissue) and increased body fat.

For a summary of selected biological changes that occur with aging after peak maturity, refer back to table 4.4 on page 136. The following is a summary of those changes and a description of associated decrements in motor performance.

Cardiorespiratory Function Cardiovascular capacity as measured by maximal oxygen consumption (maximal aerobic power) declines approximately 30% between the ages of 30 to 70 years (figure 11.2 on page 359). Closely associated with this general physiological decrement is a decrease in cardiac output (stroke volume and maximal heart rate) and respiratory (pulmonary) function. Complementing figure 11.6, research consistently shows that active individuals maintain a higher

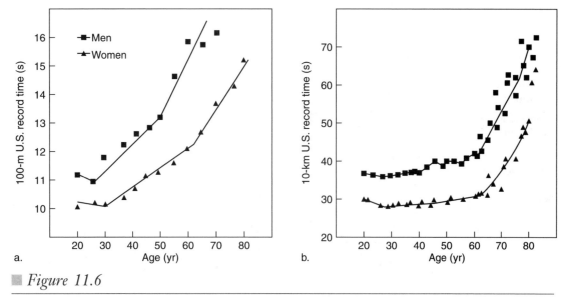

■ *Figure 11.6*

Change with age in male and female world records for (a) 100-m and
(b) 10-km runs

aerobic capacity than their sedentary counterparts. As noted in chapter 4,
sedentary persons have nearly a two-fold faster rate of decline in VO₂max as
they age (McArdle et al., 2001). In addition to diminished cardiac capacity, respiratory function decreases with advancing age, as evidenced by an
estimated 40% loss in vital capacity between the ages of 30 and 70.

Parallel to the loss in aerobic capacity after peak maturity is a slightly
greater decline in anaerobic power (about 40% by age 70). This loss is
linked, in part, to the aging body's diminishing capacity to turn over lactic acid accumulation during short bouts of intense physical activity.
Other significant cardiovascular changes include increased blood pressure and blood flow resistance. Thus aging produces significant
decreases in the body's oxygen transport and extraction capacities.

Motor performance decrements in physical work capacity tasks and
high-level aerobic activities clearly follow the general aging trend. Figures 11.3, 11.6, and 11.7 show examples of this trend. Figure 11.3 depicts changes in work capacity (exercise tolerance) in a laboratory
setting, and figures 11.6 and 11.7 illustrate age-related changes in U.S.
record 100-m and 10-km run times and masters-level freestyle swimming events. It also may be suggested from the data shown on run and
swim times that regardless of training experience, performance (aerobic
capacity) diminishes with advancing age. Wilmore and Costill (1999), in
reference to figure 11.6, note that run performance decreases by about
1% per year from age 25 to age 60. After that, the rate is approximately
2% decline per year.

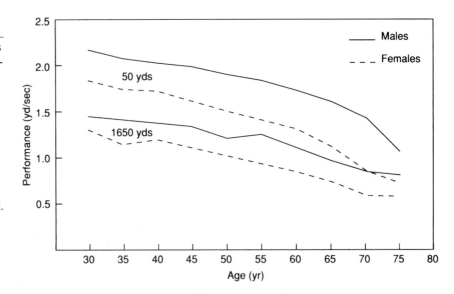

■ *Figure 11.7*

Mean performances for short- and long-distance masters-level freestyle swimming events

Source: Data from Hartley and Hartley, *Experimental Aging Research,* 10:35–42, 1984, Beach Hill Enterprises, Inc., Southwest Harbor, ME.

Muscular Strength The primary factor in the loss of muscular strength after peak performance is the decrease in muscle mass that occurs with advancing age (McArdle et al., 2001). While the average estimate is a 25% to 30% loss in muscle mass between ages 30 and 70, some reports show a loss of up to 50% by age 80. This general loss of body tissue is characterized by specific decreases in the size and number of muscle fibers, loss of biochemical capacity, increases in connective tissue and fat, and a general dehydration in body cells (Frontera et al., 2000). Concerning fiber type, it appears that type II fast twitch may be lost at a faster rate (Timiras, 1994). In addition to affecting isometric and dynamic strength, these changes also hamper mobility and speed of movement, especially among the elderly.

The general decline with advancing age in maximal muscular strength seems to parallel the loss in muscle mass. That is, there is a 25% to 30% decline in strength between the ages of 30 and 70 years. It also has been suggested that the rate of decline in leg and trunk muscles in both sexes is greater than in arm and hand-grip muscles. As evidenced in figure 11.1 on page 359, grip strength decreases slowly after peak performance and does not show a marked decline until after the approximate age of 40. For this aspect of muscular strength, the total loss from 30 to 60 years usually does not exceed 10% to 20% of maximum; the degree of decrement is somewhat greater in females than in males. However, an analysis of the literature suggests greater losses among older adults (Kallman et al., 1990; Rantanen et al., 1997). The decrement in grip-strength endurance, usually measured by the amount of force that can be held for one minute, is not as great as the decline in grip strength; estimates suggest a decrease of about 30% from age 20 to 75.

Interestingly, a study of maximal grip strength and grip-strength endurance among males, all of whom performed similar work in a machine shop, revealed no change in strength or endurance from age 22 to 62 (Petrofsky & Lind, 1975). These data suggest the changes found in a more typical population may be due largely to disuse rather than to aging. Although activity may slow the effects of aging, however, there is little question that sizable decrements occur in old age, regardless of activity level.

Neural Function As noted in chapter 7, with regard to information processing, one of the most consistently observed and significant changes with advancing age is the decline in processing (behavioral) speed, described as **psychomotor slowing.** Over the years, several theories have been proposed regarding this phenomenon; some focus on neuromuscular factors, others on a breakdown in the central nervous system (CNS). Perhaps the most compelling explanation is a general *biological degradation*. That is, with advanced aging there is a deterioration of the neural network functioning that affects processing durations (e.g., Cerella & Hale, 1994; Salthouse, 1996). Part of this degradation described earlier is the significant reduction in brain cells, increased synaptic delay, an approximate 15% decrease in nerve conduction velocity, and an estimated loss of 37% in the number of spinal cord axons. All of these are a part of the links and nodes that form the neural network. Theoretically, with aging, links in the network are broken or disrupted, which causes the decline in processing.

Evidence of age-related psychomotor slowing has been reported with several laboratory motor tasks based on reaction time and speed of movement (e.g., Desrosiers et al., 1999; Light & Spirduso, 1990; Lupinacci et al., 1993; Williams, 1990). In general, greater reductions in both reaction time and movement speed tend to occur in the lower parts of the body in contrast to the areas of most frequent use, such as the fingers. The rate of psychomotor slowing also is affected by the complexity of the motor task; tasks of greater complexity are associated with increased rates of decline. That is, as movement complexity increases, the effects of adult aging on reaction time increase.

Data reported by Williams (1990) clearly support this contention. The research showed that between the ages of 50 and 90 there was a 32% decrement in speed of simple discrete and repetitive arm/hand movements. In contrast, a 65% decrease in speed was found in the performance of complex sequential arm/hand/finger movements. The researcher also found substantial decrements of about 30% in timed bilateral and unilateral object manipulation tasks. Evidence also suggests that fine motor actions that require steadiness, such as writing digits and letters, undergo even greater decrements (68% to 78%) during the adult years. Complementing these findings are more recent comparative reports of large decrements with greater age in the performance of a variety of rapid hand aiming movements (e.g., Teeken et al., 1996; Yan et al., 2000). For a more comprehensive review of aging and eye-hand coordination refer to Williams (1990).

In general, after performance peaks during the twenties, a gradual slowing of the body occurs in relation to reaction time and speed of movement (i.e., movement time), with more marked increases occurring after the age of 60 (see figure 11.4 on page 361). Thus, the general trend is one of increasing proficiency, then peak performance, and finally the psychomotor slowing in finger, hand, and arm speed tasks with age.

The suggestion that a healthy, physically active lifestyle may reduce the decrement in psychomotor slowing (i.e., CNS deterioration) has some support in research findings. In studies that have compared groups of physically active and nonactive young and old persons on reaction and movement time tasks, similar results have been reported (Rikli & Busch, 1986; see review by Spirduso, 1995, in Suggested Readings). That is, reaction and movement time scores for the active groups (young or old) were considerably faster than the corresponding age group that was less active. As one would expect, when scores for the age groups were averaged across activity levels, the young groups were faster than their older counterparts. Studies also found that scores for the nonactive older group were substantially slower than those of the other groups. Figure 11.8 shows the movement time characteristics for simple and complex motor tasks (Spirduso, 1975).

THINK ABOUT IT

Consider how you would set up a study to test the influence of aerobic and weight training exercises on psycho-motor slowing.

What about the effects of training (practice) on reaction time and speed of movement among the elderly? Evidence has been documented that practice with videogame playing among elderly individuals who averaged 70 years of age improved the response speed (i.e., reaction time) and, in essence, reversed the age-related decline in processing (Clark, et al., 1987). This research suggested that central mechanisms (e.g., information-processing strategies), rather than neuromuscular factors, were most influenced by the practice. Unfortunately, studies that have investigated the influence of specific exercise training (i.e., aerobic and strength) on reaction time and speed of movement among the elderly have been inconclusive (Panton et al., 1990).

Balance Associated with the age-related decline in neuromuscular capacity is the loss of balance (stability). Any movement that requires balance involves the successful integration of several anatomical, muscular, and neurological functions. The deterioration of any of these functions may impede the ability to maintain equilibrium. For example, loss of brain cells (primarily in the cerebellum and brain stem) with advancing age may hinder the capacity to use proprioceptive information. That is, the kinesthetic information received concerning the position of the body's various parts is less accurate and thus inhibits precise postural control. From approximately 40 years of age there is a gradual deterioration of vestibular nerve cells. Sensory cell loss may begin as early as

■ *Figure 11.8*

Movement time
characteristics in
young (Y), old (O),
active (A), and
nonactive (NA)
subjects

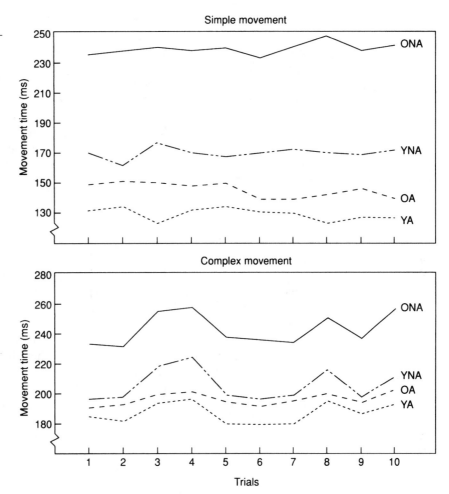

the fifth decade in the semicircular canals and may be quite marked in the saccule and utricle as well after the age of 70. In addition, with advancing age, there are deficits in the somatosensory system that involves tactile (touch) sensitivity.

Visual perception also plays a significant role in maintaining stability, especially when the body is moving. For most people the decrement in visual acuity begins around the age of 40; by 60 years the ability to focus on objects at close distance is affected greatly. A loss in the ability to judge depth is also particularly evident after age 60. Although performance (balance) and symptomatic indications of vestibular malfunction (vertigo and dizziness) in older adults are evident, the specific underlying mechanisms responsible for these responses have not been clearly defined. It is likely, however, that a number of causes may be involved with balance loss in older adults; they include disease, weak muscles, limited range of motion, abnormal reflexes, visual/vestibular deficits to central sensory integration, deficiencies in motor programming, and motor control difficulties (Manchester et al., 1989; Shumway-Cook & Woollacott, 2001).

A significant loss in the ability to establish and maintain balance can affect virtually all gross motor activities. However, the research technique most frequently used to study changes in balance is the measurement of postural sway while performing various balancing tasks in the upright position. In general, research findings suggest the magnitude of the sway tends to be greater (i.e., less stable) in the very young and the very old, and older adults are less stable than younger adults are. For example, Toupet et al. (1992) examined 500 healthy (free of pathology) adults from ages 40 to 80 and found sway increased with each decade of advancing age. Similar findings with increased sway in older compared to younger adults were reported by Shumway-Cook et al. (1997) and Era & Heikkinen (1985).

Falling is a major health concern of older adults that has been linked in part to the decrement in balance. Approximately one-third of all individuals over age 65 fall at least once each year (Sorock, 1988). With advancing age, the ability to recover from instability is slower and less efficient than in younger years. Overstall and colleagues (1977) found in their study of individuals aged 60 to 96 that the incidence of falls increases with advancing age. It also was noted that females incur about twice as many falls as males in late adulthood. Factors other than lack of balance that have been mentioned as contributors to falling include decreased levels of physical activity, stroke, arthritis, low blood pressure, muscle weakness, poor eyesight, ineffective walking pattern (especially, reduced foot raise), and adverse effects of medication (Campbell et al., 1989). Compared to males, females tend to inherit a much greater possibility of hip fracture as a result of falling due to structural and bone characteristics. The angle of insertion of the head of the femur into the hip socket creates a structural weakness more conducive to hip fracture. Females also lose considerably more bone mineral mass and have a much greater incidence of osteoporosis in late adulthood. Kreutzfeldt et al. (1984) report the annual incidence of hip fracture per 1,000 individuals of similar age (over 80 years) is 8.4 for males and 19.8 for females.

A paradox exists with regard to the difference between males and females in the frequency of falls. Information presented earlier in this text suggested females have the structural advantage (lower center of gravity and wider base relative to height) in maintaining stability. An example of this advantage is evidenced by superior scores in balance beam walking. One could speculate that, at worst, females should be no more prone to falling than males are. According to Eckert (1987), the fact that females have potentially greater stability but less balance raises the possibility of a gender difference in balance-related sensory input and/or environmental influences. The research literature provides little support for a significant gender difference in kinesthetic mechanisms (including vestibular functions) or visual processes. In fact, available information appears to favor females for balancing mechanisms. It seems plausible (though speculative) that though the female physique is more suited to balancing tasks, practice and environmental influences are also significant factors in optimal balance development. To illustrate, females generally perform better than males do on balancing tasks during childhood—a time when the female anatomical structure (a higher center of gravity and longer legs) should not provide an advantage. Based on this hypothesis, a possible explanation for the gender difference in frequency of falls in old age could be that higher participation levels by males in physical activities are conducive to maintaining efficient stability.

Included in the Rikli and Busch (1986) study of active and inactive young and old females was a difficult balancing task, the one-foot stand for time (60-second limit). The active older group performed significantly better than the inactive older group, which indicates physical activity level may influence balancing ability. It also was noted that both young groups (active and inactive) performed the task equally well and did considerably better than the active older group, which suggests a healthy, active lifestyle does not prevent the age-related decrement in balancing performance but may change the rate of decline.

Flexibility   One of the most obvious changes associated with advancing age is the loss of joint mobility (range of motion). Closely linked to this general decline are changes in the joints and muscles, and the presence of degenerative joint diseases. A smooth functioning of the joints is made possible by the strength and elasticity of the tendons and ligaments (forms of connective tissue that encompass the joint) and the synovial fluid. After the early adult years (or later adult years for some individuals), the joints become less stable and mobility diminishes. In addition, collagen fibers and synovial membranes degrade, and the viscosity of the synovial fluid decreases. As a result of these decrements, the joints become stiff, which may decrease the range of motion (flexibility). However, there is no conclusive evidence that biological aging inherently causes decreased flexibility. A considerable amount of research also links the decline in range of motion with degenerative joint diseases such as osteoarthritis and osteoarthrosis. There are indications that more than two-thirds of individuals 55 to 64 years of age have signs of osteoarthrosis in some joint.

The inherent difficulty with using a general performance curve to describe changes in flexibility across the life span is that activity level is a better indicator of flexibility than age. Though exceptions have been reported, most research suggests that general range of motion increases steadily through childhood and flexibility starts to decline around 10 years of age in males and 12 years of age in females.

Again, a strong influencing factor is individual activity level, which may vary considerably within any age group. The available information suggests, however, that after the onset of puberty (early teens), flexibility begins to decline, more so in males than in females. This trend is supported in part by evidence that indicates that as body surface area increases during adolescence, flexibility decreases; also, there is the possibility that the older population generally participates less in activities that demand a wide range of motion.

The three factors that appear to have the greatest influence on flexibility during adulthood are physical activity level, the inherent effects of aging, and degenerative joint diseases. The effects of aging on joint and muscle tissue have been verified, as well as the presence of joint diseases in the majority of elderly persons. Results of the Rikli and Busch (1986) investigation of active and inactive young and old females demonstrated clearly that physical activity level was a strong factor in maintaining flexibility in old age. In this study, the old active females performed significantly better on a sit-and-reach (trunk flexibility) test than their inactive counterparts of the same age group. In fact, the older active group demonstrated slightly greater flexibility than the young inactive group.

Changes in Skeletal Tissue and Body Fat It is typical for aging humans to increase in body weight and fat and to show a decrease in height and bone mass. The average female loses a striking 30% of bone mass between the approximate ages of 35 and 70. Bone mass loss among males generally does not begin until about age 55 and reaches a smaller total loss between 10% and 15% by age 70. With advancing age also comes a slight decrease in height, due primarily to bone mass loss, increased kyphosis (rounding of the back), compression of intravertebral disks, and deterioration of vertebrae.

For the average person, gains in body weight and fat begin gradually in the late twenties and continue to increase until approximately age of 55 or 60, when the gains show signs of decreasing. The typical increase in body weight and fat from age 20 to 60 years for both sexes is approximately 15%. This value is highly variable and may be considerably less among highly active, diet-conscious individuals. Lean body mass also tends to decrease with age. This overall effect is due primarily to bone mass loss and the reduction of muscle mass. As noted earlier, in most individuals there is a marked deterioration in muscle mass with aging.

The effects of skeletal and body composition changes on motor performance are generic; that is, rather than affecting the performance of a specific type (group) of motor activities, these changes influence the overall ability to perform a wide scope of motor skills. For example, bone mass loss results in bone with less density and tensile strength. Therefore, it is generally weaker and more prone to injury and fracture. Due to the increased likelihood of injury, many older persons limit their physical exertion levels and modify movement patterns for fear of physical harm. The presence of kyphosis (rounding of the back) also may significantly alter basic and advanced movement patterns (e.g., swimming, running, and throwing).

An increase in adult body fat of 10% to 15% may have implications for physiological functions and motor performance. In general, a significant increase in body fat impairs cardiac function by increasing the mechanical work the heart must perform and thus affects aerobic and muscular endurance activity. Numerous research studies that involve young and older adults have found percent body fat to be related inversely (negatively) to the ability to move the total body weight. This is especially true for motor performance tasks that require horizontal acceleration (e.g., running) or vertical lifting of the total body (e.g., jumping). Theoretically this relationship is based on the fact that body fat adds to the total mass of the body without contributing to the force-producing capability. Therefore, the additional body fat gained during adulthood becomes excess weight to be moved during locomotor activity.

> THINK ABOUT IT
>
> Do you know of some ways research (science) has helped curb the rate of regression?

Changing Movement Patterns

Objective 11.7 ➤ **Walking** Although the information on age-related changes in movement patterns during the adult years is limited, a number of studies have focused on walking—the most used movement pattern. In general, a deterioration in walking gait occurs with advancing age, beginning with late adulthood (over 60 years). The stereotypic gait of an elderly person normally is characterized by slow, short, shuffling steps in which there is little range of motion, and a slumping of the head, shoulders, and trunk. Differences in performance among individuals of similar age can be considerable, however.

Murray and associates have conducted several investigations on gait patterns in individuals 20 to 87 years of age (e.g., Murray et al., 1969, 1970). In summary, when males over age 65 were compared to males ages 20 to 25, the older males displayed *shorter steps* (i.e., linear distance traveled of alternate feet), *shorter stride lengths* (i.e., linear distance traveled of same foot), *increased out-toeing*, and *less pelvic rotation and ankle extension*. Out-toeing is a technique used to improve lateral stability. Similar results also were found among females. When only able-bodied older persons were compared with younger individuals, fewer differences were noted—namely, shorter steps, a shorter stride length, and increased out-toeing. A recent study using sophisticated kinetic analysis found that older adults (62 to 78) had significantly shorter stride length, longer double-support time, and less push-off power than young persons did (Winter et al., 1990).

Other significant changes noted with advancing age are *step height* (foot raise) and *walking speed* (Aniansson, 1980; Steffen et al., 2002).

Compared to the adult norm, the ability to raise each foot during walking (step height) decreases in individuals older than 70. As one might expect after reviewing the information on falling frequency, older females in particular have difficulty with step height.

By what standard should normal walking speed be judged? One suggestion of particular relevance to older adults is that the minimum velocity needed to cross a traffic intersection should be used as one criterion for measuring normal speed. Based on this criterion, Aniansson determined that the normal walking speed of the general adult population is about 1.4 meters per second. However, the average normal, functional walking speed of adults 70 and older was found to be much slower than the criterion speed; the average speed was 1.2 meters per second for males and 1.1 meters per second for females.

Another consideration among older adults in relation to gait pattern is the psychological factor. It may be speculated that many elderly persons shuffle cautiously and use short steps in fear of falling. Evidence for this speculation is supported to some degree by the findings of a study reported by Willmott (1986). The researcher found that among elderly hospital patients, gait speed and step length were significantly greater on a carpeted surface compared to a vinyl surface. More confidence and little fear were expressed about walking on the carpeted surface in comparison to the vinyl.

In an excellent review of research on walking among the elderly, Craik (1989) notes that several issues remain unclear and need to be addressed before an accurate description of the effect of aging on walking behavior can be provided. Table 11.4 summarizes gait pattern changes in the elderly, as reported by Shumway-Cook and Woollacott (2001).

THINK ABOUT IT

What are the similarities between an infant and an older adult in walking?

Running and Jumping   There are some indications that basic running and jumping patterns also change with aging. Some older persons participate in competitive sporting events (e.g., Senior Olympics, Senior Games, marathons, and triathlons) and engage in a regular routine of fitness-oriented activities, but most older individuals do not include running and jumping or other basic sport skills (e.g., throwing, catching, and kicking) in their lives. In an unpublished study by Adrian (cited in Adrian & Cooper, 1995), the kinematics (movement pattern characteristics) of healthy, active females aged 60 to 80 were identical to university track team females during a paced run. However, when the sprint patterns were compared, there was little similarity. More specifically, the younger females exhibited greater leg flexion and extension. Other information suggests that older runners do not tuck (flex) their recovery leg as completely; they display a shorter stride and take a greater number of strides to complete the distance.

Associated with the general age-related psychomotor slowing and decrements in anaerobic function and strength is a decline in running

TABLE 11.4

Summary of Gait Changes in the Older Adult

Temporal/distance factors
    Decreased velocity
    Decreased step length
    Decreased step rate
    Decreased stride length
    Increased stride width
    Increased stance phase
    Increased time in double support
    Decreased swing phase
Kinematic changes
    Decreased vertical movement of the center of gravity
    Decreased arm swing
    Decreased hip, knee, and ankle flexion
    Flatter foot on heel-strike
    Decreased ability to couple hip/knee movements
    Decreased dynamic stability during stance
Muscle activation patterns
    Increased coactivation (increased stiffness)
Kinetic changes
    Decreased power generation at push-off
    Decreased power absorption at heel-strike

Source: From Shumway-Cook & Woollacott (2001)

speed. Verification of this trend was reported by Nelson (1981) after comparing 20-year-old females and 58- to 80-year-old females on jogging and running speed. The older females were significantly slower at both jogging pace (1.85 meters per second versus 3.93 meters per second) and maximum running speed (2.60 meters per second versus 6.69 meters per second). Other evidence of an age-related decline among trained individuals can be found in the results of the U.S. National Senior Olympics (1989). Without exception, there was a decrease in speed with advancing age in the 100-meter dash in 12 age-group categories (six male and six female) for participants aged 55 to over 80 years.

With regard to jumping little has been studied among the adult population and, in particular, among the elderly. The kinematics of the vertical jump of college-aged females and females over age 60 have been compared (Klinger et al., 1980). Results suggested that, in general, the patterns of both groups were similar. However, the older persons displayed less knee flexion and could not extend their legs (at the knee joint) as quickly as the younger individuals could.

■ *Figure 11.9*

For the active older person, the decline in performance is not as great

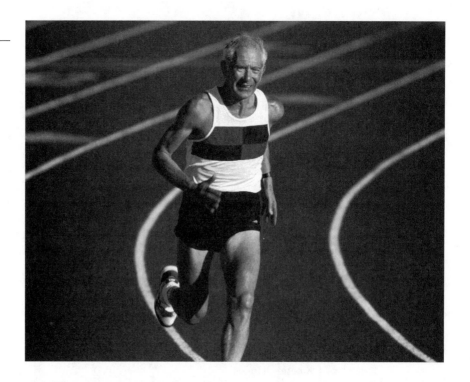

Throwing and Striking   Also included in the Klinger et al. study was a comparison of several throwing and striking patterns (tennis backhand and batting). In each case, the extension velocities older individuals achieved were slower than those of the younger group. It should be noted, however, that in many instances the older individuals had no athletic background or had gone years without practicing any of the skills. Those identified as more active displayed a more sophisticated movement pattern (e.g., better coordination, faster movement, and greater range of motion) than those in their age group who were less active.

In a more recent series of studies by Williams and colleagues (1990, 1991), similar findings were reported for the overarm throw in the elderly (ages 63 to 78 years). That is, ball velocities approximated speeds usually generated by 8- to 9-year-olds; this was accompanied by a relatively shorter backswing (i.e., less range of motion). In addition, those individuals who participated in throwing-oriented sports in their past exhibited better movements. As one might expect, men generally had better form and threw faster than the females did.

Some generalizations may be made concerning the changing of movement patterns in adulthood. In general, the average elderly person shows a definite slowing of movements and less flexion and extension compared to his or her younger counterpart. However, among active older persons the decrement in speed is not as great and the characteristics of the movement pattern are generally well maintained from younger years.

Physical Activity and Longevity

Objective 11.8 ➤ This text has presented numerous assertions with regard to the potential benefits of physical activity to growth, development, and motor performance. Discussions have affirmed that physical activity and exercise can have positive effects on bone and muscle tissue, body composition, and cardiorespiratory development. Performance characteristics in the form of strength, aerobic and anaerobic function, flexibility, coordination, balance, speed, and numerous motor skills all have been shown to progress through the psychomotor mode. Several assertions also were made in this chapter concerning the contribution of a healthy, physically active lifestyle toward delaying and modifying the effects of aging on various physiological functions and motor performance. In essence, physical activity was suggested as an important factor in the association between physiological age and chronological age.

The effects of physical activity on motor development are generally positive and, in some instances, dramatic. But what about the effects of physical activity on **longevity** (length of life)? Over the last 30 years or so, a vast amount of research has been conducted and reported to the public concerning factors associated with human health and life expectancy (e.g., smoking, high cholesterol, coronary heart disease, high blood pressure, nutrition, and exercise). More recently, several studies report convincing evidence that asserts that regular (habitual) physical activity and physical fitness of a *moderate* level is associated with increased longevity in comparison to sedentary and less active lifestyles. One of the most significant and common findings from this research is that physical activity is inversely associated with the rate of certain diseases and early mortality.

One of the most comprehensive investigations collected data on 16,936 Harvard alumni, aged 35 to 74, with 12 to 16 years of follow-up (Paffenbarger et al., 1986). The physical activity level for each subject was measured as the total amount of energy expended (in kilocalories) at physical activity (e.g., sports, yard work, and walking) per week. Results indicated that physical activity level is related inversely to total mortality. That is, death rates declined steadily as physical activity (energy expenditure) increased. This trend continued with the increase in expenditure from less than 500 kilocalories to 3,500 kilocalories per week; beyond that amount, the rates increased slightly. In males, mortality rates were one-fourth to one-third lower among those individuals who expended at least 2,000 kilocalories per week, compared to less active males.

Perhaps most important, the researchers further concluded that regardless of whether the individual smoked, had high blood pressure, experienced extreme gains or losses in body weight, or had parents who died early, mortality rates were considerably lower among the more physically active. This general finding was confirmed in a report by Powell and Blair (1994). The researchers concluded that lack of regular physical activity contributes to heart disease in a cause-and-effect relationship, with sedentary individuals almost twice as likely to develop heart disease as the most active persons. And, inadequate physical activity is responsible for about 30% of all deaths due to heart disease, colon cancer, and diabetes. Numerous studies that used general adult populations also have reported an inverse relationship between coronary heart disease, death, and regular physical activity. In addition to the inverse trends (of heart disease and mortality) with leisure-time habitual physical activity, similar results also have been associated with occupational activity.

All of the aforementioned studies used physical activity as determined by various units of measurement (e.g., kilocalories expended and hours participated) as the factor with which to compare rates of disease and death. An alternative approach perhaps more specific and objective is the use of physical fitness level. Most studies identify the level and type of physical activity, but few investigations provide the additional insight of comparing the physiological (physical fitness) state of the body to rate of disease and death.

THINK ABOUT IT

How would you use the information on physical activity and longevity to have an impact on society? That is, what strategies would you recommend?

One of the landmark investigations using the latter approach was conducted by Blair and associates (1989) and reported in the *Journal of the American Medical Association*. The study consisted of more than 13,000 males and females who ranged from 20 to over 60 years of age. They were tested for aerobic fitness, then assigned to one of five physical fitness groups (low-fit to high-fit) based on age, sex, and fitness test results. Results indicated a strong, graded, and consistent inverse relationship between physical fitness and mortality due to all causes (i.e., smoking, cholesterol level, parent history, cardiovascular disease, and cancer). When comparing least-fit to most-fit groups, the chances of a low-fit individual experiencing an early death were 3.44 times greater for males and 4.65 times more likely among females. However, one of the most important conclusions of the study was that the fitness standard associated with increased longevity may be attained by individuals who engage in regular *moderate* exercise that approximates a brisk walk of about 30 minutes several times a week. Other research by Farrell et al. (1998) shows similar results. That is, moderate cardiorespiratory fitness provides some protection from cardiovascular disease mortality.

Two disturbing statistical figures associated with these results estimate that with increasing age there is a progressive and predictable decline in exercise participation (noted in the Surgeon General's Report; Satarino et al., 2000). It was estimated that, at best, no more than 25% of adults engage in sufficient regular physical activity of an intensity to receive health benefits.

In summary, it appears from the data that regular physical activity of a moderate level of intensity can prolong life. Longevity, however, is more associated with the prevention of early mortality than with extending one's potential life span.

Summary

Motor behavior during the adult years is characterized by two distinguishing milestones: peak performance (associated with biological maturity) and regression. Peak physiological function, for the most part, occurs between the approximate ages of 25 to 30; females tend to mature at the lower end (22 to 25 years) and males at the upper end (28 to 30 years) of the range. This trend is evident in three of the most influencing factors in motor performance: muscular strength, cardiorespiratory efficiency, and processing speed. Closely associated with peak physiological function is maximal motor performance in several activities.

A basic fact of development during the adult years is the difference between chronological and physiological age. However, it appears that no matter how well people take care of themselves, some degree of regression in physiological processes and associated motor performance is inevitable. After peak maturity, most physiological functions begin to show decrements at a general rate of 0.75% to 1% per year. The decline is characterized by decrements in cardiorespiratory function, muscular strength, neural function, balance, and flexibility. Other major forms of biological regression include bone tissue loss (especially for females), an increase in body fat, and a decrease in muscle mass. There is some suggestion that much of the loss in physiological aging may be attributed to inactivity and poor health habits.

During late adulthood a deterioration in specific movement patterns (e.g., walk, run, and jump) also may occur. Although wide differences in performance exist, in general, elderly persons exhibit a definite slowing of movements with less flexion and extension compared to younger persons.

Physical activity, especially habitual participation, has been shown to have positive effects on several aspects of growth, development, and motor performance. In recent years, several research studies have verified that habitual health-related physical activity of moderate intensity is positively associated with a prolonged life span in comparison to sedentary and less active lifestyles.

Think about It

1. Speculate on a secular trend for peak physiological function and performance 50 years from now. Relate your projections to specific types of activities.

2. What does the environment have to do with the discussion on race?
3. How much do genetics influence the regression of motor behavior?
4. Consider how you would set up a study to test the influence of aerobic and weight training exercises on psychomotor slowing.
5. Do you know of some ways research (science) has helped curb the rate of regression?
6. What are the similarities between an infant and an older adult in walking?
7. How would you use the information on physical activity and longevity to have an impact on society? That is, what strategies would you recommend?

Suggested Readings

Birren, J. E., & Schaie, K. W. (Eds.). (1996). *Handbook of the phychology of aging*. 4th ed. San Diego: Academic Press.

McArdle, W. D., Katch, F. I., & Katch, V. L. (2001). *Exercise physiology*. 5th ed. Philadelphia: Lea & Febiger.

Shepard, R. J. (1997). *Aging, physical activity, and health*. Champaign, IL: Human Kinetics.

Shumway-Cook, A. & Woollacott, M. (2001). *Motor control*. 2nd ed. Baltimore: Lippincott Williams & Wilkins.

Spirduso, W. W. (1995). *Physical dimensions of aging*. Champaign, IL: Human Kinetics.

WebLinks

Aamerican College of Sports Medicine
www.acsm.org

American Heart Association
www.americanheart.org

American Senior Fitness Association
www.seniorfitness.org

Centers for Disease Control and Prevention
www.cdc.gov

Duke University Center for the Study of Aging and Human Development
www.geri.duke.edu/aging/aging.html

Biomechanics (Gait and locomotion)
www.per.ualberta.ca/biomechanics/sections.htm#loco

Fifty-plus Fitness Association
www.50plus.org

Healthy People 2010
www.health.gov/healthypeople

Institute on Aging and Environment
www.uwm.edu/Dept/IAE

International Society for Aging and Physical Activity
www.isapa.org

National Institute on Aging
www.nih.gov/nia

National Senior Games Association (Senior Olympics)
www.nsga.com

Osteoporosis Online
www.osteoporosis.ca

The National Council on Aging
www.nccoa.org

Assessment

PART FIVE consists of a single chapter that provides insight into the concepts and techniques associated with motor assessment. Along with a discussion of the purposes and considerations for selecting and implementing a wide variety of instruments, this chapter features examples of the most widely used and contemporary instruments available.

chapter

12 Assessment

12   *Assessment*

OBJECTIVES

Upon completion of this chapter, you should be able to

12.1 Discuss the general scope of motor assessment.

12.2 List and define the basic terms associated with motor assessment.

12.3 Describe the purposes of motor assessment.

12.4 Identify the considerations for selecting an assessment instrument.

12.5 Provide examples of product-oriented assessment instruments.

12.6 Provide examples of process-oriented assessment instruments.

KEY TERMS

assessment

measurement

evaluation

norm-referenced standards

criterion-referenced
  standards

product-oriented assessment

process-oriented assessment

THE OPERATIONAL DEFINITION of motor development in this text is the study of the process of change in growth, development, and motor behavior (performance) across the life span. Assessment, in general, provides the opportunity to observe, document, and interpret this change, as well as to determine the growth and developmental status of the individual at that particular time in the life span. Motor assessment can be as diverse as the field of motor development itself. Table 12.1 presents items that may be used in a comprehensive physical-motor assessment. They are grouped according to each of the different perspectives of growth, development, and performance from which motor development may be observed and assessed. An aspect that could be added to the assessment of performance is the evaluation of either the process (qualitative) or product (quantitative) characteristics of the movement action. Chapter 9

TABLE 12.1

Comprehensive Physical-Motor Assessment

Biological Growth	Development (Level of Functioning)	Motor Behavior (Performance)
Body mass	Cardiorespiratory	Reflex behavior
Height	Muscular strength/endurance	Spontaneous movement behavior
Body weight	Flexibility	Rudimentary behavior
Physique (body build)	Coordination	Fundamental movement behavior
Posture	Speed	Sport skill behavior
Anthropometric measures	Agility	
Circumference	Power	
Breadth/Length	Visual	
Skeletal maturity (age)	Balance	
Body composition	Reaction time	
Body fat	Kinesthetic	
Lean body mass	Temporal (Rhythm) timing	
Secondary sex characteristics	Menarche	

THINK ABOUT IT

Describe how you could apply table 12.1 to assess lifelong motor development (developmental continuum).

described these perspectives under the discussion of fundamental movement skills.

An example of the dynamic nature and potential for assessment through motor performance may be illustrated using the skill of running. From a development, or level of functioning perspective, running may be used as an indicator of cardiorespiratory function, speed, agility, general coordination, and reaction time. From the viewpoint of motor performance, running may be judged by its process characteristics (movement pattern), or by the product produced (e.g., performance times in the 50-yard dash or the marathon).

Numerous component-specific and task-specific tests are available for assessing the physical and motor behavior characteristics of individuals at virtually all ages. Unfortunately, no assessment batteries include norms that reflect the lifelong perspective. Most batteries were developed to assess a diversity of age-span characteristics (e.g., motor, mental, and social) displayed during the primary growth and development years of infancy through childhood.

This chapter provides an understanding of the basic terms, purposes, and considerations for motor assessment. Also presented are a description and review of selected popular and contemporary assessment instruments. For additional information refer to the Suggested Readings at the end of this chapter.

Basic Terminology of Assessment

Objective 12.2 ➤ Before the student of motor development can grasp a functional understanding of motor assessment with regard to the purpose, selection, and administration of assessment instruments, a review of basic terminology is warranted.

Assessment is a process that involves both measurement and evaluation. **Measurement** refers to the collection of information on which a decision is based. In measurement, various instruments and techniques are used to collect data. A *test* is a specific type of measurement. These instruments may take the form of requested motor performance, observation of behavior, or questions asked on paper or in an interview setting. Height, body weight, and leg length are examples of measurements that are not tests.

Evaluation is the process of decision making with regard to the value or worth of collected information. Support for such judgments commonly is based on norm-referenced or criterion-referenced standards. For cases in which such standards are not available or an overall judgment is needed for several measurements that represent a diverse spectrum of traits, evaluation frequently is thought of as the process that qualitatively (subjectively) appraises the quantitative data. For example, the results of three groups of tests (e.g., physical growth, fundamental motor skill process characteristics, and motor performance product results) may be combined to produce a single assessment score.

Criterion-referenced and norm-referenced standards are the two most widely used types of standards. **Norm-referenced standards** involve the hierarchical ordering of individuals. Assessment instruments that use this form of evaluation are basically quantitative evaluations designed to compare an individual's characteristics with those of other persons of similar sex, age, and socioeconomic group. Quality norm-referenced tests are based on statistical samplings of hundreds or, ideally, thousands of individuals.

The most common descriptors used to communicate norm-referenced standards are *percentile norms*. This type of norm describes the percentage of a given group that can be expected to score above or below a given value. For example, 40 modified sit-ups in a 1-minute period for a boy 10 years of age is at the 75th percentile. This means that only 25% of the boys in this age group did more sit-ups, and about 75% did less. For purposes of practical interpretation, the 50th percentile mark (and above) often is used as the level of acceptability. Norm-referenced standards are particularly useful for making comparisons among individuals when the situation requires a degree of selectivity, such as in identifying excellence or extremely low status values. Most assessment batteries are based on norm-referenced standards.

Criterion-referenced standards are concerned with the degree to which an individual achieves a specified level of development, motor performance, or physical status. This type of standard has received considerable attention in recent years, as evidenced by its use with most national physical fitness assessment batteries. In this case, the value of the criterion standard represents the acceptable level of performance, which is usually based on normative data and expert judgment. For example, the criterion standard for sit-ups for a 10-year-old boy is 34, and the acceptable level of flexibility on the sit-and-reach test is 25 centimeters, or 2 centimeters beyond the toes. In contrast to norm-referenced standards, individuals are compared to the criterion value and not to others of the same sex and age. Criterion-referenced standards are useful for setting performance standards for all individuals. However, a limitation of its use is that the tester knows only when an individual has met an acceptable performance level, not to what degree the person actually performed.

Some assessments are specific to motor behavior, such as fundamental movement skill performance; these are referred to as product-oriented or process-oriented instruments. With the **product-oriented assessment,** the examiner is primarily interested in the performance outcome, or the product of the behavior. Product values are described as quantitative data such as the yards a ball is thrown, running velocity in seconds, and feet and inches jumped.

In contrast, **process-oriented assessment** involves the measurement and evaluation of the characteristics of the process, or form, such as those used in rudimentary actions and fundamental movement patterns. These types of data are most often qualitative rather than quantitative. Although product-oriented data can be used with either norm-referenced or criterion-referenced standards, they commonly are associated with population norms. On the other hand, process-oriented assessment instruments are most often criterion-referenced; that is, individuals are compared to themselves in relation to established criteria. This chapter highlights such examples based on contemporary motor development theory.

▪ *Purposes of Assessment*

Objective 12.3 ➤ Assessment instruments are employed for many reasons, and the applications of the information obtained are varied. Whether the setting is in schools, child care centers, university laboratories, or in the home, assessment provides vital services in the areas of teaching, learning, and science. Although most people associate measurement and evaluation with grading, as is practiced in the schools, this is perhaps one of the least useful reasons to assess. Regardless of the setting and type of program, the most important factor is to conduct assessment with a specific purpose. The following discussion explains some of the more widely accepted purposes for assessment.

Diagnosis/screening. Some of the frequently used assessment instruments are known as diagnostic/screening tools (e.g., Apgar scale and Denver Developmental Screening Test). Assessments such as these provide a means of differentiating normal-functioning individuals (usually newborns to middle childhood) from those who may not be developing normally. If weaknesses are detected, this information is then used to determine whether the individual should be referred for additional testing or remedial work. Basic screening procedures at the beginning of any physical education or motor development program are an excellent means of identifying individuals who may have special needs.

Determine status. Perhaps the most commonly stated purpose of assessment is to determine individuals' status, progress, or achievement. This information may be used for a multitude of reasons related to more specific purposes. One indispensable practice of any instructional program is to determine whether objectives have been reached. Assessment is also essential for providing feedback on the individual's physical status or level of performance.

Placement. The results of assessment instruments frequently are used to place individuals in classes or groups according to their motor abilities. A common practice within instructional programs is to arrange individuals into homogeneous groups. In several cases this practice enhances the teaching or learning process (e.g., swimming, gymnastics, and fitness classes).

Program content. After student behaviors and characteristics have been assessed, results can be used to plan program content and guide individual progress. Assessment information is a considerable aid in writing student and program objectives that are reasonable and challenging.

Program evaluation. Program directors and administrators frequently use assessment results to evaluate the program and thereby determine the possible need for change. A common change that occurs is a modification of program standards.

THINK ABOUT IT

Explain how you could use these purposes if you were a director of an early childhood learning center with a motor development program.

Construction of norms and performance standards. Measurement, especially among large populations, provides data that can be used in establishing norms and performance standards. Group norms enable comparisons with other groups, such as those based on a nationwide sample. When criterion standards for specific performance tasks are not available, local norms (or a combination of local and national) can be used to establish them. Norms and performance standards are instrumental in providing motivation and interest within a program.

Research. Measurement and evaluation conducted scientifically can add significantly to the body of motor development research and provide information upon which educational programs can improve. Research is an important responsibility of any outstanding program.

Prediction. Theoretically, some aspects of assessment may be used to a limited degree to predict future performance. That is, specific information may be useful to directors in selecting activities individuals are most likely to master. For example, an individual with a high maximal oxygen consumption may decide to participate in triathlons or other endurance events.

Motivation of individuals. Assessment instruments can be used as motivational tools. Individuals who know how well they are performing and how they can improve are likely to be better motivated than those who receive no feedback.

Considerations for Proper Assessment

Objective 12.4 ➤ After the purposes for assessment have been established, additional considerations are warranted, especially with regard to instrument selection. Along with deciding what physical and motor characteristics are to be measured (which usually accommodate program objectives), a review of available instruments should be conducted. In addition to including the desired assessment items, only instruments that have an acceptable level of validity, reliability, and objectivity should be selected.

Validity refers to the degree to which an assessment item measures that which it is intended to measure. For example, if the purpose of the assessment is to measure aerobic capacity, experts have determined that a 1-mile run or 12-minute run is a valid indicator of this characteristic, while a half-mile run is not a valid indicator.

Reliability is a measure of the repeatability of assessment results. An individual's scores should not differ markedly on repeated administrations of the same assessment. Factors related to repeatability are consistency (dependability) of the instrument used to measure the individual's status (e.g., skinfold calipers and grip dynamometers), the examiner's instructions, and the subject's effort. One also should be aware that a test can be reliable without being valid, whereas a valid test must also be reliable.

The *objectivity* of a test refers to the degree of agreement among examiners. That is, a test that is completely objective will be scored identically by different examiners. The level of acceptability of these basic test characteristics can vary widely, even among the most popular assessment instruments. The statistical term related to the comparison of test characteristics and repeated occurrences is a *correlation;* a correlation coefficient of .80 or above generally is deemed quite acceptable.

Additional considerations for the selection of an assessment instrument include the following:

1. Is the instrument norm-referenced or criterion-referenced? Care should be taken to determine if the sampled population is representative of the population of individuals in the program.

2. Is the instrument feasible to administer? This consideration may involve several things, including time, cost, equipment, space requirements, and personnel needed. Since time is often a perpetual problem facing program administrators who have large and small numbers of participants, instruments should be evaluated in terms of time economy.

3. Are the funds available? Some assessment instruments cost hundreds of dollars and require expensive equipment, whereas others may accomplish the basic objectives with only minor compromises at a much lower price. For example, the best measurement of aerobic capacity is maximal oxygen consumption. However, thousands of dollars worth of equipment are needed to carry it out, and each test requires about 45 minutes to administer. Less accurate but acceptable and more feasible measures (field tests) are the 1-mile walk/run and 12-minute walk/run (using norm-referenced or criterion-referenced standards). In general, however, the cost factor should consider accuracy, durability, and long-term use.

4. What levels of training and expertise are required to administer the items and interpret the data? Additional training and practice may be needed. In the interest of time economy, more than one examiner is usually imperative. This may call for considerable planning in order to provide reliable and objective assessment.

For a more thorough treatment of test development as a science, refer to *Psychological Testing* (Kaplan & Saccuzzo, 2001) and Salvia & Ysseldyke (2001) in the Suggested Readings. Both are excellent sources of information and guidance.

■ *Assessment Instruments*

The possibilities of assessing the various aspects of physical growth, development, and motor behavior are numerous (see table 12.1 on page 389). In the areas of physical growth and physiological assessment alone, there are hundreds of instruments. Many of these have been mentioned or described throughout the text (e.g., skinfolds, anthropometric measures, and various physiological tests). This discussion will focus on some of the more widely used product-oriented motor assessment batteries and process-oriented instruments. An *assessment battery* is a group of several tests standardized on the same population.

Motor behavior assessment items have been included in general child development batteries, along with mental, language, and social entries, since the 1920s (Gesell, 1925). Since that time numerous instruments have been developed. However, while the quantity of instruments seems sufficient, the quality has been suspect. Most motor behavior items have minimal, if any, rationale for development and are based on generalized product (quantitative) characteristics (i.e., how far, how fast, how many, etc). Other global assessment items merely ask if the child can throw a ball, kick a ball forward, stack cubes, or balance on one foot. Although some of these types of assessments may have an acceptable level of validity and reliability, they are limited from a motor development perspective, especially in describing the process of change. In recent years greater focus has centered on the qualitative characteristics of motor behavior as evidenced by the development of process-oriented assessment instruments based on contemporary motor development theory.

The following pages describe only a selected number of assessment instruments. The intent of this discussion is to provide the student of motor development with a glimpse into the diversity of assessment items and formats available. For additional information on specific instruments, the latter part of this chapter provides a list of recommended sources. Refer to Suggested Readings for in-depth descriptions of these and other physical and motor assessment tests.

The following examples represent standardized and accessible instruments that have received considerable recognition for the assessment of newborns, infants, and school-age populations.

Newborn Assessment

Objective 12.5 ➤ **The Apgar Scale** *The Apgar scale* (Apgar, 1953) is used in delivery rooms all over the world to test the physical health of newborns. The scale typically is administered to newborns 1 minute and 5 minutes after delivery and measures the appearance (skin color), pulse, grimace (reflex irritability), activity (muscle tone), and respiratory effort (APGAR) of the infant. Each characteristic is rated on a scale of 0 to 2 in which 2 denotes normal function, 1 denotes reduced function, and 0 denotes seriously impaired function (see table 12.2 on page 396). Thus, a total score of 10 is perfect.

Approximately 90 percent of all newborns score 7 or higher. A score of 4 or less is generally an indication that immediate medical assistance is needed. The most controversial assessment item on the scale is skin color. Few newborns receive a 2 at one minute, and of course, the measure is invalid with dark-skinned babies. Despite these limitations the Apgar scale is noted as a reliable and accurate indicator of later neuromuscular difficulties.

Standardization of the instrument showed newborns with the lowest scores had the highest mortality rates, and the device was useful in predicting infant death rate. A high percentage of infants found to have neuromuscular or developmental problems by 1 year of age had low Apgar scores at birth (Drage et al., 1966).

The Brazelton Behavioral Assessment Scale Among the unique characteristics of the *Brazelton Behavioral Assessment Scale* (Brazelton,

TABLE 12.2

The Apgar Scale

	0	1	2
Appearance (skin color)	White or blue	Limbs blue, body pink	Pink
Pulse (rate)	No pulse	100 beats/min	More than 100 beats/min
Grimace (reflexive grimace initiated by stimulating the plantar surface of the foot)	No response	Facial grimaces, slight body movement	Facial grimaces, extensive body movement
Activity (muscle tone)	No movement, muscles flaccid	Limbs partially flexed, little movement, poor muscle tone	Active movement, good muscle tone
Respiratory effort (amount of respiratory activity)	No respiration	Slow, irregular respiration	Good, regular respiration, strong cry

Source: From V. A. Apgar, "A Proposal for a New Method of Evaluation of a Newborn Infant" in *Anesthesia and Analgesia: Current Research,* 32:260–267. Copyright © 1953 Williams & Wilkins, Baltimore, MD. Reprinted by permission.

1984) is that it provides an assessment two or three days after the baby is born, then another assessment on day 9 or 10 after the baby is home from the hospital and has had the opportunity to relax from the stress of delivery. The Brazelton was designed to measure three primary items: subtle central nervous system functions, temperamental differences, and the capacity for interaction. Typically the scale is administered to at-risk babies or those for whom there is a concern about development.

The instrument generates results in three areas. One consists of 20 reflex items designed to screen for neurological soundness. The second is the neonate's interactive behavioral repertoire, which is assessed with 26 items (table 12.3). The third area of assessment, which is not as closely linked to motor behavior, is a rating of attractiveness behavior (i.e., the baby's contribution to and readiness for interaction) and need for stimulation (i.e., the need for and use of stimulation as it relates to organizing responses).

In the reflex assessment, each reflex is scored 0 (no response), 1 (low), 2 (medium), or 3 (high level of response). Babies with three or more low scores typically are referred for additional neurological assessment.

The 26 behavioral items are considered the most important assessment area. These items may be grouped into four dimensions:

1. Interaction capacities: the capacity to attend to and process environmental events.

TABLE 12.3

Reflex and Behavioral Items for the Brazelton Neonatal Behavioral Assessment Scale

	BEHAVIORAL ITEMS	
Reflex Behaviors	**Specific**	**General**
1. Plantar grasp	1. Response decrement to light	1. Alertness
2. Hand grasp	2. Response decrement to rattle	2. General tonus
3. Anal colonus	3. Response decrement to bell	3. Motor maturity
4. Babinski	4. Response decrement to pinprick	4. Cuddliness
5. Standing	5. Inanimate visual orientation response (focusing and following an object)	5. Consolability with intervention
6. Stepping		6. Peak to excitement
7. Placing		7. Rapidity of buildup
8. Incurvation	6. Inanimate auditory orientation response (reaction to an auditory stimulus)	8. Irritability
9. Crawling		9. Activity (alert states)
10. Glabulla	7. Animate visual orientation (reaction)	10. Tremulousness
11. Tonic deviation of head and eyes		11. Startle
12. Nystagmus	8. Animate auditory orientation (reaction to a voice)	12. Liability of skin color
13. Tonic neck	9. Animate visual and auditory orientation (reaction to a person's face and voice)	13. Liability of states
14. Moro		14. Self-quieting activity
15. Rooting (intensity)		15. Hand-to-mouth facility
16. Sucking (intensity)	10. Pull-to-sit	
17–20. Passive movements (right arm, left arm, right leg, left leg)	11. Defensive movements	

2. Motoric capacities: the ability to maintain muscle tone, control motor behavior, and accomplish integrated acts, such as placing the thumb in the mouth and sucking.
3. Organizational capacities with respect to state control: the ability to maintain a calm, alert state when facing increased stimulation from events such as a light, bell ring, or pinprick.
4. Organizational capacities in the physiologic response to stress: the capacity to master the physiologic demands of immaturity, such as the ability to inhibit startles and tremors while attending to stimuli.

Each item is scored on a continuum of 1 to 9. A score of 1 represents the lowest state, while the ideal state varies from item to item and lies somewhere between 1 and 9 (table 12.3). The baby's performance also may be rated on each item with a more simplistic "good," "adequate," or "deficient."

Although evidence of the Brazelton's validity has been verified (Als et al., 1979), its test-retest reliability and standardization have been questioned. The reliability problem is due primarily to the fact that the instrument assesses the neonate's current status, which can change rapidly. One problem plaguing standardization is that newborns from different cultures tend to behave differently. There are two primary reasons that the Brazelton scale is not used extensively. First, only highly trained examiners normally found at large medical centers are deemed competent to administer the instrument. Second, it is recommended not to use the instrument with premature babies (which excludes a large risk group). However, there is evidence the instrument has utility as a research device and in identifying high-risk infants (Wodrich, 1997).

Infant Assessment

The Bayley Scales of Infant Development   Originally published in 1933, the Bayley Scales of Infant Development (Bayley, 1969, 1993) are regarded as having outstanding psychometric properties for infant assessment. The Bayley-II (1993) is a norm-referenced, standardized instrument designed for use with children from 1 to 42 months. It consists of three sections: the Mental Scale, Motor Scale, and Behavior Rating Scale.

The Behavioral Rating Scale contains 30 ratings completed after the evaluation of the mental and motor items. The record is a systematic way of summarizing such behavioral observations as attention/arousal, orientation/engagement, emotional regulation, and motor quality.

The Motor Scale (psychomotor development index) includes items related to the progression of postural control; gross motor abilities such as sitting, standing, walking, and stair climbing; and abilities involving fine motor control. In Bayley's words the Motor Scale was "designed to provide a measure of the degree of control of the body, coordination of the large muscles and finer manipulative skills of the hands and fingers" (Bayley, 1969, 3). Table 12.4 lists Bayley-II Motor Scale items.

As noted earlier, the Bayley scales are known as one of the best infant assessments available. They can make accurate, reliable, and valid measures of an infant's current ability status. Their use as a research instrument also has received wide support. The scales are relatively expensive. Because they are somewhat difficult to administer, a significant amount of training is required to do so. Thus, use of the scales is confined mostly to specialists who work extensively with infants.

In 1995, the *Bayley Infant Neurodevelopmental Screener (BINS)* was introduced as a companion screener to the Bayley-II. It was designed to quickly assess the auditory and visual receptive functions, verbal and motor expressive functions, and cognitive processes in infants ages 3 to 24 months. Its psychometric properties appear sound, with comparative scores based on a large sample of clinical and normal infants. Scores identify (screen) infants as low, moderate, or high-risk, in relation to

TABLE 12.4

Bayley-II Motor Scale Items

Group	Motor Area (Number of Items)
Gross motor	Head control (10)
	Hands posture (2)
	Turning (3)
	Imitative behavior (2)
	Preambulatory skills (4)
	Body positioning (10)
	Sitting (8)
	Stairs (6)
	Balance (9)
	Walking (16)
	Jumping (5)
	Throwing (1)
Fine motor	Grasping (9)
	Drawing (4)
	Pencil grasp/Writing (6)
Ungrouped (e.g., retains ring, buttons one button, tactile discrimination)	(16)
Motor quality (behavioral rating scale)	(8)

developmental delays or neurological impairment. As with the Bayley-II, this test is designed for use by professionals trained in early childhood assessment.

The Alberta Infant Motor Scale The *Alberta Infant Motor Scale (AIMS)* (Piper & Darrah, 1994) is an observational assessment designed to evaluate the motor development of infants from 2 weeks through independent walking (18 months). The authors identify two purposes of the AIMS: (1) to identify infants delayed or impaired in their motor development, and (2) to evaluate motor development over time. This uniquely qualitative test consists of 58 developmentally sequenced pictorial items that describe the infant's posture, weight bearing, and spontaneous antigravity movements while in four postural positions: prone, supine, sitting, and standing (figure 12.1 on page 400 provides an example). To score the items (observed/not observed), the infant is observed in an

■ *Figure 12.1*

Example of an
AIMS item

Sitting with Propped Arms

Weight bearing	Weight on buttocks, legs, and hands
Posture	Head up, shoulders elevated
	Hips flexed, externally rotated, and abducted
	Knees flexed
	Lumbar and thoracic spine rounded
Antigravity movement	Maintains head in midline
	Supports weight on arms briefly

Prompt: Examiner places the infant in sitting position. To pass this item, the infant must maintain the position independently without the examiner's support.

unobtrusive environment with minimal handling. The total test easily is completed in 20 to 30 minutes. Normative data are available, and the raw scores can be converted to percentile ranks from monthly age levels.

The AIMS has demonstrated excellent psychometric properties with high test-retest and inter-rater reliability, and concurrent validity with the Bayley-II and Peabody Scales (see pages 398 and 405) (Darrah et al., 1998). Complementing the qualitative nature of the assessment, it also has been reported that the descriptive indicators are consistent with functional movement. For example, the infant's skill level is represented by a developmental window (range of skills), which hypothetically depicts the dynamic nature of movement in transition (Case-Smith, 1996).

Posture and Fine Motor Assessment of Infants   Based on contemporary dynamic systems theory, the *Posture and Fine Motor Assessment of Infants (PFMAI)* (Case-Smith & Bigsby, 2000) measures qualitative aspects of motor skill development by using systems that rate the dynamic quality of postural control and grasping/manipulation (fine-motor) patterns in infants in the first year of postnatal life (2 to 12 months). The PFMAI is sensitive to small increments of change in individual infants. A 4-point criterion referenced scale is used to rate the specific aspects of movement believed to be important in attaining functional mobility and manipulation. An additional purpose of the PFMAI is to measure progress or developmental change. Figure 12.2 presents an example of a PFMAI assessment item.

The Fine Motor section has 41 items that measure accuracy and quality of reach and grasping patterns, precision of release, and control of arm and hand movements when specific objects are presented. In

■ *Figure 12.2*

Example of a PFMAI assessment item (posture: ages 2 to 6 months)

Posture in Prone

Observe the infant in a prone position with a toy placed in front of him or her.

1. **Stability of posture**
   1. Lies flat on the supporting surface.
   2. Assumes an upright posture momentarily.
   3. Maintains an upright posture for less than 10 seconds.
   4. Maintains an upright posture for more than 10 seconds.

2. **Movement against gravity**
   1. Lies flat on the supporting surface.
   2. Infrequently and momentarily moves against gravity.
   3. Lifts head and chest from surface in the vertical plane.
   4. Moves side to side.

3. **Trunk stability and extension**
   1. Does not lift head or demonstrates neck extension only.
   2. Trunk extension through the scapular region.
   3. Trunk extension to the lumbar spine.
   4. Trunk extension to pelvis.

addition to its qualitative merits, the PFMAI Fine Motor section is unique because it provides a method for assessing the influence of object affordances in eliciting a range of manipulative movements. This is accomplished by presenting the infant with objects of different size and action potential, which thereby facilitates different movement patterns.

The Posture Scale consists of 31 items designed to measure postural control and proximal stability/mobility, and the infant's ability to move within and between postures. According to the authors, psychometric properties include high inter-rater reliability (.86 to .99), moderate test-retest reliability (.58 to .96), and a high correlation with chronologic age ($r = .94$).

Toddler and Infant Motor Evaluation   The stated purposes of the *Toddler and Infant Motor Evaluation (TIME)* are (1) to diagnose motor delays, (2) to plan intervention, and (3) to evaluate change due to intervention and/or maturation (Miller & Roid, 1994). The TIME was designed to assess the quality of movement in children 4 to 42 months of age. The qualitative assessment includes standard scores on eight subtests, five of which have been standardized: Mobility, Stability, Motor Organization, Social/Emotional Abilities, and Functional Performance.

Holding to the dynamic systems perspective, the TIME identifies the components of specific actions and assesses the infant's ability to organize those components. For example, the Mobility subtest assesses the infant's ability to move within and from five starting positions (supine, prone, sitting, quadruped, and standing) that complement his/her developmental age. The scale analyzes the maturity and number of variations within and between positions, and the highest developmental level obtained. The test provides a measurement of the patterns of transitional movements observed over a 20-second time period.

Standardized with a sample ($n = 144$) of children with motor delays and children ($n = 731$) developing normally, the TIME has good test-retest and inter-rater reliability (.89 to .99). It is reported to have excellent sensitivity in identifying infants with motor dysfunction (Miller & Roid, 1994).

Test of Infant Motor Performance   The *Test of Infant Motor Performance (TIMP)* (Campbell et al., 1994) is an assessment of motor function in infants at risk for developmental disabilities. The test was designed for use by physical therapists and occupational therapists who assess and treat infants from 32 weeks gestational age through 4 to 5 months past term-equivalent age. The concepts underlying the test include the notion that movement assessment must be based contextually, must reveal the development of postural control synergies that lead to functional movement in daily life, and must reflect the hypothesis that development of postural control may be a rate-limiting factor in motor development and motor learning. The TIMP assesses the infant's ability to sustain postures in a variety of spatial orientations; regain postural stability following perturbations; and make transitions between postures for orienting to interesting events and people, changing positions, and self-comforting. The test consists of two scales. The infant's ability to make coordinated postural responses when positioned in a variety of spatial orientations is rated with the *Elicited Scale* (for example, "Head turn in prone position to sound"). The *Observed Scale* assesses the infant's attempt to change positions, orient head and trunk, and selectively initiate individual body segments into action (for example, "Reaches for person or object" and "Reciprocal kicking").

Recent studies indicate the test discriminates among children with varying degrees of risk for motor dysfunction in the first year of life, is reliable in the hands of experienced clinicians, and has test-retest stability (Campbell, 1999; Campbell & Kolobe, 2000). An independent review of the test by Case-Smith concludes that the TIMP is a "sensitive measure of motor development in the first 4 months of life (1996, 36).

Assessment of (up to) School-Age Populations

The Denver Developmental Screening Test The *Denver Developmental Screening Test (DDST)* is one of the most extensively used screening instruments for children from birth to 6 years of age (DDST, 1990). As a screening device, the instrument's purpose is to identify quickly those individuals likely to have significant developmental delays. The instrument is not an IQ test or an in-depth assessment device. The DDST consists of 125 items divided into four assessment areas:

1. Personal/social. Assesses the child's ability to get along with people and to provide personal care. Sample items: smiles spontaneously at 3 months, drinks from cup at 11½ months, and dresses without supervision by 4 years.
2. Language. Assesses the ability to hear, understand, and use language. Sample items: laughs at 2 months, combines two different words at 20 months, and gives first and last name by 2½ years.
3. Fine motor/adaptive. Assesses the child's ability to use vision and the hands to pick up objects and draw.
4. Gross motor. Assesses the ability to perform rudimentary and fundamental gross motor skills.

Table 12.5 on page 404 shows a sample of gross motor and fine motor/adaptive items from the DDST.

A unique and interesting characteristic of the DDST form is the bar graph for each item that represents the age at which the standardization population (norm group) performed the specific task (see figure 12.3 on page 405). As shown, the bar indicates the ages at which 25%, 50%, 75%, and 90% of the norm group performed the task. Consistent with its stated purpose, the DDST looks for delays rather than producing a

TABLE 12.5

Sample Motor Items from the DDST

Area	Items
Gross motor	Rudimentary posture control: of head, neck, trunk; rolling over, sitting, standing with support, pulling to stand, cruising, standing alone, walking Fundamental manipulative behaviors: kicking, throwing, tricycle riding, catching Fundamental locomotor behaviors: jumping in place, long jumping, hopping Fundamental stability abilities: balancing on one foot, heel-toe walk
Fine motor/ adaptive	Rudimentary manipulative behaviors: visual tracking, reaching, grasping and releasing, cube stacking, scribbling, copying, draw a person

numerical score. A developmental delay is described as any item that is completely to the left of the age line, which indicates the child failed an item passed by 90% of the norm group.

Research concerning the DDST's reliability and validity has been generally supportive, but the fact that the norm group was limited to children from Denver, Colorado, has been suggested as a limitation. The concern is that the DDST norms may not reflect the country's racial and socioeconomic levels. However, the DDST generally is recognized as a valuable screening instrument capable of providing a great deal more insight than clinical observation or global descriptions from parents in the search for children who may have developmental problems.

A short form of the DDST, the *Revised-Prescreening Developmental Questionnaire (R-PDQ)*, consists of 24 to 25 questions designed for four age groups: 0 to 9 months, 9 to 24 months, 2 to 4 years, and 4 to 6 years (R-PDQ, 1986). The instrument can be administered by the parent or caregiver. It is designed primarily to make guardians more aware of the development of their children and to screen out those children likely to have problems with the longer DDST.

The Basic Motor Ability Tests-Revised   The *Basic Motor Ability Tests-Revised (BMAT-R)* was designed to assess motor behavior in children 4 to 12 years of age (Arnheim & Sinclair, 1979). The assessment battery consists of 11 tests for evaluating the general areas of fine and gross motor ability, coordination, balance, and selected physical fitness components (table 12.6).

Advantages of this instrument are that it is easy to administer and requires little training to do so. The authors of the test point out that a single examiner can test one child in about 15 to 20 minutes and a group of up to five children in approximately 30 minutes. Norms were

■ *Figure 12.3*

Percentage of
normal children
passing the item

established on children from diverse backgrounds, and the retest reliability for the entire battery is high (.93). However, inadequate information is available concerning validity, and the instrument consists of a
relatively few general items (as is the case with most motor assessment
instruments). Thus, its use is limited, except perhaps as a screening
device to discriminate between normal children and those with physical
and motor deficiencies.

Peabody Development Motor Scales II The *Peabody Development
Motor Scales II (PDMS-2)* (Folio & Fewell, 2000), a revision of the 1983
version, assesses the gross- and fine-motor ability of children from birth

TABLE 12.6

BMAT-R Test Items

Item	Stated Purpose of Test
Bead stringing	Bilateral eye-hand coordination and dexterity
Target throwing	Eye-hand coordination as associated with throwing
Marble transfer	Finger dexterity and speed of hand movement
Back and hamstring stretch	Flexibility of back and hamstring muscles
Standing long jump	Strength and power in the thigh and lower leg muscles
Face down to standing	Speed and agility
Static balance	Static balance with eyes open and closed
Basketball throw	Arm and shoulder girdle explosive strength
Ball striking	Coordination associated with striking
Target kicking	Eye-foot coordination
Agility run	Ability to rapidly move the body and alter direction

through 6 years of age. The Fine Motor section consists of test items that measure (1) controlled use of the fingers and hands under the general heading of Grasping (26 items), and (2) Visual-Motor Integration (72 items), using such test items as reaching and grasping an object, building with blocks, and copying designs.

The normative sample for the PDMS-2 consisted of 2,003 persons who resided in 46 states and were considered to be representative of the current U.S. population. The manufacturer claims that with regard to psychometrics, this version is an improvement over the original. For example, it has good reliability and validity within a variety of subgroups as well as with the general population. According to the manual for the 1983 version, the test has acceptable test-retest reliability (.95 and .80, for the gross- and fine-motor scales), inter-rater reliability (.99 for both scales), and is a valid assessment of motor development. An outside review of the test's psychometric properties by Palisano et al. (1995) was supportive.

The Bruininks-Oseretsky Test of Motor Proficiency Of the available product-oriented motor assessment instruments, the *Bruininks-Oseretsky Test of Motor Proficiency (BOT)* is heralded as one of the best. Since its introduction, the BOT has undergone substantial review from the psychological and motor development community (Bruininks, 1978). This has resulted in the general conclusion that it is a well-normed, technically acceptable measure of gross and fine motor ability for children 4½ to 14½ years of age (e.g., Haubenstricker & Sapp, 1985; Sabatino, 1985).

The BOT consists of 46 items that yield a comprehensive index of motor proficiency and separate composite scores for fine and gross motor abilities. These items are clustered into eight subtests designed to measure running speed and agility, balance, bilateral coordination, strength, upper limb coordination, response speed, visual-motor control, and upper limb speed and dexterity (table 12.7). An acceptable 14-item BOT short form that provides a brief survey of the child's motor proficiency is also available.

The BOT is an individually administered test that takes 45 to 60 minutes to complete; the short form takes about 15 to 20 minutes to complete. Among its several merits as an assessment instrument is that its norms are provided in the form of standard scores, percentile ranks, stanines, and age equivalents for the complete battery. Interpretation tables that represent age intervals of six months permit the conversion of subtest scores into subtest standard scores. Practitioners have noted one disadvantage of the BOT is that results are not too helpful for programming.

In summary, though the BOT has limitations in overall motor assessment because it is not capable of detecting developmental change as process-oriented instruments do, it is a well-developed, well-standardized test battery of value as a research tool and diagnostic device.

THINK ABOUT IT

Have you noticed any commonalties among the product-oriented tests? Describe some of them.

TABLE 12.7

Test Items from the BOT

General Category	Subtest Area	Items
Gross motor skills	1. Running—Designed to measure running speed	Shuttle run
	2. Balance (8 times)—Designed to measure static and dynamic balance abilities	Static balance (3 items) Dynamic balance (5 items)
	3. Bilateral coordination (8 items)—Designed to measure simultaneous coordination of upper and lower limbs	Foot and finger tapping (3 items) Jumping in place (4 items) Drawing lines and crosses simultaneously (1 item)
	4. Strength (3 items)—Designed to measure upper arm and shoulder girdle strength, abdominal strength, and leg strength	Standing broad jump Sit-ups Knee push-ups (boys under 8; all girls) Full push-ups (boys 8 and older)
Gross and fine motor skills	5. Upper limb coordination (9 items)—Designed to measure gross and fine eye-hand coordination	Ball bounce and catch (2 items) Catching tossed ball (2 items) Throwing a ball (1 item) Touching swinging ball (1 item) Precise upper limb movements (3 items)
Fine motor skills	6. Response speed (1 item)—Designed to measure response to a moving object	Yardstick drop (1 item)
	7. Visual-motor control (8 items)—Designed to measure coordination of eye-hand movements	Cutting (1 item) Drawing and copying (7 items)
	8. Upper limb speed and dexterity (8 items)—Designed to measure hand and finger dexterity, hand speed, and arm speed	Penny placing (2 items) Card sorting (1 item) Bead stringing (1 item) Peg displacing (1 item) Lines and dots (3 items)

Process-Oriented (Fundamental Movement) Assessment Instruments

Objective 12.6 ➤ A variety of assessment instruments are designed to examine the process (i.e., qualitative) characteristics of movement. Inherent in these instruments is the intent to identify an individual's current movement qualities and compare the actions to an established developmental sequence.

(Chapter 9 discussed the research and applied information concerning developmental sequence with regard to specific fundamental movement skills. It may be helpful to review that information. Particularly relevant are the discussions related to stage theory and Roberton's intratask component theory of identifying change in motor behavior.) Generally accompanying process-oriented instruments are criterion-referenced standards that compare individuals to themselves as well as to the criterion standard rather than to others as with norm-referenced standards.

Keep in mind the instruments described in the following pages represent practical attempts to observe, measure, and assess the process characteristics of movement. Research endeavors in this field are relatively recent; not a great deal has been established concerning the validity of several developmental movement pattern sequences. To more accurately assess the developmental change of an individual's movement pattern characteristics, film analysis over time is desirable (though it is generally not practical). For additional information regarding movement analysis using film, various scientific instruments, and computers, refer to Adrian and Cooper (1994).

Since the use of sophisticated instrumentation and film analysis are needed to detect precise changes, most process-oriented instruments use a global analysis. That is, the developmental sequence of a specific skill is identified using three to five total body stages (e.g., immature, elementary, and mature), rather than making a developmental level analysis of specific body segments. There are also instruments that use identifiers considered to be relatively subjective; these are useful primarily as global screening and diagnostic devices.

Test of Gross Motor Development #2   The *Test of Gross Motor Development (TGMD-2)* (Ulrich, 1999) is one of the best examples, to date, of a practical, easily administered instrument developed to assess the sequence and qualitative aspects of motor skill behavior. Designed for use with children 3 to 11 years of age, the TGMD-2 provides assessment of 12 of the most commonly practiced locomotor and manipulative motor skills. The locomotor skill assessment includes running, leaping, horizontal jumping, hopping, galloping, skipping, and sliding. The manipulative skill section includes two-handed striking, stationary ball bouncing, catching, kicking, and overhand throwing. Table 12.8 presents a sample of the qualitative assessment format.

The TGMD-2 is considered quite comprehensive in the number and diversity of the motor skills that it assesses; it also can be administered with a minimum amount of special training and takes only about 15 minutes to complete per child. Another attractive characteristic is that it provides both norm-referenced and criterion-referenced interpretations. The instrument has well-established validity and reliability characteristics and, for an instrument of this type, is standardized on a diverse and relatively large normative sample.

TABLE 12.8

The TGMD-2 Assessment Format

LOCOMOTOR SKILLS					
Skill	Equipment	Directions	Performance Criteria	1st	2nd
Run	50 feet of clear space and tape or other marking device	Mark off two lines 50 feet apart Instruct student to "run fast" from one line to the other	1. Brief period where both feet are off the ground 2. Arms in opposition to legs, elbows bent 3. Foot placement near or on a line (not flat-footed) 4. Nonsupport leg bent approximately 90 degrees (close to buttocks)	1 0 1 0	
Horizontal jump	10 feet of clear space and tape or other marking device	Mark off a starting line on the floor, mat, or carpet Have the student start behind the line Tell the student to "jump far"	1. Preparatory movement includes flexion of both knees with arms extended behind the body 2. Arms extend forcefully forward and upward, reaching full extension above head 3. Take off and land on both feet simultaneously 4. Arms are brought downward during landing	1 0 1 0	
OBJECT CONTROL SKILLS					
Kick	8–10 inch plastic or slightly de-flated playground ball, 30 feet of clear space, tape or other marking device	Mark off one line 30 feet away from a wall and one that is 20 feet from the wall Place the ball on the line nearest the wall and tell the student to stand on the other line	1. Rapid continuous approach to the ball 2. The trunk is inclined backward during ball contact 3. Forward swing of the arm opposite kicking leg 4. Follow-through by hopping on the nonkicking foot	1 0 0 0	
Overhand throw	3 tennis balls, a wall, 25 feet of clear space	Tell the student to kick the ball "hard" at the wall Tell student to throw the ball "hard" at the wall	1. A downward arc of the throwing arm initiates the windup 2. Rotation of hip and shoulder to a point where the nondominant side faces an imaginary target 3. Weight is transferred by stepping with the foot opposite the throwing hand 4. Follow-through beyond ball release diagonally across body toward side opposite throwing arm	0 0 0 0	

1 = performs task correctly 2 of 3 trials
0 = does not perform task correctly 2 of 3 trials
Source: From Ulrich, 1999, the Test of Gross Motor Development.
Reprinted by permission of Pro-Ed, Inc., Austin, TX.

TABLE 12.9

Sample of Body Action Assessment of the FMPAI

	RUNNING		
	Initial	**Elementary**	**Mature**
Leg action (side view)	—Leg swing is short, limited —Stiff, uneven stride —No observable flight phase —Incomplete extension of support leg	—Length, swing, and speed increase —Limited but observable flight phase —Support leg extends more completely at takeoff	—Length of stride is at its maximum; speed of stride is fast —Definite flight phase —Support leg extends completely —Recovery thigh is parallel to ground
Arm action	—Stiff, short swing; varying degrees of elbow flexion —Tend to swing outward horizontally	—Arm swing increases —Horizontal swing is reduced on backswing	—Swing vertically in opposition to the legs —Arms are bent in approximate right angles
Leg action (rear view)	—Swinging leg rotates outward from the hip —Swinging foot, toes outward —Wide base of support	—Swinging foot crosses midline at height of recovery to rear	—Little rotary action of recovery leg and foot

Source: From *Fundamental Movement* by Bruce A. McClenaghan and David L. Gallahue, Copyright © 1978 by Saunders College Publishing, a division of Holt, Rinehart and Winston, Inc. Reprinted by permission of David L. Gallahue.

Fundamental Movement Pattern Assessment Instrument Originally developed by McClenaghan and Gallahue (1978), the *Fundamental Movement Pattern Assessment Instrument (FMPAI)* (Gallahue & Cleland, 2003), of the more established process-oriented instruments, is one of the easiest to use. It was designed to measure the present developmental status of children and to assess movement pattern change over time. The instrument includes assessment of five fundamental movement skills: running, horizontal jumping, throwing, catching, and kicking. After the individual's movement pattern is observed, it is analyzed by body segment action and classified according to one of three stages (for that body action) to depict the developmental continuum. These stages are the initial stage, the elementary stage, and the mature stage (table 12.9). In essence, this is a form of the component approach to movement pattern assessment.

The instrument includes good visual illustrations of each stage and easy-to-use scoring aids. In contrast to the TGMD-2, the developmental sequences of the FMPAI were not developed from or standardized on a population sample but are based on a review of the biomechanical literature. Nonetheless, the authors report acceptable validity and reliability. In summary, the FMPAI is a carefully developed observation instrument that allows for the documentation of change over time and by individual comparison.

Developmental Sequence of Fundamental Motor Skills Inventory
The *Developmental Sequence of Fundamental Motor Skills Inventory (DSFMSI)* also provides process analysis of the commonly practiced fundamental locomotor and manipulative motor skills of children (Seefeldt & Haubenstricker, 1976). Included in the assessment are locomotor-walking, running, jumping, hopping, and skipping, and manipulative-throwing, catching, striking, kicking, and punting. Each motor skill is described within a developmental sequence that includes four or five stages ranging from immature (stage 1) to mature (stage 4 or 5). During the evaluation process children are matched to both visual and verbal descriptions of each stage.

Though the psychometric properties of the test have not been reported, the developmental sequences are based on longitudinal and cross-sectional data collected as part of the ongoing Michigan State University Motor Performance Study.

Recall that chapters 8 and 9 provide useful information of assessing rudimentary behaviors and fundamental movement patterns. For example, in chapter 9 the information related to the mature characteristics and developmental sequence of each skill may be used to create a useful observation instrument.

Other Commonly Used Instruments

Hughes Basic Gross Motor Assessment Known for its practical application in the field, the Hughes Basic Gross Motor Assessment is a process/product-oriented assessment designed for use with children 5½ to 12½ years of age (Hughes, 1979). The test consists of items intended to evaluate a selection of locomotor, balance, throwing, dribbling, and other ball-handling skills. Although the norm population did not include children from various ethnic groups, overall reliability has been reported as good and the validity acceptable. The test is scored with a four-point rating scale based on quality of movement using stated deviations from normal performance. Inter-rater reliability also is reported to be quite good (.97). The test is administered individually and uses commonly available equipment for several tasks. In summary, the Hughes test is useful in the field for evaluating minor motor problems and identifying those children who require further assessment and possible remediation.

TABLE 12.10

Sample Process Analysis Format of SIGMA

SKILL OF STAIR CLIMBING			
Test Eqipment: Series of Stairs			
Level I	**Level II**	**Level III**	**Level IV**
When positioned at the bottom of a series of steps, the child demonstrates one of the following behaviors: 1. creeps up five steps and slides down from step to step on buttocks 2. creeps up and down five steps 3. walks up and back down while in a hands-feet position like animal walking	When standing at the bottom of a series of steps, the child, with or without the aid of the railing or wall, walks up and down five steps and demonstrates the following behaviors in two out of three trials: 1. walks up using two-foot landing (mark time pattern) 2. walks down either in the same manner or by sliding from step to step on the buttocks	When standing at the bottom of a series of steps, the child, with the aid of the railing or wall, walks up and down five steps and demonstrates the following behaviors in two out of three trials: 1. walks up using an alternate-stepping pattern 2. walks down in the same manner or by using a two-foot landing (mark time pattern)	When standing at the bottom of a series of steps, the child independently walks up and down five steps and demonstrates the following behaviors in two out of three trials: 1. walks up using an alternate-stepping pattern 2. walks down using an alternate-stepping pattern

Source: Reprinted by permission of Mike Loovis.

Note: Examiner cannot serve as an aid in place of railing or wall.

Ohio State University Scale of Intra-Gross Motor Assessment

The *Ohio State University Scale of Intra-Gross Motor Assessment (SIGMA)* is a criterion-referenced instrument designed to assess fundamental motor skills of children of preschool to 14 years of age (Loovis & Ersing, 1979). The motor skills included are walking, running, jumping, hopping, skipping, throwing, catching, striking, and kicking. Also included are ladder and stair climbing. Each skill is described on a separate sheet in four levels of developmental sequence. Table 12.10 shows a sample of this format for the skill of stair climbing.

Aside from face validity with the literature, the instrument's other psychometric properties have been questioned. However, the authors report that the SIGMA can be administered with acceptable accuracy in a formal as well as in an informal free play setting. An additional strength of the SIGMA is the accompanying Performance Base Curriculum

(PBC). The PBC provides the much-needed link between assessment and program intervention. The curriculum is an objective-based instructional program that provides activities to accommodate each developmental level within each skill.

McCarthy Scales of Children's Abilities   Of the numerous instruments known primarily for their assessment of children's cognitive abilities, the *McCarthy Scales of Children's Abilities* warrants mention with regard to its perceptual and motor components. The McCarthy is designed for children ages 2½ to 8½ years of age, but it is known primarily as a preschool assessment device of considerable value with good psychometric properties (Wodrich, 1997).

The instrument offers three general indexes of behavior: a general cognitive index, which consists of verbal, perceptual/performance, and quantitative subareas; a memory index; and a motor index. The memory and motor indexes are interpreted separately from the general cognitive index. The perceptual/performance and motor index components have specific relevance to motor behavior, in general, and include the following task behaviors:

1. Perceptual/Performance: block building, puzzle solving, tapping sequence, right-left orientation, draw-a-design, draw-a-child, and conceptual grouping
2. Motor: leg coordination, arm coordination, imitative action, draw-a-design, and draw-a-child

Compared with similar measurement instruments, the objective scoring for the motor tasks on the McCarthy scales has been well received. The tasks approximate the motor screening given by a specialist but offer the advantage of objective scoring and derived scores. It is perhaps due at least in part to this advantage that researchers in recent years have used parts of the McCarthy motor index as variables in several scientific studies. The entire battery takes approximately 45 to 60 minutes per child. It is suggested that individuals with specific training and background administer the instrument.

Tests for Older Persons

Since physical function can differ considerably in the elderly, a wide range of tests is needed. Test categories correspond to general capability level and range from physically elite and fit, to the physically independent (low-level function), to the physically frail and dependent (Spirduso, 1995). Tests for the frail and dependent typically include items that assess function of basic daily living activities (e.g., feeding, tying shoelaces, and basic mobility). Physically fit individuals can be tested using routine laboratory items with some or no modification (e.g., treadmill, bicycle ergometer, and dynamometer). (For a description of testing the elderly at this level, see McArdle et al., 2001.) The highlights of two attractive test batteries follow; each is appropriate for the physically independent.

AAHPERD Test for Adults Over 60   Revised in 1996, the *American Alliance for Health, Physical Education, Recreation and Dance (AAHPERD)* Test is designed to specifically assess selected physical function capabilities in adults over age 60. The field-based battery includes measures of aerobic fitness (half-mile walk), muscular strength/endurance (timed, sit-and-stand; elbow flexor test), agility/dynamic balance (chair agility test), coordination (manipulative, can placement test), balance (one-legged stand), and flexibility (sit-and-reach). Part of its attractiveness is that it is a norm-referenced test (age/gender) designed for use by personnel not necessarily trained for such responsibilities. An excellent administering video is available to help explain testing procedures.

Williams-Greene Test of Physical and Motor Function   While the AAHPERD Test is a good example of general physical function, the *Williams-Greene Test* (1990) assesses several aspects of motor behavior in the elderly. Based on a theory of movement classification schema, test items have been identified by categories of upper-extremity function and

> **THINK ABOUT IT**
>
> In contrast to being physically elite as an older person, a minimal level of physical function is essential to daily living. Provide some specific examples of the latter.

TABLE 12.11

Williams-Greene Test Areas

General Classification Subclassification Function	Test Aspects
Upper-Extremity Function	
Underlying components	strength, steadiness
Simple arm/hand movements	rapid-, repetitive-, and sequential movements
Distal extremity control: object manipulation	simple unilateral and bilateral dexterity, fine unilateral and bilateral dexterity, finger dexterity
Distal extremity control: self-help actions	object and implement usage
Mobility	
Underlying components	strength and flexibility, general mobility maneuvers, balance
Gait and mobility functions	simple and precise gait control, maximum speed, body agility

TABLE 12.12

Summary Information on Selected Instruments

Instrument	Age Range (Yr)	Type of Items	Source
AIMS	2 wks–18 mos	Process (rudimentary motor behaviors)	Saunders, Philadelphia, PA *http://www.harcourthealth.com*
Bayley-II	1–42 mos	Product (comprehensive, including motor scale)	The Psychological Corporation *http://www.psychcorp.com*
BOT	4.5–14.5	Product (gross motor, coordination, motor fitness, balance, visual-motor)	American Guidance Service Circle Pines, MN 55014 *www.agsnet.com*
DDST	Birth–6	Product (screening: fine motor; adaptive: gross motor)	DDM, Inc. P.O. Box 20037 Denver, CO 80220-0037
PDMS-2	Birth–7	Product (fine and gross motor)	PRO-ED 8700 Shoal Creek Blvd. Austin, TX 78757-6897 *www.proedinc.com*
PFMAI	2–12 mos	Process (posture and manipulative)	The Psychological Corporation
TGMD-2	3–11	Process (basic locomotor and manipulative skills)	PRO-ED
Williams-Greene Test of Physical and Motor Function	Elderly	Upper-extremity functions Mobility functions	Motor Development Laboratory Department of Exercise Science University of South Carolina Columbia, SC 29208

mobility (table 12.11). An attractive feature of the test is that items within each classification are designed to measure (and understand) aspects of physical function and motor behavior important to the elderly. For example, test items include measures of strength and steadiness as reflected in actions of practical manual control of objects and self-help activities. Components important to gait and postural control that often are limited in the elderly, such as strength, flexibility, and balance, are also measured. Specific test items for the battery were developed by the researchers or selected from the literature.

Table 12.12 provides some information about a few of the more recommended and available motor assessment instruments. Table 12.13 lists

TABLE 12.13

Fitness Assessment Batteries

Name	Level	Components	Web Address
AAHPERD Physical Best	Ages 5–18	Cardiovascular Body composition Strength/endurance Flexibility	*www.aahperd.org*
AAHPERD Functional Fitness Test For Older Adults	Ages 60+	Cardiovascular Strength/endurance Flexibility Agility/dynamic balance Coordination	*www.aahperd.org*
Fitnessgram	Grades K–12	Cardiovascular Strength/endurance Flexibility Body composition Agility	*www.humankinetics.com*
Presidential Physical Fitness Award Program	Ages 6–17	Cardiovascular Flexibility Strength/endurance Agility	*www.fitness.gov*

selected field-oriented tests in physical fitness test batteries. Refer to Baumgartner et al. (2003) in the Suggested Readings for single test and laboratory-oriented recommendations.

Summary

Assessment provides the opportunity to observe, document, and interpret change across the life span, as well as to determine the growth and developmental status of an individual at a particular time. The possibilities for physical and motor assessment as associated with growth, development, and motor performance are vast.

Assessment involves both measurement (collection of information) and evaluation (process of judgment). The two most widely used types of standards by which performance is judged are norm-referenced standards (which order individuals on a quantitative basis) and criterion-referenced standards (which specify a level by which individuals are judged). The assessment of movement skill performance usually is conducted with process-oriented (form characteristics) or product-oriented (performance outcome) assessment instruments.

After the purpose for conducting the assessment has been established, additional considerations are warranted with regard to instrument selection. Considerations should include a review of the instrument with regard to its psychometric properties (e.g., validity, reliability, and norm sample), feasibility (e.g., cost, equipment, space, personnel needed, and time), and level of training and expertise needed.

Although motor assessment items have been included in general child development batteries for more than 60 years, their general quality has been suspect. Most instruments are based on generalized product (quantitative) characteristics and provide little insight into the process of developmental change. These shortcomings have been addressed to some degree in recent years, as evidenced by the introduction of several process-oriented instruments and motor-specific, product-oriented assessment batteries.

Think about It

1. Describe how you could apply table 12.1 to assess lifelong motor development (developmental continuum).
2. Explain how you could use these purposes if you were a director of an early childhood learning center with a motor development program.
3. Have you noticed any commonalties among the product-oriented tests? Describe some of them.
4. In contrast to being physically elite as an older person, a minimal level of physical function is essential to daily living. Provide some specific examples of the latter.

Suggested Readings

General Assessment
Bracken, B. (2000). *The psychoeducational assessment of preschool children.* 3rd ed. Boston: Allyn & Bacon.
Kaplan, R. M., & Saccuzzo, D. P. (2001). *Psychological testing.* 4th ed. Belmont, CA: Wadsworth.
Salvia, J., & Ysseldyke, J. E. (2001). *Assessment.* 8th ed. Boston: Houghton Mifflin.
Wodrich, D. L. (1997). *Children's psychological testing: A guide for nonpsychologists.* 3rd ed. Baltimore, MD: Brookes.

Physical and Motor Assessment

Adrian, M. J., & Cooper, J. M. (1994). *Biomechanics of human movement.* 2nd ed. Madison, WI: Brown & Benchmark. (See chapter 8.)

Baumgartner, T. A., Jackson, A. S., Mahar, M., & Rowe, D. (2003). *Measurement for education: In physical education and exercise science.* 6th ed. New York: McGraw-Hill.

Burton, A. W., & Miller, D. E. (1998). *Movement skill assessment.* Champaign, IL: Human Kinetics.

WebLinks

American Fitness Alliance (Fitnessgram health-related fitness test)
www.americanfitness.net

Health Status Internet Assessments (Body Mass Index Calculator)
health status.com/bmi.htm

PE Central (Discussion on movement assessment issues)
http://pe.central.vt.edu/assessment/assessment.html

PE Central (Review of several assessment instruments for adapted physical education)
http://pe.central.vt.edu/adapted/adaptedinstruments.html

President's Council on Physical Fitness and Sports
www.fitness.gov

The Cooper Institute (Aerobics research)
www.cooperinst.org

The President's Challenge (Physical activity and fitness awards program)
www.indiana.edu/~preschal

part six

Sociocultural Influences on Motor Development

THE FINAL CHAPTER of this text describes the role of sociocultural factors in motor development. This information addresses the primary sociocultural factors from infancy to old age that may influence the individual's participation in sport and physical activity.

c h a p t e r

13 Sociocultural Influences on Motor Development

13 *Sociocultural Influences on Motor Development*

OBJECTIVES

Upon completion of this chapter, you should be able to

13.1 List and identify the basic terminology associated with socialization.

13.2 Describe the processes involved in socialization.

13.3 Define *socializing agent* and provide primary examples of those agents.

13.4 Explain Bronfenbrenner's ecological systems model.

13.5 Briefly discuss the importance of socialization to motor development.

13.6 Identify and elaborate on the primary sociocultural influences that may affect motor development during childhood and adolescence.

13.7 Describe Parten's four categories of play.

13.8 Define *gender roles* and *gender-role stereotyping* and discuss their influence on motor development.

13.9 Explain the role of self-esteem in motor development.

13.10 Explain the possible influences of race on socialization into physical activity and sport.

13.11 Identify the primary sociocultural influences that can affect physical activity involvement during adulthood.

13.12 Describe the social views of aging that have implications for socialization into physical activity.

■ **KEY TERMS**

socialization	Parten's play model
culture	peers
status	gender roles
social class	gender-role stereotyping
social role	self-esteem
norm	age-related stereotyping
socializing agent	activity theory
Bronfenbrenner's ecological systems model	

AT BIRTH, newborns are very much alike in that they have similar needs for nurturing, progress through the same general sequence in developing locomotion and speech, and must learn appropriate social behavior. However, children become different due to sociocultural influences, experience, and their biological uniqueness. Chapter 5 addressed factors that affect growth and development: maternal and external influences on prenatal development, nutrition, hormones, and the effects of physical activity (and exercise) on lifelong human development. This chapter focuses specifically on the influences and importance of sociocultural factors on lifelong motor development.

■ *Basic Terminology of Socialization*

Objective 13.1 ➤ Although socialization commonly is linked with child and adolescent development, it is a lifelong process. As individuals vary their social environment, they must learn to adapt to new situations. **Socialization** refers to a set of events and processes by which individuals acquire the beliefs and behaviors of the particular society and subgroup in which they live and, in most cases, are born into. Many goals of socialization are common to all societies, but each society and subgroup develops its own unique practices and goals to maintain itself in its particular ecological context.

Culture, which is generally thought of as a subset of society, is the collection of specific attitudes, behaviors, and products that characterize an identifiable group of people. Since societies and cultures frequently differ, it is reasonable to assume that expectations would vary from culture to culture. Though differences exist between our society and those of other countries, differences exist *within* our society between cultural groups. Some cultures place a higher priority on leisure, recreation, and sports than do others; this will have an effect on the motor development of its members.

Four general concepts frequently used to describe the structure of socialization are status, class, role, and norm. **Status** refers to an individual's position in society. One individual can hold many positions—father, brother, coach, mentor, friend, athlete, and so on. Some positions are conferred on individuals due to their experience or expertise, whereas others are simply a function of sex (e.g., mother, wife) or age (e.g., family leader and grandparent). Individuals learn to assume the role associated with the established position of status.

A complementary term to one's status in society is *social class.* **Social class,** also called socioeconomic status, refers to a grouping of people with similar economic, educational, and occupational characteristics. Cross-cultural studies often use terms like *lower-, middle-,* and *upper-socioeconomic class* as a factor for making comparisons.

Accordingly, a **social role** is the particular behavior an individual uses to fulfill a position of status. One may describe a role as the set of dynamics and expectations that complements the status; in essence, it is the job description that goes with a position. For example, a quarterback holds the status of team leader on the field. With that status, the individual is expected to do such things as organize the group and carry out the game plan. As role expectations for a specific position of status are developed and a relatively predictable set of characteristics are formed, norms are established.

A **norm** refers to a standard of behavior that would be expected from members of a similar group of society. For instance, common and expected behaviors are associated with specific groups of teachers and coaches in addition to their individual personalities.

Cultural socialization should be viewed as an interactive process between society and the individual, with one intricately influencing the other. Socialization is a lifelong dynamic process that allows people to use their individual differences to make unique contributions.

■ *Socializing Processes and Agents*

Objective 13.2 ➤ Socialization involves acquiring knowledge and various types of skills, including those related to the motor domain. According to one of the dominant cognitive-social learning perspectives associated with child development (Ladd & Mize, 1983), there are three principal modes of socialization: direct instruction, shaping, and modeling. All three are used to teach individuals about social roles they and others can play in the culture. Each also is mediated by the individual's social cognition, or understanding of the social world.

Direct instruction deals primarily with concepts and ideas conveyed through language. This mode of socialization includes specific or general information about how to act and what to say, and when to act and speak. *Shaping* refers to the social learning processes that allow an individual to benefit from experience. The concept that individuals can learn social behaviors by observing others who serve as models is known as *modeling*. Frequently associated with cognitive-social learning theory and the works of Bandura (refer to chapter 1), it is suggested that individuals cognitively represent the behavior of others through observational learning and then possibly adopt, or model, this behavior themselves. Modeling can have a profound effect on the development of motor skills, especially during childhood and adolescence when individuals frequently attempt to model the behavior of famous athletes.

Objective 13.3 ➤ Socialization depends on the contexts and settings in which it occurs. Individuals may be influenced by the overlapping factors of society at large, one or more subcultures, socioeconomic class, institutions, and individuals. Each can play a significant role in the socialization process. Complementary to the processes of socialization are the various agents influential in affecting social behavior and motor development.

A **socializing agent** is an individual, group, or institution that interprets culture to the individual. Although there are numerous subagents, the major socializing influences are the family, school, peer group, church, and community. Of this group, it is generally acknowledged that the family is the primary socializing agent that transmits cultural content during the early developmental years. The family not only passes on its attitudes, prejudices, and health habits, but also determines social class, ethnic origin, race, and religious beliefs. As individuals grow older, the school and peer group characteristically become stronger influences in socialization. More specific to motor development, teachers and coaches are in positions of powerful influence in the school and community. Other potentially strong agents (medium) through which individuals may be socialized are play and sports involvement. Subsequent discussions of the primary factors that influence development during childhood, adolescence, and adulthood will incorporate these primary agents.

Objective 13.4 ➤ One of the few comprehensive frameworks for understanding sociocultural influences on socialization was developed by Bronfenbrenner (refer to chapter 1). **Bronfenbrenner's ecological systems model** places the individual at a theoretical center surrounded by five environmental systems: microsystem, mesosystem, exosystem, macrosystem, and chronosystem. The most direct interactions are with the *microsystem*, the environment in which the person lives. Influential agents include the family, school, peers, church, and neighborhood play area. Within these contexts the individual is viewed as one who helps construct the environment.

Influences that occur as a result of relationships between different microsystems are part of the *mesosystem*. For example, the relation of family experiences to school experiences, or church training to family experiences, falls within the mesosystem. Developmentalists suggest it is important to observe the individual's behavior in multiple contexts to provide a more complete picture of social development.

The *exosystem* involves indirect influences from another social context that affect what the person experiences in an immediate setting. This would include, for instance, the school board and city government, both of which have control over the quality of physical education and recreational facilities available to individuals.

The *macrosystem* incorporates the broad-based attitudes and ideologies of the society and specific culture in which the individual lives. It is suggested these influences may permeate virtually all of the other systems within the individual's ecological world. As mentioned earlier, different societies and cultures place varying levels of importance on such influential factors as education, leisure time, sports, and health promotion, all of which may have a powerful impact on motor development across the life span.

The final influence is the *chronosystem*, which involves the patterning of environmental events and transitions over the life span—that is, the sociohistorical contexts. For example, females today are much more likely to participate in athletic activities than they were in the 1950s.

THINK ABOUT IT

How could you use Bronfenbrenner's ecological systems model to study environmental effects on motor behavior?

Objective 13.5   ➤ Socialization affects behaviors that include values, knowledge, social skills, and traits and is vital for optimal physical and motor development. Societies, cultures, or parents who do not expose their members or their children to physical activities, sports, and proper health practices are limiting the human potential for optimal development.

The following discussion focuses on the primary sociocultural influences that can affect motor development through involvement in sports and other physical activity across the life span. Although it has been shown that sociocultural factors begin to show their influence on growth and development in the prenatal stages (when the mother's health practices may be affected by socioeconomic status) and become more direct after birth, this discussion will focus on the primary factors associated with early childhood through adulthood.

▧ *Primary Influences during Childhood and Adolescence*

Objective 13.6   ➤ The primary sociocultural influences that have been shown to influence sports involvement and physical activity during childhood and adolescence are the family, peer relations in play and sport participation, and the relationship to coaches and teachers in the school and community. Additional factors to be discussed are gender-role expectations, self-esteem, and race.

Parental beliefs and attitudes toward a healthy lifestyle are important in socializing the child

The Family

The family is the socializing agent most directly responsible for the communication of cultural content to the growing child. This observation is relevant not only to socialization in general, but also with regard to the child's movement endeavors (e.g., Pargman, 1997; Weiss & Barber, 1996). Significant changes in the family unit have taken place in recent decades, brought about by an increase in the number of working mothers and single-parent homes. In fact, the majority of mothers of children and youth now work outside of the home (Hoffman, 1989). In today's society, about 60% of American children spend some time in a single-parent family, usually with their mother (Hetherington et al., 1999). Despite all of these changes and their ramifications, the family is still the primary caregiver and socializing agent during infancy and childhood.

Of the many influences associated with the family, perhaps the most dominant are *parental beliefs and attitudes.* Parents who believe in the importance of an active, healthy lifestyle usually share it with their children. Many parents take their young offspring along to such settings as tennis courts, swimming pools, health clubs, and other recreational areas. With this positive attitude and the knowledge that physical activity is beneficial, it is usually the parent's wish that their children adopt these characteristics. Consequently, these parents usually provide their children with early experiences (figure 13.1).

The first contact young children have with motor activities and sports normally takes place with the family. Along with taking their children to fitness and sporting activities, parents may give sport equipment and clothing as presents and introduce the basic skills and concepts of selected activities. All of this may begin at a very young age. As children grow older, they are encouraged to participate in more formal settings (e.g., youth sports) and to maximize their abilities. Sports involvement for the vast majority of eventual participants normally begins by the age of 8; if parental interest is high, the likelihood of participation is much greater.

As a result of early experiences and watching their parents participate in physical activity regularly over the years, children also may develop a positive attitude about physical activity and thus become socialized into an active physical lifestyle. Participation in sport activities in later years (i.e., older childhood through adulthood) reflects, at least to some degree, their parent's beliefs, attitudes, and encouragement during earlier years. Although other influences are likely to be present, research findings indicate that the best predictor of participation in sports by adults is childhood and adolescent involvement (Greendorfer, 1979; Weiss & Barber, 1996).

Research findings with regard to *individual family member influence*, though somewhat inconsistent, indicate that specific members of the unit likely play differential roles in play and sport socialization. One body of literature suggests that the same-gender parent has the most influence on the extent of the child's involvement (DiLorenzo et al., 1998; Lewko & Ewing, 1980; McPherson, 1978). In the Lewko and Ewing study that involved children 9 to 11 years of age, the investigators found girls seemed to require a higher level of encouragement than boys did to become involved. This perhaps reflects traditional gender-role expectations regarding sport involvement, which appear to be changing. There is also evidence that the opposite-gender parent influences involvement, but that fathers are the primary influencing agent for both girls and boys (Greendorfer & Lewko, 1978). Evidence from this investigation also found the mother's role in influencing sport participation of either gender child was minimal, which supports the more traditional view that the father is responsible for initiating sport involvement of the offspring, especially for the male child.

The literature concerning sibling influence seems to be inconsistent. However, it appears that older brothers and sisters may be important agents in the sport socialization of younger siblings (Lewko & Ewing, 1980; Weiss & Knoppers, 1982). Overall, it is clear that the family, especially the father, is the significant agent in the socialization of their children to physical activity and sport.

Along with determining religious beliefs, race, and ethnic origin, the family also serves as the economic unit. Economic factors can affect nutritional practices and corresponding physical growth and development. There are also indications that socioeconomic status may be an influential factor in motor development. Although research on this topic is gravely lacking, it appears as though children from low-income families (especially single-parent homes) may be limited in motor development experiences due at least in part to lack of financial resources, parental involvement time, and the parents' experience. Living on a tightly budgeted low income may present a shortage of funds for such items as toys, sport equipment, and activity program enrollment fees.

There are also indications that children in low-income or single-parent homes may have limited exposure to different kinds of play activities and sports in comparison to children of higher income families. For instance, Greenspan (1983) found that age-group skiers, gymnasts, and swimmers come primarily from homes of upper-middle class socioeconomic status, whereas young boxers, wrestlers, and baseball players derive from less economically endowed families. Empirical evidence also would suggest that activities such as golf and tennis are associated with higher income families.

Another consideration is socioeconomic status as it relates to education and knowledge of the importance of motor activities in child and adolescent development. Low-income families, who generally lack higher education, may be less knowledgeable about the importance of physical activity to health and thus may be less apt to consider motor activities important to their children's development. On the other hand, some highly educated people may view the time spent on motor activities as detrimental to optimal cognitive development.

Peer Relations

The influence of peers and participation in play and sport activities become increasingly powerful socializing influences through the childhood years. As the effects of these factors increase through later childhood and adolescence, family dominance tends to decrease on several socialization issues. From a motor development perspective, the influence of both of these agents are intertwined. Although research has not shown that participation in play and sport activities systematically produces positive social characteristics, it does suggest that when good consequences occur, they are tied to the social relationships found in these settings (Coakley, 1987).

Play, as it relates to socialization and other aspects of human behavior, has been one of the most extensively studied areas of child development. In addition to stimulating peer relations, play also has been shown to advance cognitive development, increase exploration, release tension, enhance self-esteem, influence attitude formation, and stimulate moral growth. As mentioned earlier, Piaget viewed play as a medium that advances the child's cognitive development. Several traditional and contemporary theorists share the general notion that play is a positive influence in child development. Play and sport activities take up a sizable amount of time during childhood and adolescence, and provide many opportunities for enhancing physical and motor development.

■ *Figure 13.2*

Play is considered a primary mode of social development during childhood

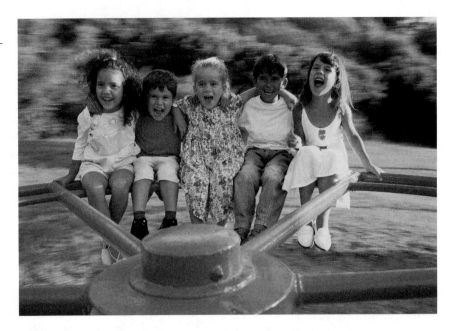

Although numerous research papers have been written on the topic, the term *play* remains an elusive concept. Descriptions of play range from an infant's simple display of a newly discovered perceptual-motor talent, to a parent and child catching a ball, to an older child's involvement in organized youth sports. In general, play can be described as a pleasurable activity engaged in for its own sake.

Objective 13.7   ➤ Many years ago Parten (1932) identified categories of play **(Parten's play model)** still recognized by developmentalists today as relevant forms of social development (figure 13.2). These include the categories of solitary, parallel, associative, and cooperative play. In *solitary play* the child plays alone or independently of those around him or her. Solitary play is characteristic of 2- and 3-year-olds. *Parallel play* is similar to solitary play in that the child still plays independently but plays with toys like those other children are using. Thus, parallel play mimics the behavior of children who are playing alongside. Although this type of play decreases in frequency with age, older preschool children can be observed in this behavior often.

Social interaction in the form of play with little or no organization is described as *associative play*. At this time in social development children seem to be more interested in associating with each other than they are in the tasks around them. Specific characteristic behaviors include follow-the-leader and invitation-type activities, along with borrowing and sharing toys. This type of play often is observed between the ages of 3½ to 5 years.

Around the age of 5 marks the beginning of purposeful, *cooperative play*, which represents social interaction in a group with a sense of group identity and organization. This category is characterized by formal games, competitive group activities, and activities in which children must work together to achieve a common goal. Cooperative play at this level is the precursor to forms of movement activities and sport observed during older childhood and adolescence. Observation also suggests that as children grow older, they tend to form more complex and larger social structures when at play.

There are indications that play behavior, as described by these categories, has changed over the last half century. Some of this change has implications for motor development. It would appear that children do not engage in as much associative and cooperative play as they did in the past. In addition to being less physically active in general, it has been suggested that children may be expressing more passive solitary and parallel play behavior as a reflection of the extended periods of time they spend watching television, operating computers, and playing video games. Related to this is the notion that play items are more attractive today and parents seem to encourage this type of play behavior. Children spend about 25 hours per week viewing television, which is more time spent than on any other activity except sleep (Huston et al., 1990). By the time the average adolescent completes high school, the individual will spend more time watching television (approximately 20,000 hours) than in the classroom (Santrock, 2002). Obviously, this type of social behavior can have strong implications for motor development.

Beginning at approximately age 5, individuals engage in physical activities that are more cooperative and complex (i.e., group oriented). The need for this type of play appears to increase with age (and peak during adolescence) due in part to the individual's strong social desire to be a part of a peer group. Cooperative play may take the form of informal or formal games (and sports). In informal activities, children usually get together on their own to play with equipment at hand, and use makeshift or flexible rules.

Organized activities such as youth sport and school athletic programs often demand significant time commitments by the participant and family. It is not uncommon for parents to adjust meal and work schedules and weekend plans to get their children to practices and games. Along with probable financial requirements, these considerations, when compared to other family commitments and priorities, can be important factors in the degree of organized sport socialization. In addition to being influential in developing social behaviors and stimulating peer relations, sport settings also provide excellent opportunities for advancing motor development and physical fitness (refer to chapter 10).

One of the most frequently cited reasons for involvement in play and sport activities is the desire to interact with peers (e.g., Brown et al., 1990; Weiss & Barber, 1996). **Peers** are individuals of about the same age or maturity level and, in some instances, social class. A common characteristic of the peer group during childhood and adolescence is that its members are usually of the same sex. This provides an extremely powerful socialization environment. Most peer relations arise from associations made in the school, particularly if the schools are attended by individuals from the same neighborhood. The desire to fit in and the need to belong and be identified as part of a group, team, or club can be compelling socialization forces. Adolescent peer groups are often organized around *cliques*—small groups with similar interests. As individuals enter later childhood and adolescence, influence from the peer group becomes increasingly important, while that of the family and other social agents may diminish.

Coakley (1987) notes that children's involvement in informal or organized sports is influenced by (a) the availability of opportunities, (b) support from the family, peers, role models, and the general community, and (c) the child's self-perception as a participant. Of these influences, there are strong indications that the peer group is a dominant factor with respect to socialization into physical activity and sport from childhood through early adulthood. Peers have the potential to reinforce family influence concerning socialization into physical activity and sport and to provide new considerations not stressed at home. There also may be situations when peer influence challenges those values set by other social agents (e.g., family, school, and church).

Through childhood and adolescence this influence seems to be stronger with regard to involvement in team (group) activities rather than individual sport endeavors. However, regardless of the type of activity in which the individual is drawn by peer influence to participate, peer relations can be a powerful social agent in enhancing motor development.

Coaches and Teachers

THINK ABOUT IT

Using your experience, describe how the various socializing agents (family members, peers, coaches, and teachers) have influenced your participation in physical activity.

Usually associated with the school and community social structures, teachers and coaches have the potential for being influential agents with regard to sport involvement. In fact, in some situations where few other influential adults are available, these agents may become significant others for the child. Although some suspicion has been cast regarding the primary motives of coaches (e.g., too much emphasis on winning), research shows that in most cases these agents are genuinely concerned with helping members of the team to experience positive socialization outcomes (Weiss & Sisley, 1984). Unfortunately, no evidence has been presented on the extent to which coaches affect behaviors that transcend sport situations and influence individuals in later life.

In general, coaches and teachers appear to influence males more than females with regard to involvement in sport and physical activity (Greendorfer & Lewko, 1978). In 1976 female athletes reported that coaches and teachers influenced their involvement during adolescence but not in the earlier years or as young adults. In another early investigation, male athletes reported they benefited from these influences before, during, and after adolescence (Kenyon & McPherson, 1973). Empirical evidence would suggest these characteristics have not changed significantly over the years for males, but those for females may be outdated considering more recent views and opportunities (e.g., university scholarships).

Gender-Role Expectations and Stereotyping

Objective 13.8 ➤ **Gender roles** are social expectations of how individuals should act and think as males and females. Along with being influenced by biological factors (primarily sex hormones), socializing agents such as family members, schools, peers, and the media can have a significant effect on this aspect of human behavior. With regard to family influence, fathers seem to play an especially important part in gender-role development and are more likely to act differently toward opposite-gender children than mothers do (Fagot & Leinbach, 1987; Lamb, 1986). In general, however, parents tend to encourage boys and girls to engage in different types of play and activities (e.g., Campbell & Eaton, 2000; McBride-Chang & Jacklin, 1993).

Related to this aspect of sociocultural influence is **gender-role stereotyping,** the use of different methods to introduce boys and girls to physical activities and sports. Even as infants, girls tend to be handled more gently and protectively than boys are. Infant boys, on the other hand, are perceived as tougher, stronger, and more athletic, and are more often given toys that require active play and the use of motor skills.

Toy selection and marketing traditionally are based on gender-role stereotyping and tied to socialization into physical activity and sport. For example, when a parent gives a basketball to a young boy, the gesture usually promotes physical activity in the form of shooting and dribbling, and introduces the child to the sport. Although basketball also is considered a female sport, there seem to be few promotion products that use females as gender-role models. By about 3 years of age, most children have a firmly established preference for gender-appropriate play items. Although biological disposition cannot be completely ruled out, early preferences for play items probably are influenced strongly by parents and significant others. Social learning theory (chapter 1) provides some insight into this phenomenon by suggesting that gender development occurs primarily through observation and imitation of behavior, and through reward and punishment with experience.

As children enter school they also tend to be treated differently. For instance, males are more likely to receive strong support from family, relatives, peers, teachers, and coaches to begin and continue in sports. For boys, sport involvement is viewed as part of the young man's path to manhood, whereas such endeavors are traditionally not linked to becoming a woman. Because many girls are not encouraged to participate in skilled, vigorous motor activities, many never develop their skills to full potential. These attitudes also have an effect on the motivation to get involved seriously in sports and to train to achieve maximum performance.

THINK ABOUT IT

Explain your view of gender-role behavior.

During adolescence, gender-role expectations can be of primary influence in the individual's decision to get involved in sport activities. *Gender-role conflict* may be created when adolescents decide to participate in certain sport activities. Anthrop and Allison (1983) found in a survey of female high school athletes that 17% indicated they had a significant problem with role conflict in that they were concerned their participation in games may be viewed as a masculine endeavor. Once again, this reflects the traditional view of females in sport. A survey of high school graduates of the 1980s reported indications of less traditionalism (Suitor & Reavis, 1995). That is, compared to younger cohorts, those that graduated in the late 1980s noted an increase in gaining prestige through sports and a decrease through cheerleading.

For males, however, involvement in sport seems to cause little gender-role conflict and is viewed as stereotypic of ideal male characteristics. Related research findings also suggest males are more easily socialized into sports than females (Ostrow et al., 1981). Two reasons were given for this finding. First, there are relatively few female role models. Second, the majority of the sports surveyed were considered to be masculine. Participation in these sports can cause more gender-role conflict in females, and therefore decrease the likelihood of their involvement.

However, society's view that females are the weaker gender appears to be changing. In more recent years, female participation in sports has increased not only at the youth sport level, but also in school and university programs (due in part to Title IX legislation). As a result, participation levels have increased, which has decreased the performance differences between the genders.

Self-Esteem

Objective 13.9   ➤ Also referred to as self-image and self-concept, **self-esteem** is the evaluative and personal judgment of one's self. The judgment does not necessitate accuracy so much as one's belief that it is correct. Self-esteem is included in this section as a sociocultural factor because it is considered, in large part, a reflection of social support in the form of parents, peers, teachers, and coaches, etc. For example, a child highly praised by a teacher for her physical ability and preferred by peers as a teammate for games generally has a good sense of worth for this particular endeavor. Self-esteem is considered by some to be a critical index of mental health; a high sense of worth during childhood is linked to satisfaction in later life. However, global self-esteem judgments should be viewed with caution, for an individual's sense of worth may vary according to different skill domains and areas of competence. For example, an individual may perceive that he or she is quite intelligent but inadequate in athletic and social abilities. Variation within skill domains is not uncommon. Some individuals may have a strong sense of self-worth in, for example, basketball but not in baseball or track. Indications are that feelings about self-esteem are relatively well established by middle childhood (Harter, 1987).

Within the context of youth sports involvement, researchers have found that such participation generally is associated with higher self-esteem (e.g., Anthrop & Allison, 1983; Hall et al., 1986; Kirshnit et al., 1988). It would seem reasonable to expect a person with a good self-esteem regarding physical ability to be more likely to engage in complementary activities such as youth sports. On the other hand, research confirms that a person with a low sense of physical competence is more likely to avoid these opportunities (Weiss, 1993). Along with the internal factors associated with personality type and emotions, social interactions play a vital role in the development of self-esteem.

Whereas children under the age of about 10 years depend primarily on parents and the outcomes of contests for appraisals, those who are older tend to rely more on comparison to and appraisals their peers provide (Horn & Weiss, 1991). In addition, feedback from teachers and coaches also may be influencing factors. For example, young athletes tend to exhibit higher self-esteem while playing for coaches who give frequent encouragement and corrective feedback, especially if the individual begins the sport with a relatively low sense of worth. As one would expect, the type of feedback given to young athletes is also a factor in their state of self-esteem. With some participants, general comments and appraisals may not be as effective as corrective feedback, even if delivered in the form of criticism (Horn, 1985). Obviously, mental maturity, emotional state, manner of delivery, and rapport between athlete and coach are critical factors in effectiveness of communication and development of self-esteem.

THINK ABOUT IT

From your perspective, what are the positives and negatives of youth sports?

Individuals with a high self-esteem in their physical abilities may be more apt to join in sport programs. Nevertheless, a large portion of children and youth, especially females, drop out (Gould, 1987; Kirshnit et al., 1989). There are two prominent theories that address this issue. One suggests that during adolescence, interest in sports conflicts with other opportunities more than it did in childhood (Petlichkoff, 1996). That is, adolescents have a greater number of desirable options during leisure time and more demands on how they use their time. This drop-out dilemma may reflect a normal trial-and-error sampling done in research of an enjoyable activity or achievement domain. A second (general) perspective emphasizes the negative aspects of youth sports and disenchantment with participation. Such experiences as loss of interest, not having fun, lack of playing time, dislike for the coach, pressure to perform (or win), and lack of success have been suggested as factors in dropping out (e.g., Athletic Footwear Association, 1990).

Although different age groups may state different reasons for participating and continuing in youth sport programs, the most commonly stated reasons include to have fun; to improve skills; to demonstrate competency; and the desire to compete; pleasing family and friends, affiliate with or make new friends, and be part of a team (e.g., Athletic Footwear, 1990; Brodkin & Weiss, 1990).

There have been critics who suggest that much of youth sport is emotionally stressful due, for example, to an overemphasis on winning and maximum performance. However, in a thorough review of studies of state anxiety and associated symptoms in young athletes, Gould and Eklund (1996) estimated that only a small percent (5–10) were experiencing high levels of stress (e.g., loss of sleep and appetite).

Possible Influences of Race

Objective 13.10 ➤ Although the research on this topic is sparse and the effects of socioeconomic factors are difficult to separate, there are indications that African-American and Caucasian children are socialized into sports differently (Braddock, 1980; Greendorfer & Ewing, 1981; Oliver, 1980). A generalization is that possible success in sports appears to take on more importance for black youths compared to their white counterparts, especially for males from lower socioeconomic homes.

Encouragement from family members, same-sex peers, coaches, teachers, and the community may be more influential for blacks than for whites. It is suggested that some of this encouragement originates from the somewhat misleading perception that sports offer blacks more opportunities than other careers in society, and therefore provide a more readily conceivable means for increasing social status. Harris and Hunt (1984) found that encouragement for involvement in sports among black youth gets stronger as they move through adolescence and begin to perceive major obstacles to success in careers outside of sports and entertainment. Adding to this view is the fact that although professional black athletes are strong role models for young blacks and whites, blacks have fewer role models from other occupations to emulate. Research also indicates that encouragement in sport involvement among lower socioeconomic black families is stimulated by the wish for their child's fame and fortune (Snyder & Spreitzer, 1983). Although little research on this topic is available and much needs to be learned concerning the effects of such influences on several aspects of human development, one could speculate that positive motor development benefits could arise from such encouragement and parental involvement.

■ *Primary Influences during Adulthood*

Objective 13.11 ➤ Just as society and various cultures have expectations for individual behavior from infancy through adolescence, numerous sociocultural influences and expectations are also present through adulthood. Whereas home and school settings were dominant socializing factors prior to adulthood, these agents become less of a primary influence in establishing or changing behavior characteristics as individuals attain independence from the family and complete formal schooling. For the remainder of life, the primary agents are usually the media, peers, spouses, and other individuals in the community (e.g., doctors and class instructors). In addition to these influences, seasonal, personal, and situational factors that are continuous and dynamic over the life cycle (e.g., marriage, children, and employment situation) play an important role in adult sport socialization (Mihalik et al., 1989). Just as there are varying sociocultural views and expectations for behavior concerning health practices and physical activity in earlier years, a variety of views and trends are evident during adulthood. Society in general, as expressed through various media, places a premium on youth and good looks. The idea of living a zestful, active lifestyle while at the same time eating and drinking things that allow one to remain slim has been one of the central themes in advertising. In today's world, advertising is a powerful socializing agent. During early adulthood individuals can still be quite impressionable; the need for self-esteem and peer acceptance has led many to take up or continue physical activity in some form. This is also the period in the life span when most individuals are at their healthiest and reach peak physical performance (around age 30). For many individuals, the notion that they are at their best and not slowing down physically needs to be tested on a regular basis. Obviously, however, many young adults have not been influenced or do not have the desire to engage in physical activities as part of their lifestyle. In fact, empirical evidence suggests that due at least in part to their relatively healthy status during this period in their lives, many individuals do not think about how their lifestyles will affect their health in later years. College students specifically seem to have unrealistic and overly optimistic views about their future health and longevity. Unfortunately, many of those who are not healthy (e.g., overweight and unfit) at this time have established attitudes concerning physical activity that are difficult to overcome.

As individuals approach middle age (ages 35 to 40), concern for health and physical appearance becomes more evident. For most individuals this is a time when the regression of physical skills and signs of physical aging begin, which causes more attention to be drawn to these characteristics. Part of the stimulus for personal concern is likely related to two sociocultural influences. As mentioned earlier, our society places a premium on a healthy, youthful physical appearance. This factor alone is responsible for millions of dollars spent nationally each year on health and beauty items and classes to help preserve youthfulness. Many individuals begin dying gray hair, undergoing cosmetic surgery, and enrolling in weight reduction and conditioning classes, all in effort to maintain a healthy, youthful appearance.

Another major influence that has drawn attention and concern to health status and promoted physical activity is the flood of educational information that comes by way of the media. This information also is conveyed by physicians, peers, spouses, and various community agents (e.g., class instructors and pharmacists). For several years there has been a national effort to make the general public aware of such health concerns as obesity, cardiovascular disease, high blood pressure, too much salt, high cholesterol, and lack of exercise.

Although recent trends seem to suggest that attitudes have changed with regard to involvement in physical activity and active sports among the middle-aged and elderly, many adults still decrease their level of involvement as they age (McArdle et al., 2001; Centers for Disease Control and Prevention [CDC], 2000). These views may be described as a form of **age-related stereotyping.** Although such activities as swimming, jogging, and tennis currently are encouraged as lifelong pursuits, there are sociocultural forces that expect aging adults (especially the elderly) to become more sedentary with age.

Objective 13.12 ➤ Although several social views of aging have been proposed, few have received more support than **activity theory.** Most research studies have found that when individuals continue to live active and productive lives as older adults, their satisfaction with life, in general, does not decline and may even go up (Takkinen et al., 2001; Schaie & Willis, 1991; Rook, 2000). According to activity theory, an active lifestyle during later adulthood increases the likelihood for life satisfaction (Neugarten et al., 1968). That is, the more active older people are, the less likely they are to age and show discontent with life. This theory suggests that middle-aged adults continue their roles and practices through late adulthood, and that if activities cease for some reason (e.g., retirement), it is important to find comparable substitutes.

In addition to this general view of aging, several theories related to exercise motivation in older adults have been proposed. One of the more interesting perspectives proposes that Bandura's social cognitive theory may be an appropriate framework to study this behavior (Dzewaltowski, 1989; Resnick, 2001). Using the triadic causation concept (the person, behavior, and context) as the basis for affecting change across the life span, three mechanisms are suggested as important mediators in influencing exercise motivation. Foremost is *self-efficacy*, defined as the individual's judgment of his or her capabilities to complete courses of action. Older adults who lack this characteristic usually drop out of or do not participate in exercise programs. As with younger populations, a strong

THINK ABOUT IT

If you were presenting a speech on physical activity to senior adults, what would you say? Consider other chapter topics also.

An active lifestyle during later adult-hood increases the likelihood of life satisfaction.

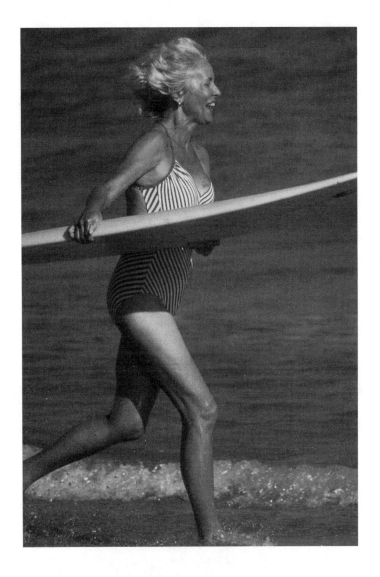

influence in self-efficacy is interaction with various social agents. Mental and physical health directly influence this factor (Resnick, 2001). A second factor is the value older persons place on the outcome and the provision of incentives, which is associated with *outcome expectations*. The third mechanism, *self-evaluated dissatisfaction*, is illustrated by individuals who are motivated to exercise because they are not satisfied with their current level of performance (e.g., muscular strength and flexibility). Many older persons will continue exercising to avoid becoming dissatisfied if they quit. This perspective in general recognizes that in addition to psychological factors, social contexts and biological constraints are strong influences in exercise motivation in the elderly.

Summary

Sociocultural influences have been shown to have a lifelong effect on involvement in physical activity and motor development. Socialization is a lifelong process that refers to a set of events and processes by which individuals acquire the beliefs and behaviors of a particular society and subgroup (culture). The general concepts of status, class, role, and norm commonly are used to describe components of the social structure.

Socialization involves acquiring knowledge and skills, including those related to the motor domain. Individuals may be taught these skills and information by direct instruction, shaping (experience), and modeling (observing others). Socialization strongly is influenced by various sociocultural agents that interpret culture to the individual. The major socializing agents are the family, school (teachers and coaches), peers, church, and the community. Within these agents are the influences of play and sport participation. During the early developmental years, the family is the primary socializing agent responsible for the transmission of cultural content. A good systems approach to studying sociocultural influences is the Bronfenbrenner ecological model.

Gender-role stereotyping, introducing boys and girls to physical activities and sport differently, is practiced by several social agents. Traditionally, male children tend to be given more active, sports-oriented play items and are encouraged early to be involved in vigorous physical activity and sports. On the other hand, females normally are introduced to more passive play items and are not expected to strongly pursue athletic endeavors. As a result of these and other influences, young males and females develop a preference for gender-appropriate play items and physical activities. When individuals decide to get involved in physical activities that are not gender-appropriate in their view, a gender-role conflict can occur. However, society's view of gender-appropriate behavior for females does appear to be changing.

Self-esteem influences participation in play and sports involvement. Children who are praised by others generally have good self-esteem and are more likely to participate in organized activities.

Although research on the issue of race and its influence on physical activity and sport involvement is sparse and difficult to separate from socioeconomic factors, there are indications that African-American and Caucasian children are treated differently. Generalizations contend that possible success in sports seems to take on more importance among black youths (compared to white youths), especially males from low-income homes, and that encouragement from several social agents may be more influential. It is speculated that many black youths view sports as a more readily conceivable means for increasing social status, due in part to perceived barriers to other careers. There are also indications that blacks have fewer role models from other occupations to emulate.

The adulthood years are also a time of much social learning with the presence of several sociocultural influences and expectations. Beginning with early adulthood, the primary social agents are the media (education), peers, spouses, and individuals in the community. Other influences include personal, seasonal, and situational factors. Society in general, as expressed predominantly through the media, places a premium on youth and physical appearance. This influence, along with the positive habits formed in earlier years, causes many young adults to continue, improve on, or take up a physically active lifestyle.

As individuals approach middle age and enter later adulthood, concern for health status and physical appearance normally receives more attention. This is a time when physical skills are regressing and physical aging is becoming more evident. Society's emphasis on good health and youthfulness stimulates many to become involved in physical activity. Another strong agent is the extensive media promotion of information concerning the need for good health practices. Similar information may also be transmitted through peers, spouses, and members of the community.

Although recent trends seem to suggest that attitudes have changed with regard to involvement in physical activity among the middle-aged and elderly, many older adults still decrease their level of involvement as they age. However, of the various social views of aging, activity theory seems to have the most support. According to this view, an active lifestyle during later adulthood increases the likelihood for life satisfaction. Implications include continuing or beginning a physically active lifestyle.

Think about It

1. How could you use Bronfenbrenner's ecological systems model to study environmental effects on motor behavior?
2. Using your experience, describe how the various socializing agents (family members, peers, coaches, and teachers) have influenced your participation in physical activity.
3. Explain your view of gender-role behavior.
4. From your perspective, what are the positives and negatives of youth sports?
5. If you were presenting a speech on physical activity to senior adults, what would you say? Consider other chapter topics also.

Suggested Readings

Goldstein, J. H. (Ed.). (1994). *Toys, play, and child development.* New York: Cambridge University Press.
Golombok, S., & Fivush, R. (1994). *Gender development.* New York: Cambridge University Press.
Shields, D. L. L., & Bredenmeir, B. J. L. (1995). *Character development & physical activity.* Champaign, IL: Human Kinetics.

WebLinks

American Psychological Association (aging issues)
www.apa.org/pi/aging/homepage.html

The Institute for the Study of Youth Sports
http://ed-web3.educ.msu.edu/ysi

National Alliance for Youth Sports
www.nays.org

References

AAHPERD (American Alliance for Health, Physical Education, Recreation, and Dance). (1985). Norms for college students health-related physical fitness test. Reston, VA: AAHPERD Publications.

Adams, J. A. (1971). A closed theory of motor learning. *Journal of Motor Behavior* 3:111–150.

Adolph, K. E., Eppler, M. A., & Gibson, E. J. (1993a). Development of perception of affordances. In C. Rovee-Collier & L. P. Lipsitt (Eds.), *Advances in infancy research* (Vol. 8). Norwood, NJ: Ablex.

Adolph, K. E., Eppler, M. A., & Gibson, E. J. (1993b). Crawling versus walking infants' perception of affordances for locomotion over sloping surfaces. *Child Development* 64:1158–1174.

Adrian, M. J., & Cooper, J. M. (1995). *Biomechanics of human movement.* 2nd ed. Indianapolis: Benchmark Press.

Als, H., Tronick, E., Lester, B. M., & Brazelton, T. B. (1979). Specific neonatal measures: The Brazelton Neonatal Assessment Scale. In J. D. Osofsky (Ed.), *Handbook of infant development.* New York: John Wiley & Sons.

Ama, P. F. M., Simoneau, J. A., Boulay, M. R., Seresse, O., Theriault, G., & Bouchard, C. (1986). Skeletal muscle characteristics in sedentary Black and Caucasian males. *Journal of Applied Physiology* 61:1758–1761.

American Academy of Pediatrics. (1990). Strength training, weight and power lifting, and body building by children and adolescents. *Pediatrics* 86:801–803.

American Academy of Pediatrics. (2002). Intensive Training and Sports Specialization in Young Athletes. *Pediatrics* 106 (1):154–157.

American Diabetes Association. (2000). As quoted in *USA Today*, Tests urged to fight diabetes' surge in obese kids, by M. Elias (February 22).

Andersen, R. E., Carlos, J. C., Bartlett, S. J., Cheskin, L. J., & Pratt, M. (1998). Relationship of physical activity and television watching with body weight and level of fatness among children. *Journal of the American Medical Association* 279 (12):938–942.

Aniansson, A. (1980). *Muscle function in old age with special reference to muscle morphology, effect of training and capacity in activities of daily living.* Goteborg, Sweden: Goteborg University.

Annett, M. (1970). The growth of manual performance and speed. *British Journal of Psychology* 61:545–558.

Annett, M. (1985). *Left, right, hand, and brain: The Rightshift theory.* London: Lawrence Erlbaum Associates.

Annett, M. (1996). In defence of the right shift theory. *Perceptual and Motor Skills* 82:115–137.

Anthrop, J., & Allison, M. T. (1983). Role conflict and the high school female athlete. *Research Quarterly for Exercise and Sport* 54:104–111.

Apgar, V. A. (1953). A proposal for a new method of evaluation of the newborn infant. *Current Research in Anesthesia and Analgesia* 32:260–267.

Arendt, R. E., Angelopoulos, J., Salvator, A., & Singer, L. (1999). Motor development of cocaine-exposed children at age two years. *Pediatrics* 103 (1):86–92.

Armitage, M., & Larkin, D. (1993). Laterality, motor asymmetry and clumsiness in children. *Human Movement Science* 12:155–177.

Arnheim, D. D., & Sinclair, W. A. (1979). *The clumsy child: A program of motor therapy.* 2nd ed. St. Louis: Mosby.

Astrand, P-O., & Rodahl, K. (1986). *Textbook of work physiology: Physiological bases of exercise.* 3rd ed. New York: McGraw-Hill.

Athletic Footwear Association (1990). *American youth and sports participation.* North Palm Beach, FL: Athletic Footwear Association.

Baddeley, A. (2000). Short-term and working memory. In E. Tulving & F. I. M. Craik (Eds.), *The Oxford handbook of memory.* New York: Oxford University Press.

Bandura, A. (1986). *Social foundations of thought and action: A social cognitive theory.* Englewood Cliffs, NJ: Prentice Hall.

Bandura, A. (2000). Social Cognitive Theory. In A. Kazdin (Ed.), *Encyclopedia of psychology.* Washington, DC and New York: American Psychological Association and Oxford University Press.

Banks, M. S., & Salapatek, P. (1981). Infant pattern vision: A new approach based on the contract sensitivity function. *Journal of Experimental Child Psychology* 31:1–45.

Baranowski, T., Thompson, W. O., Durant, R. H., Baranowski, J., & Puhl, J. (1993). Observations on physical activity in physical locations: Age, gender, ethnicity, and month effects. *Research Quarterly for Exercise and Sport* 64 (2):127–133.

Bar-Or, O. (1983). *Pediatric sports medicine for the practitioner: From physiologic principles to clinical applications.* New York: Springer-Verlag.

Bar-Or, O., Foreyt, J., Bouchard, C., Brownell, K. D., Dietz, W. H., Ravussin, E., Salbe, A. D., Schwenger, S., Jeor, S. S., & Tourun, B. (1998). Physical activity, genetic, and nutritional considerations in childhood weight management. *Medicine and Science in Sports and Exercise* 30 (1):2–10.

Barr, H. M., & Streissguth, A. P. (2001). Identifying maternal self-reported alcohol use associated with fetal alcohol disorders. *Alcoholism: Clinical and Experimental Research* 25:283–287.

Barr, H. M., Streissguth, A. P., Darby, B. L., & Sampson, P. D. (1990). Prenatal exposure to alcohol, caffeine, tobacco, and aspirin: Effects on fine and gross motor performance in 4-year-old children. *Developmental Psychology* 26 (3):339–348.

Barsch, R. H. (1965). *Achieving perceptual-motor efficiency*. Seattle: Special Child Publications.

Bartlett, F. C. (1932). *Remembering: A study in experimental and social psychology*. Cambridge, MA: Cambridge University Press.

Bayley, N. (1969). *Manual for the Bayley Scales of infant development*. New York: The Psychological Corporation.

Bayley Scales of Infant Development (Bayley II). (1993). San Antonio, TX: The Psychological Corporation.

Becker, P., Grunwald, P., & Brazy, J. (1999). Motor organization in very low birth weight infants during caregiving: Effects of a developmental intervention. *Developmental and Behavioral Pediatrics* 20:344–354.

Bemben, M. G., Massey, B. H., Bemben, D. A., Boileau, R. A., & Misner, J. E. (1995). Age-related patterns in body composition for men aged 20–79 yr. *Medicine and Science in Sports and Exercise* 27:264–269.

Bennell, K., Khan, K., Matthews, B., Cook, E., Holzer, K., McKay, H., Wark, J. (2000). Activity-associated differences in bone mineral are evident before puberty: A cross-sectional study of 130 female novice dancers and controls. *Pediatric Exercise Science* 12:371–381.

Berg, K. M., & Smith, M. C. (1983). Behavioral thresholds for tones during infancy. *Journal of Experimental Child Psychology* 35:409–425.

Bernstein, N. (1967). *The coordination and regulation of movements*. London: Pergamon Press.

Bertenthal, B. I., & Clifton, R. K. (1998). Perception and action. In W. Damon (Ed.), *Handbook of child psychology: Vol. 2. Cognition, perception and language*: 51–102. New York: John Wiley & Sons.

Bertenthal, B. I., & Von Hofsten, C. (1998). Eye, head and trunk control: The foundation for manual development. *Neuroscience and Biobehavioral* 22 (4):515–520.

Berthier, N. E. (1996). Learning to reach: A mathematical model.

Developmental Psychology 32 (5): 811–823.

Berthier, N. E., DeBlois, S., Poirier, C. R., Novak, M. A., & Clifton, R. K. (2000). Where's the Ball? Two- and three-year-olds reason about unseen events. *Developmental Psychology* 36 (3):394–401.

Bjorklund, D. F. (1995). *Children's thinking: Developmental function and individual differences*. 2nd ed. Pacific Grove, CA: Brooks/Cole.

Bjorklund, D. F., & Rosenbaum, K. (2000). Middle childhood: Cognitive development. In A. Kazdin (Ed.), *Encyclopedia of psychology*. Washington, DC and New York: American Psychological Association and Oxford University Press.

Blair, S. N., Kohl, H. W., Paffenbarger, R. S., Jr., Clark, D. G., Cooper, K. H., & Gibbons, L. W. (1989). Physical fitness and all-cause mortality: Prospective study of healthy men and women. *Journal of American Medical Association* 262:2395–2401.

Blote, A. W., & Van Haastern, R. (1989). Developmental dimensions in the drawing behavior of preschool children. *Journal of Human Movement Studies* 17:187–205.

Boileau, R. A. (1996). Body composition assessment in children and youths. In O. Bar-Or (Ed.), *The child and adolescent athlete*. Cambridge, MA: Blackwell Science.

Bornstein, M. H., & Sigman, M. D. (1986). Continuity in mental development from infancy. *Child Development* 57:251–274.

Bosch, A., Goslin, B. R., Noakes, T. D., & Dennis, S. T. (1990). Physiological differences between black and white runners during a treadmill marathon. *European Journal of Applied Physiology* 61:68–72.

Botwinick, J., & Storandt, M. (1974). *Memory, related functions and age*. Springfield, IL: Charles C. Thomas.

Bouchard, C., & Perusse, L. (1994). Heredity, activity level, fitness, and health. In *Physical Activity, Fitness, and Health*. Champaign, IL: Human Kinetics.

Bourass, D. C., McManu, I. C., & Bryden, M. P. (1996). Handedness and eye-dominance: A meta-analysis of their relationship. *Laterality* 1 (1):5–34.

Bower, T. G. R. (1976). Repetitive processes in child development. *Scientific American* 235 (5):38–47.

Bower, T. G. R. (1989). *The rational infant: Learning in infancy*. New York: Freeman.

Braddock, J. (1980). Race, sports, and social nobility: A critical review. *Sociological Symposium* 30:18–38.

Branta, C. F., Painter, M., & Kiger, J. E. (1987). Gender differences in play patterns and sport participation of North American youth. In D. Gould & M. R. Weiss (Eds.), *Advances in Pediatric Sport Sciences: Vol. 2. Behavioral Issues*: 25–42. Champaign, IL: Human Kinetics.

Brazelton, T. B. (1984). *Neonatal behavioral assessment scales*. 2nd ed. Philadelphia: J. B. Lippincott.

Broadhead, G. D., & Church, G. E. (1985). Movement characteristics of preschool children. *Research Quarterly for Exercise and Sport* 56:208–214.

Broca, P. (1865). Sur la faculté du langage articulé. *Bulletin of Social Anthropology* 6:493–494.

Brodkin, P., & Weiss, M. R. (1990). Developmental differences in motivation for participating in competitive swimming. *Journal of Sport and Exercise Psychology* 12:248–263.

Broekhoff, J. (1986). The effect of physical activity on physical growth and development. In G. A. Stull & H. M. Eckert (Eds.), *The academy papers: Effects of physical activity on children*. Champaign, IL: Human Kinetics.

Bronfenbrenner, U. (1986). Ecology of the family as a context for human development: Research Perspectives. *Developmental Psychology* 22:723–742.

Bronfenbrenner, U. (2000). Ecological theory. In A. Kazdin (Ed.), *Encyclopedia of psychology*. Washington, DC and New York: American Psychological Association and Oxford University Press.

Bronson, G. W. (1982). Structure, status and characteristics of the nervous system at birth. In P. Stratton (Ed.), *Psychobiology of the human newborn*. New York: John Wiley & Sons.

Brooks, G. A., & Fahey, T. D. (1985). *Exercise physiology: Human bioenergetics and its applications*. New York: Macmillan.

Brown, B., Frankel, G., & Fennell, M. (1990). Hugs and shrugs: Parental and peer influences on continuation of involvement in sport by female adolescents. *Sex Roles* 20:397–412.

Brown-Sequard, C. E. (1877). Dual character of the brain: The Toner lectures (Lecture II). *Smithsonian miscellaneous collections:* 1–21. Washington, DC: Smithsonian Institute.

Bruininks, R. H. (1978). *Bruininks-Oseretsky test for motor proficiency.* Circle Pines, MN: American Guidance Service.

Bukatko, D., & Daehler, M. (2001). *Child Development, A Thematic Approach.* 4th ed. Boston, New York: Houghton Mifflin Company.

Burfoot, A. (1992). White men can't run. *Runner's World* (August): 90–95.

Bushnell, E. W. (1982). The ontogeny of intermodal relations: Visions and touch in infancy. In R. Walk & H. Pick (Eds.), *Intersensory perception and sensory integration:* 5–36. New York: Plenum.

Bushnell, E. W. (1985). The decline of visually guided reaching during infancy. *Infant Behavior and Development* 8:139–155.

Campbell, A. J., Borrie, M. J., & Spears, G. F. (1989). Risk factors for falls in a community-based prospective study of people 70 years and older. *Journal of Gerontology,* 44 (4):112–117.

Campbell, D., & Eaton, W. (2000). Sex differences in the activity level of infants. *Infant and Child Development* 8:1–17.

Campbell, S. K. (1999). Test-retest reliability of the test of infant motor performance. *Pediatric Physical Therapy* 11:60–66.

Campbell, S. K., & Kolobe, T. H. A. (2000). Concurrent validity of the Test of Infant Motor Performance with the Alberta Infant Motor Scale. *Pediatric Physical Therapy* 12:1–8.

Campbell, S. K. & Kolobe, T. H. A., Osten, E., Girolami, G. L., & Lenski, M. (1994). *Test of Infant Motor Performance.* Chicago, IL: Department of Physical Therapy, University of Illinois.

Carson, L., & Wiegand, R. L. (1979). Motor schema formation and retention in young children: A test of Schmidt's schema theory. *Journal of Motor Behavior* 11: 247–251.

Carter, J. E. L., & Heath, B. H. (1990). *Somatotyping—development and applications.* Cambridge: Cambridge University Press.

Case, R. (Ed.). (1992). *The mind's staircase: Exploring the conceptual underpinnings of children's thought and knowledge.* Hillsdale, NJ: Lawrence Erlbaum Associates.

Case-Smith, J. (1996). Analysis of current motor development theory and recently published infant motor assessments. *Infants and Young Children* 9 (1):29–41.

Case-Smith, T., Bigsby, R. (2000). *Posture and fine-motor assessment of infants.* San Antonio, TX: The Psychological Corporation.

Cassell, J., Bickmore, T., Campbell, L., Vilhjalmsson, H., & Yan, H. (2001). More than just a pretty face: conversational protocols and the affordances of embodiment. *Knowledge-Based Systems* 14:55–64.

Centers for Disease Control and Prevention (CDC). (1996). *A report of the Surgeon General: Physical activity and health.* Atlanta: U.S. Department of Health and Human Services.

Centers for Disease Control and Prevention (CDC). (2000). *Physical activity and good nutrition.* U.S. Department of Health and Human Services.

Cerella, J. (1990). Aging and information-processing rate. In J. E. Birren & K. W. Schaie (Eds.), *Handbook of the psychology of aging.* 3rd ed. New York: Academic Press.

Cerella, J., & Hale, S. (1994). The rise and fall in information-processing rates over the life span. *Acta Psychologica* 86:109–197.

Chasnoff, I. J. (1991). *Cocaine versus tobacco: Impact on infant and child outcome.* Paper presented at the biennial meeting of the Society for Research in Child Development, Seattle.

Cherry, E. C. (1953). Some experiments on the recognition of speech with one and with two ears. *Journal of the Acoustical Society of America* 25:975–979.

Chi, M. (1977a). Age differences in memory span. *Journal of Experimental Child Psychology* 23:266–281.

Chi, M. (1977b). Age differences in the speed of processing: A critique. *Developmental Psychology* 13:543–544.

Chi, M. (1978). Knowledge structures and memory development. In R. Siegler (Ed.), *Children's thinking: What develops?* Hillsdale, NJ: Lawrence Erlbaum Associates.

Chugani, H. T. (1996). As quoted in Your child's brain. *Newsweek* (February 19): 55–62.

Chugani, H. T. (1997). Neuroimaging of developmental nonlinearity and developmental pathologies. *Developmental Neuroimaging:* 187–195.

Chugani, H. T. (1998). A critical period of brain development. *Preventive Medicine* 27:184–188.

Claessens, A. L., Lefevre, J., Beunen, G., & Malina, R. M. (1999).The contributions of anthropometric characteristics to performance scores in elite female gymnasts. *Journal of Sports Medicine and Physical Fitness* 39:355–360.

Clark, J. E., Lanphear, A. K., & Riddick, C. C. (1987). The effects of videogame playing on the response selection processing of elderly adults. *Journal of Gerontology* 42:82–85.

Clark, J. E., & Phillips, S. J. (1993). A longitudinal study of intralimb coordination in the first year of independent walking: A dynamical systems analysis. *Child Development* 64 (4):1143–1157.

Clarke, H. H. (Ed.). (1975). Joint and body range of movement. *Physical Fitness Research Digest* 5:16–18.

Clifton, R. K., Morrongiello, B. A., Kulig, J. W., & Dowd, J. M. (1981). Developmental changes in auditory localization in infancy. In R. N. Aslin, J. R. Alberts, & M. R. Petersen (Eds.), *Development of perception, Vol. 1.* Orlando: Academic Press.

Clifton, R. K., Muri, D. W., Ashmead, D. H., & Clarkson, M. G. (1993). Is visually guided reaching in early infancy a myth? *Child Development* 64 (4):1099–1110.

Coakley, J. J. (1987). Children and the sport socialization process. In *Advances in pediatric sport sciences.* Champaign, IL: Human Kinetics.

Corballis, M. C. (1983). *Human laterality.* New York: Academic Press.

Corballis, M. C., & Morgan, M. J. (1978). On the biological basis of human laterality: I. Evidence for a maturational right-left gradient. *Behavioral and Brain Sciences* 2:261–269.

Corbetta, D., Thelen, E., & Johnson, K. (2000). Motor constraints on the development of perception-action matching in infant reaching. *Infant Behavior and Development* 23 (3–4): 351–374.

Coren, S. (1993). The lateral preference inventory for measurement of handedness, footedness, eyedness, and earedness: Norms for young adults. *Bulletin of the Psychonomic Society* 31 (1):1–3.

Corso, J. F. (1987). Sensory-perceptual processes and aging. *Annual Review of Gerontology and Geriatrics* 7:29–55.

Cotman, C., & Engesser-Cesar, C. (2002). Exercise enhances and protects brain function. *Exercise and Sport Sciences Reviews* 30 (2): 75–79.

Coveney, P., & Highfield, R. (1995). *Frontiers of complexity: The search for order in a chaotic world.* New York: Fawcett Columbine.

Craik, R. (1989). Changes in locomotion in the aging adult. In M. H. Woollacott & A. Shumway-Cook (Eds.), *Development of posture and gait across the life span.* Columbia, SC: University of South Carolina Press.

Cratty, B. (1986). Perceptual and motor development in infants and children. 3rd ed. Englewood Cliffs, NJ: Prentice Hall.

Cummings, M. F., Van Hof-van Duin, J., Mayer, D. L., Hansen, R. M., & Fulton, A. B. (1988). Visual fields of young children. *Behavioral Brain Research* 29:7–16.

Damsgaard, R., Bencke, J., Matthiesen, G., Petersen, J. H., & Muller, J. (2000). Is prepubertal growth adversely affected by sport? *Medicine and Science in Sports and Exercise* 32 (10):1698–1703.

Dargent-Paré, C., De Agnostini, M., Mesbah, M., Dellatolas, G. (1992). Foot and eye preferences in adults: Relationship with handedness, sex, and age. *Cortex* 28:343–351.

Darrah, J., Redfern, L., Maguire, T. O., Beaulne, P., & Watt, J. (1998). Intra-individual stability of rate of gross motor development in full-term infants. *Early Human Development* 52:169–179.

David, K., Bennett, S., Kingsbury, D., Jolley, L., & Brian, T. (2000). Effects of postural constraints on children's catching behavior. *Research Quarterly for Exercise and Sport* 71 (1):69–73.

Day, N. (1991). *Effects of alcohol and marijuana on growth and development.* Paper presented at the biennial meeting of the Society for Research in Child Development, Seattle.

Deach, D. (1950). *Genetic development of motor skills in children two through six years of age.* Unpublished doctoral dissertation, University of Michigan, Ann Arbor.

Delacato, C. H. (1966). *Neurological organization and reading.* Springfield IL: Charles C. Thomas.

Dempster, F. N. (1981). Memory span: Sources of individual and developmental differences. *Psychological Bulletin* 89:63–100.

Denver Developmental Screening (Denver II). (1990). W. K. Frankenburg & J. B. Dodds. Denver: DDM.

DeOreo, K. L., & Keogh, J. (1980). Performance of fundamental motor tasks. In C. B. Corbin (Ed.), *A textbook of motor development.* 2nd ed. Dubuque, IA: Wm. C. Brown.

Desrosiers, J., Hebert, R., Bravo, G., & Rochette, A. (1999). Age-related changes in upper extremity performance of elderly people: A longitudinal study. *Experimental Gerontology* 34:399–405.

deVries, H., & Housh, T. (1994). *Physiology of exercise.* 5th ed. Madison, WI: Brown & Benchmark.

Diamond, A. (1998). Understanding the A-not-B error: Working memory vs. reinforced response, or active trace vs. latent trace. *Developmental Science* 1:185–189.

Diamond, M. (1988). *Enriching heredity.* New York: Free Press/Macmillan.

Dietz, W. (1997). Periods of risk in childhood for the Development of Adult Obesity—What do we need to learn. *Journal of Nutrition* 127:1884S–1886S.

DiLorenzo, T., Stucky-Ropp, R., Vander Wal, J., & Gotham, H. (1998). Determinants of exercise among children: II. A longitudinal analysis. *Preventive Medicine* 27:470–477.

Drage, J. S., Kennedy, C., Berendes, H., Schwartz, B. K., & Weiss, W. (1966). The Apgar score as an index of infant morbidity. *Developmental Medicine and Child Neurology* 8:141–148.

Dunkel-Schetter, C., Gurung, R. A. R., Lobel, M., & Wadhwa, P. D. (2001). Stress processes in pregnancy and birth. In A. Baum, T. A. Revenson, & J. E. Singer (Eds.), *Handbook of Health psychology.* Mahwah, NJ: Lawrence Erlbaum Associates.

Dzwaltowski, D. A. (1989). A social cognitive theory of older adult exercise motivation. In A. C. Ostrow (Ed.), *Aging and motor behavior.* Indianapolis: Benchmark Press.

Easton, T. A. (1972). On the normal use of reflexes. *American Scientist* 60:591–599.

Eckert, H. M. (1987). *Motor development.* 3rd ed. Indianapolis: Benchmark Press.

Edleman, G. M. (1987). *Neural darwinism.* New York: Basic Books.

Edleman, G. M. (1989). *The remembered present.* New York: Basic Books.

Einkauf, D. K., Gohdes, M. L., Jensen, G. M., & Jewell, M. J. (1987). Changes in spinal mobility with increasing age in women. *Physical Therapy* 67:370–375.

Eisenberg, R. B. (1976). *Auditory competence in early life.* Baltimore: University Park Press.

Era, P., & Heikkinen, E. (1985). Postural sway during standing and unexpected disturbance of balance in random examples of men of different ages. *Journal of Gerontology* 40:287–295.

Erbaugh, S. J. (1984). The relationship of stability performance and the physical growth characteristics of pre-school children. *Research Quarterly for Exercise and Sport* 55:8–16.

Eriksson, P. S., Perfilieva, E., Bjork-Eriksson, T., Alborn, A., Nordborg, C., Peterson, D. A., & Gage, F. H. (1998). Neurogenesis in the adult human hippocampus. *Nature Medicine* 4 (11):1313–1317.

Espenschade, A. (1960). Motor development. In W. R. Johnson (Ed.), *Science and medicine of exercise and sport.* New York: Harper & Row.

Eveleth, P. B., & Tanner, J. M. (1990). *Worldwide variation in human growth.* 2nd ed. Cambridge, England: Cambridge University Press.

Fagan, J. W. (1984). Infants' long-term memory for stimulus color. *Developmental Psychology* 20:435–440.

Fagard, J., & Jacquet, A. Y. (1996). Changes in reaching and grasping objects of different sizes between 7 and 13 months of age. *British Journal of Developmental Psychology* 14:65–78.

Fagot, B. I., & Leinbach, M. D. (1987). Socialization of sex roles within the family. In D. B. Carter (Ed.), *Current conceptions of sex roles and sex typing: Theory and research.* New York: Praeger.

Fahey, T. D. (1990). The development of respiratory capacity during exercise in children and adolescents. In E. Meisami & P. S. Timiras (Eds.), *Handbook of human growth and developmental biology* (Vol. III, Part B: 209–218). Boca Raton: CRS Press.

Farrell, S. W., Kampert, J. B., Kohl, H. W., Barlow, C. E., Macera, C. A., Paffenbarger, R. S., Gibbons, L. W., & Blair, S. N. (1998). Influences of cardiorespiratory fitness levels and other predictors on cardiovascular disease mortality in men. *Medicine and Science in Sports and Exercise* 30 (6):899–905.

Fiatarone, M. A., et al. (1994). Exercise training and nutritional supplementation for physical frailty in very elderly people. *New England Journal of Medicine* 330:1769.

Field, T. (1990). *Infancy.* Cambridge, MA: Harvard University Press.

Finegan, J. K., Niccols, G. A., & Sitarenios, G. (1992). Relations between prenatal testosterone levels and cognitive abilities at 4 years. *Developmental Psychology* 28 (6): 1075–1089.

Fiorentino, M. R. (1981). *A basis for sensorimotor development: The influence of the primitive, postural reflexes on the development and distribution of tone.* Springfield, IL: Charles C. Thomas.

Fischman, M. G., Moore, J. B., & Steele, K. H. (1992). Children's one-hand catching as a function of age, gender, and ball location. *Research Quarterly for Exercise and Sport* 63 (4):349–355.

Fisk, A. D., & Rogers, W. A. (2000). Influence of training and experience on skill acquisition and maintenance in older adults. *Journal of Aging and Physical Activity* 8:373–378.

Fitts, P. M. (1954). The information capacity of the human motor system in controlling the amplitude of movement. *Journal of Experimental Psychology* 47:381–391.

Flavell, J. H., Miller, P. H., & Miller, S. A. (1993). *Cognitive development.* 3rd ed. Englewood Cliffs, NJ: Prentice Hall.

Folio, R., & Fewell, R. (2000). *Peabody Developmental Motor Scales.* Austin, TX: Pro-ed.

Forfar, J. O., & Arneil, G. C. (Eds.). (1998). *Textbook of pediatrics.* 5th ed. London: Churchill Livingstone.

Freedland, R. L., & Bertenthal, B. I. (1994). Developmental changes in interlimb coordination: Transition to hands-and-knees crawling. *Psychological Science* 5 (1):26–32.

Fried, P. A., & Watkinson, B. (1990). 36- and 48-month neurobehavioral follow-up of children prenatally exposed to marijuana, cigarettes, and alcohol. *Developmental and Behavioral Pediatrics* 11:49–58.

Frisancho, A. R. (1990). *Anthropometric standards for the assessment of growth and nutritional status.* Ann Arbor: University of Michigan Press.

Frisch, R. E. (1991). Puberty and body fat. In R. M. Lerner, A. C. Petersen, & J. Brooks-Gunn (Eds.), *Encyclopedia of adolescence.* New York: Garland.

Frontera, W. R., Hughes, V. A., Fielding, R. A., Fiatarone, M. A., Evans, W. J., & Roubenoff, R. (2000). Aging of skeletal muscle: a 12-yr longitudinal study. *Journal of Applied Physiology* 88:1321–1326.

Gabbard, C. (1982). Comparison and relationships of selected upper limb and anthropometric measurements to strength and endurance among children aged 4–6 years. *Journal of Human Movement Studies* 8:55–91.

Gabbard, C. (1985). Children's striking force characteristics. *Journal of Human Movement Studies* 11:53–63.

Gabbard, C., Goncalves, V., & Santos, D. (2001). Visual-motor integration problems in low birth weight infants. *Journal of Clinical Psychology in Medical Settings* 8 (3):199–204.

Gabbard, C., & Hart, S. (1996). Probing Previc's theory of postural control. *Brain and Cognition* 30 (3):351–353.

Gabbard, C., & Iteya, M. (1996). Foot laterality in children, adolescents, and adults. *Laterality* 1 (3):199–205.

Gallahue, D. L., & Cleland, F. (2003). *Developmental Physical Education for Today's Children.* 4th ed. Champaign, IL: Human Kinetics.

Gentilucci, M., Chieffi, S., Scarpa, M., & Castiello, U. (1992). Temporal coupling between transport and grasp components during prehension movements. *Behavioural Brain Research* 47:71–82.

Geschwind, N., & Galaburda, A. S. (1985). Cerebral lateralization: Biological mechanisms, associations, and pathology: A hypothesis and program for research, I, II, III. *Archives of Neurology* 42:426–457, 521–552, 634–654.

Gesell, A. (1925). *The mental growth of the preschool child.* New York: Macmillan.

Gibson, E. J. (2001). *Perceiving the affordances.* Mahwah, NJ: Lawrence Erlbaum Associates.

Gibson, E. J., & Spelke, E. J. (1983). The development of perception. In P. H. Mussen (Ed.), *Handbook of child psychology.* New York: John Wiley & Sons.

Gibson, E. J., & Walk, R. D. (1960). The "visual cliff." *Scientific American* 202:64–71.

Gibson, E. J., & Walker, A. S. (1984). Development of knowledge of visual-tactile affordances of substance. *Child Development* 55:453–460.

Gibson, J. J. (1979). *The ecological approach to visual perception.* Boston: Houghton Mifflin.

Gilbert, A. N., & Wysocki, C. J. (1992). Hand preference and age in the United States. *Neuropsychologia* 30 (7):601–608.

Goldfield, E. (1995). *Emergent forms: Origins and early development of human action and perception.* New York: Oxford University Press.

Gottfried, A. W., & Bathurst, K. (1983). Hand preference across time is related to intelligence in young girls, not boys. *Science* 221:1074–1076.

Gottlieb, G. (1992). *Individual development and evolution: The genesis of novel behavior.* New York: Oxford University Press.

Gould, D. (1987). Understanding attrition in children's sport. In D. Gould & M. R. Weiss (Eds.), *Advances in Pediatric Sport Sciences, Vol. 2, Behavorial Issues*: 61–85. Champaign, IL: Human Kinetics.

Gould, D., & Eklund, R. C. (1996). Emotional stress and anxiety in the child and adolescent athlete. In O. Bar-Or (Ed.), *The child and adolescent athlete*: 383–398. Osney Mead, Oxford: Blackwell Science Ltd.

Grattan, M. P., DeVos, E., Levy, J., & McClintock, M. K. (1992). Asymmetric action in the human newborn: Sex differences in patterns of organization. *Child Development* 63: 273–289.

Greendorfer, S. L. (1979). Children sport socialization influences of male and female track athlete. *Arena Review* 3:39–53.

Greendorfer, S. L., & Ewing, M. E. (1981). Race and gender differences in children's socialization into sport. *Research Quarterly for Exercise and Sport* 52:301–310.

Greendorfer, S. L., & Lewko, J. H. (1978). Role of family members in sport socialization of children. *Research Quarterly* 49:146–182.

Greenough, W. T. (1996 February). As quoted in Your child's brain. *Newsweek* (February 19): 55–62.

Greenspan, E. (1983). *Little winners: Inside the world of the child sport star*. Boston: Little Brown.

Greulich, W. W., & Pyle, S. I. (1959). *Radiographic atlas of skeletal development of the hand and wrist*. 2nd ed. Stanford: Stanford University Press.

Guyton, A. C. (1991). *Basic neuroscience* 2nd ed. Philadelphia: Saunders.

Hack, M. H., Klein, N. K., & Taylor, H. G. (1995). Long-term developmental outcomes of low birth weight infants. *Future of Children* 5:176–196.

Hadders-Algra, M. (2000). The neuronal group selection theory: An attractive framework to explain variation in normal motor development. *Developmental Medicine & Child Neurology* 42:566–572.

Hager, A., Sjostrom, L., & Arvidsson, B. (1977). Body fat and adipose tissue cellularity in infants: A longitudinal study. *Metabolism* 26:607–614.

Haith, M. M., Wentworth, N., & Canfield, R. L. (1993). The formation of expectations in early infancy. In C. Rovee-Collier & L. P. Lipsitt (Eds.), *Advances in infancy research* (Vol. 8). Norwood, NJ: Ablex.

Hale, S. (1990). A global developmental trend in cognitive processing speed. *Child Development* 61:653–663.

Hale, S., Fry, A., & Jessie, K. A. (1993). Effects of practice on speed of information processing in children and adults: Age sensitivity and age invariance. *Developmental Psychology*, 29:880–892.

Hall, E. G., Durborow, B., & Progen, J. (1986). Self-esteem of female athletes and nonathletes relative to sex role type and sport type. *Sex Roles* 15:379–390.

Halverson, L. E., Roberton, M. A., & Langendorfer, S. (1982). Development of the overarm throw: Movement and ball velocity changes by seventh grade. *Research Quarterly for Exercise and Sport* 53:198–205.

Halverson, L. E., Roberton, M. A., Safrit, M. J., & Roberts, T. W. (1977). Effect of guided practice on overhand throw ball velocities of kindergarten children. *Research Quarterly* 48:311–318.

Halverson, L. E., & Williams, K. (1985). Developmental sequences for hopping distance: A prelongitudinal screening. *Research Quarterly for Exercise and Sport* 56:37–44.

Hart, S., & Gabbard, C. (1996). Brief communication: Bilateral footedness and task complexity. *International Journal of Neuroscience* 88: 141–146.

Hata, E., & Aoki, K. (1990). Age at menarche and selected menstrual characteristics in young Japanese athletes. *Research Quarterly for Exercise and Sport* 61 (2):178–183.

Haubenstricker, J., Branta, C., Seefeldt, V., Forsblom, L., & Kiger, J. (1990). *Prelongitudinal screening of a developmental sequence of skipping*. Paper presented at the annual meeting of the North American Society for the Psychology of Sport and Physical Activity, Houston.

Haubenstricker, J., & Sapp, M. (1985). A brief review of the Bruininks-Oseretsky test of motor proficiency. *Motor Development Academy Newsletter* (NASPE) 5 (1):1–2.

Haubenstricker, J., & Seefeldt, V. (1986). Acquisition of motor skills during childhood. In V. Seefeldt (Ed.), *Physical activity and well-being*: 41–102. Reston, VA: AAHPERD.

Haubenstricker, J. L., et al. (1997). Gender differences and mixed-longitudinal norms on selected motor skills for children and youth. *Journal of Sport & Exercise Psychology: 1997 NASPSPA Abstracts* 19:S63.

Head, H. (1926). *Aphasia and kindred disorders of speech*. Cambridge, MA: Cambridge University Press.

Hellerstedt, W. L., Himes, J. H., Story, M., Alton, I. R., & Edwards, L. E. (1997). The effects of cigarette smoking and gestational weight change on birth outcomes in obese and normal-weight women. *American Journal of Public Health* 87 (4):591–596.

Hellige, J. B. (1993). *Hemispheric asymmetry: What's right and what's left*. Cambridge, MA: Harvard University Press.

Hepper, P. G., McCartney, G. R., & Shannon, E. A. (1998). Lateralised

behaviour on first trimester human foetuses. *Neuropsychologia* 36 (6): 531–534.

Hepper, P. G., Shahidullah, S., & White, R. (1991). Handedness in the human fetus. *Neuropsychologia* 29 (11):1107–1111.

Himes, J. (1988). Racial variation in physique and body composition. *Canadian Journal of Sport Science* 13 (2):117–126.

Hirata, K. (1979). *Selection of Olympic champions* (Vol. 1). Santa Barbara: Institute of Environmental Stress.

Hodgkins, J. (1962). Influence of age on the speed of reaction and movement in females. *Journal of Gerontology* 17:385–389.

Hoffman, L. W. (1989). Effects of maternal employment in the two-parent family. *American Psychologist* 44:283–292.

Hofsten, C. (1991). Structuring of early reaching movements: A longitudinal study. *Journal of Motor Behavior* 23:280–292.

Hofsten, C. & Rönnqvist, L. (1988). Preparation for grasping an object: A developmental study. *Journal of Experimental Psychology: Human Perception and Performance* 14:610–621.

Hofsten, C., & Rönnqvist, L. (1993). The structuring of neonatal arm movements. *Child Development* 64 (4):1046–1057.

Hoptman, M. J., & Davidson, R. J. (1994). How and why do the two cerebral hemispheres interact? *Psychological Bulletin* 116 (2):195–219.

Horn, T. S. (1985). Coach's feedback and changes in children's perceptions of their physical competence. *Journal of Educational Psychology* 77: 174–186.

Horn, T. S., & Weiss, M. R. (1991). A developmental analysis of children's self-ability judgments in the physical domain. *Pediatric Exercise Science* 3:310–326.

Howe, M. L., & Courage, M. L. (1993). On resolving the enigma of infantile amnesia. *Psychological Bulletin* 113: 305–326.

Hughes, F. P., & Noppe, L. D. (1991). *Human development across the lifespan*. New York: Macmillan.

Hughes, J. E. (1979). *Manual for the Hughes basic motor assessment*. Golden, CO: University of Colorado.

Huston, A. C., Wright, J. C., Rice, M. C., Kerkman, D., & St. Peters, M. (1990). Development of television viewing patterns in early childhood: A longitudinal investigation. *Developmental Psychology* 26:409–420.

Huttenlocher, P. R. (1994). Synaptogenesis, synapse elimination, and neural plasticity in human cerebral cortex. In C.A. Nelson (Ed.), *Threats to optimal development: Integrating biology, psychology, and social risk factors.* Minnesota symposium of child psychology 20:35–54. Mahwah, NJ: Lawrence Erlbaum Associates.

Huttenlocher, P. R., & Dabhholkar, A. S. (1997). Regional differences in synaptogenesis in human cerebral cortex. *The Journal of Comparative Neurology* 387:167–178.

Ille, A., & Cadopi, M. (1999). Memory for movement sequences in gymnastics: Effects of age and skill level. *Journal of Motor Behavior* 31:290–300.

Inbar, O. (1996). Development of anaerobic power and local muscular endurance. In O. Bar-Or (Ed.), *The child and adolescent athlete*: 538–742. Osney Mead, Oxford: Blackwell Science Ltd.

Issacs, L. (1980). Effects of ball size, ball color, and preferred color on catching by young children. *Perceptual and Motor Skills* 51:583-586.

Jackson, A. S., et al. (1995). Changes in aerobic power of men, ages 25–70 yr. *Medical Science Sports Exercise* 27:113.

James, W. ([1890]1950). *The principles of psychology.* New York: Dover.

Jersild, A. T., & Bienstock, S. F. (1935). Development of rhythm in young children. *Child Development Monographs* (No. 22).

Johnson, R. (1962). Measurements of achievement in fundamental skills of elementary school children. *Research Quarterly* 33:94–103.

Jones, T., & Greenough, W. T. (1996). Ultrastructural evidence for increased contact between astrocytes and synapses in rats reared in a complex environment. *Neurobiology of Learning & Memory* 65 (1):48–56.

Kail, R. (1991). Developmental change in speed of processing during childhood and adolescence. *Psychological Bulletin* 109 (3):490–501.

Kail, R., & Salthouse, T. A. (1994). Processing speed as a mental capacity. *Acta Psychologica* 86:199–225.

Kallman, D. A., Plato, C. C., & Tobin, J. D. (1990). The role of muscle loss in the age-related decline of grip strength: Cross-sectional and longitudinal perspectives. *Journal of Gerontology: Medical Sciences* 45:M82–88.

Kaplan, R. M., & Saccuzzo, D. P. (1993). *Psychological testing.* Pacific Grove, CA: Brooks/Cole.

Kasch, F. W., et al. (1990). The effect of physical activity and inactivity on aerobic power in older men (a longitudinal study). *The Physician and Sportsmedicine* 18:73.

Katsarka, A., Smith, H., & Galiana, H. (1994). Postural instability on one foot in patients with loss of unilateral peripheral vestibular function. *Journal of Vestibular Research* 4 (2):153–160.

Kavale, K., & Matson, P. D. (1983). One jumped off the balance beam: Meta analysis of perceptual motor training. *Journal of Learning Disabilities* 16:165–173.

Kellogg, R. (1969). *Analyzing children's art.* Palo Alto, CA: National Press Books.

Kelso, J. A. S., & Norman, P. E. (1978). Motor schema formation in children. *Developmental Psychology* 14:153–156.

Kelso, J. A. S., Tuller, B. H., Vatikiotis-Bateson, E., & Fowler, C. A. (1984). Functionally specific articulatory cooperation following jaw perturbations during speech: Evidence for coordinative structures. *Journal of Experimental Psychology: Human Perception and Performance* 10:812–832.

Kempermann, G., & Gage, F. H. (1999). New nerve cells for the adult brain: Contrary to dogma, the human brain does produce new nerve cells in adulthood. Can our newfound capacity lead to better treatments for neurological disease? *Scientific American* (May):48–53.

Kenyon, G. S., & McPherson, B. D. (1973). Becoming involved in physical activity and sport: A process of socialization. In G. L. Rarick (Ed.), *Physical activity: Human growth and development*: 301–332. New York: Academic Press.

Keogh, J. (1965). *Motor performance of elementary school children* (U.S. Public Health Service grants MH08319-01 and HD01059). Los Angeles: University of California, Dept. of Physical Education.

Keogh, J., & Sugden, D. (1985). *Movement skill development.* New York: Macmillan.

Kephart, N. C. (1971). *The slow learner in the classroom.* 2nd ed. Columbus, OH: Charles E. Merrill.

Kerr, R., & Booth, B. (1978). Specific and varied practice of motor skill. *Perceptual and Motor Skills* 46:385–401.

Kirshnit, C. E., Ham, M., & Richards, M. H. (1989). The sporting life: Athletic activities during early adolescence. *Journal of Youth and Adolescence* 18:601–615.

Kirshnit, C. E., Richards, M. H., & Ham, M. (1988). *Athletic participation and body image during early adolescence.* Paper presented at the meeting of the American Psychological Association, Atlanta, GA.

Klinger, A., Masataka, T., Adrian, M., & Smith, E. (April 1980). *Temporal and spatial characteristics of movement patterns of women over 60.* (Cited in Adrian, 1982). American Alliance for Health, Physical Education, Recreation and Dance Research Consortium Symposium, Detroit.

Knobloch, H., & Pasamanick, B. (Eds.). (1974). *Gesell and Amatruda's developmental diagnosis.* 3rd ed. New York: Harper & Row.

Konczak, J., Borutta, M., & Dichgans, J. (1997). The development of goal-directed reaching infants: Learning to produce task-adequate patterns of joint torque. *Experimental Brain Research* 113:465–474.

Kreutzer, M., Leonard, C., & Flavell, J. (1975). An interview study of children's knowledge of memory. *Monographs of the Society for Research in Children Development* 40 (1, serial no. 159).

Kreutzfeldt, J., Haim, M., & Bach, E. (1984). Hip fracture among the elderly in mixed urban and rural population. *Age and Aging* 13:111–119.

Kugler, P. N., Kelso, J. A. S., & Turvey, M. T. (1980). On the concept of coordinative structures as dissipative structures. I. Theoretical lines of convergence. In G. E. Stelmach & J. Requin (Eds.), *Tutorials in motor behavior*:1–47. New York: North-Holland, Amsterdam.

Kugler, P. N., Kelso, J. A. S., & Turvey, M. (1982). On the control and coordination of naturally developing systems. In J. A. S. Kelso & J. E. Clark (Eds.), *The development of movement control and coordination:* 5–78. New York: John Wiley and Sons.

Kuhlman, J. S., & Beitel, P. A. (1997). Development/Learning of coincidence anticipation. *Journal of Sport & Exercise Psychology: 1997 NASPSPA Abstracts* 19:S76.

Ladd, G. W., & Mize, J. A. (1983). A cognitive social learning model of social-skill training. *Psychological Review* 90:127–157.

Landreth, C. (1958). *The psychology of early childhood.* New York: Alfred A. Knopf.

Lang, G. J., & Luff, A. R. (1990). Skeletal muscle growth, hypertrophy, repair, and regeneration. In E. Meisami & P. S. Timiras (Eds.), *Handbook of human growth and developmental biology* (Vol. 3). Boca Raton, FL: CRS Press.

Ledebt, A. (2000). Changes in arm posture during early acquisition of walking. *Infant Behavior and Development* 23 (1):79–89.

Lerner, R. M. (2002). *Concepts and theories of human development.* 3rd ed. Mahwah, NJ: Lawrence Erlbaum Associates.

Lewis, M. D. (2000). The promise of dynamic systems approaches for an integrated account of human development. *Child Development* 71 (1):36–43.

Lewko, J. H., & Ewing, M. E. (1980). Sex differences and parental influences in sport involvement of children. *Journal of Sport Psychology* 2:62–68.

Liberty, C., & Ornstein, P. A. (1973). Age differences in organization and recall: The effects of training in categorization. *Journal of Experimental Child Psychology* 15:169–186.

Light, K. L., & Spirduso, W. W. (1990). Effects of adult aging on the movement complexity factor or response programming. *Journal of Gerontology* 45 (3):107–109.

Lockman, J. J., & Thelen, E. (1993). Developmental biodynamics: Brain, body and behavior connections. *Child Development* 64 (4):953–959.

Lohman, T. G. (1989). Assessment of body composition in children. *Pediatric Exercise Science* 1:19–30.

Lohman, T. G. (1992). *Advances in body composition assessment.* Champaign, IL: Human Kinetics.

Londeree, B. R., & Moeschberger, M. L. (1982). Effects of age and other factors on maximal heart rate. *Research Quarterly for Exercise and Sport* 53:297–304.

Loovis, E. M., & Ersing, W. F. (1979). *Assessing and programming gross motor development for children.* 2nd ed. Loudonville, OH: Mohican Textbook Publishing.

Lorton, J. W., & Lorton, E. L. (1984). *Human development through the life span.* Pacific Grove, CA: Brooks/Cole.

Lowrey, G. H. (1986). *Growth and development of children.* 8th ed. Chicago: Year Book Medical Publishers.

Lund, R. D. (1978). *Development and plasticity of the brain.* New York: Oxford University Press.

Lupinacci, N. S., Rikli, R. E., Jones, J., & Ross, D. (1993). Age and physical activity effects on reaction time and digit symbol substitution performance in cognitively active adults. *Research Quarterly for Exercise and Sport* 64 (2):144–150.

MacNeilage, P. R. (1991). The postural origins theory of primate neurobiological asymmetries. In N. Krasnegor, D. Rumbaugh, M. Studdert-Kennedy, & R. Schiefelbusch (Eds.), *The biological foundations of language development.* Hillsdale, NJ: Lawrence Erlbaum Associates.

Magill, R. A. (2001). *Motor learning: Concepts and application.* 6th ed. Dubuque, IA: Wm. C. Brown. (undergraduate)

Malina, R. M. (1984). Human growth, maturation, and regular physical activity. In R. A. Boileau (Ed.), *Advances in Pediatric Sport Sciences: Biological Issues* (Vol. 1). Champaign, IL: Human Kinetics.

Malina, R. M., & Bouchard, C. (1991). *Growth, maturation, and physical activity.* Champaign, IL: Human Kinetics.

Manchester, D., Woollacott, M., Zederbauer-Hylton, N., & Marin, O. (1989). Visual, vestibular and somatosensory contributions to balance control in the older adult. *Journal of Gerontology* 44 (4): 118–127.

Mandler, J. M, & McDonough, L. (1995). Long-term recall in infancy. *Journal of Experimental Child Psychology* 59:457–474.

Manis, F. R., Keating, D. P., & Morrison, F. J. (1980). Developmental differences in the allocation of processing. *Journal of Experimental Child Psychology* 29:156–169.

Marker, K. (1981). Influence of athletic training on the maturity process. In J. Borms, M. Hebbelinck, & A. Venerando (Eds.), *The female athlete:* 117–126. Basel, Switzerland: Karger.

McArdle, W. D., Katch, F. I., & Katch, V. L. (2001). *Exercise physiology: Energy, nutrition, and human performance.* 5th ed. Philadelphia: Lea & Febiger.

McBride-Chang, C., & Jacklin, C. (1993). Early play arousal, sex-typed play and activity level as precursors to later rough-and-tumble play. *Early Education and Development* 4:99–108.

McClenaghan, B. A., & Gallahue, D. L. (1978). *Fundamental movement: A developmental and remedial approach.* Philadelphia: W. B. Saunders.

McDonnell, P. M. (1979). Patterns of eye-hand coordination in the first year of life. *Canadian Journal of Psychology* 33:253–267.

McManus, I. C., Sik, G., Cole, D. R., Mellon, A. F., Wong, J., & Kloss, J. (1988). The development of handedness in children. *British Journal of Developmental Psychology* 6:257–273.

McPherson, B. D. (1978). The child in competitive sport: Influences of the social milieu. In R. A. Magill, M. J. Ash, & F. L. Smoll (Eds.), *Children in sport: A contemporary anthology:* 219–249. Champaign, IL: Human Kinetics.

Meeuwsen, H. J., Tesi, J. M., & Goggin, N. C. (1992). Psychophysics of arm movements and human aging. *Research Quarterly for Exercise and Sport* 63 (1):19–24.

Meltzoff, A. N., & Moore, M. K. (1977). Imitation of facial and manual gestures by human neonates. *Science* 198:75–78.

Milani-Comparetti, A. (1981). The neurophysiologic and clinical implications of studies on fetal motor behavior. *Seminars in Perinatology* 5:183–189.

Milani-Comparetti, A., & Gidoni, E. A. (1967). Pattern analysis of motor development and its disorders. *Developmental Medicine and Child Neurology* 9:625.

Miller, L. J., & Roid, R. G. (1994). The TIME: Toddler and infant motor evaluation: A standardized assessment. Tucson, AZ: Therapy Skill Builders.

Molnar, G. (1978). Analysis of motor disorder in retarded infants and young children. *American Journal of Mental Deficiency* 83:213–222.

Monk, C., Fifer, W. P., Sloan, R. P., & Myers, M. M. (2000). *Individual differences in fetal cardiac reactivity are associated with maternal anxiety and infant birth weight.* Paper presented at joint meeting of the Pediatric Academic Societies and the American Academy of Pediatrics, Boston.

Morgane, P. J., Austin-LaFrance, R., Bronzino, J., Tonkiss, J., Diaz-Cintra, S., Cintra, L., Kemper, T., & Galler, J. R. (1993). Prenatal malnutrition and development of the brain. *Neuroscience and Biobehavioral Reviews* 17:91–128.

Morris, A. M., Williams, J. M., Atwater, A. E., & Wilmore, J. H. (1982). Age and sex differences in motor performance of 3 through 6 year old children. *Research Quarterly for Exercise and Sport* 53:214–221.

Moxley, S. E. (1979). Schema: The variability of practice hypothesis. *Journal of Motor Behavior* 11:65–70.

Murray, M. P., Kory, R. C., & Clarkson, B. H. (1969). Walking patterns in healthy old men. *Journal of Gerontology* 24:169–178.

Murray, M. P., Kory, R. C., & Sepic, S. B. (1970). Walking patterns of normal women. *Archives of Physical Medicine and Rehabilitation* 51: 637–650.

Nachshon, I., Denno, D., & Aurand, S. (1983). Lateral preferences of hand, eye and foot: Relation to cerebral dominance. *International Journal of Neuroscience* 18:1–10.

National Center for Health Statistics. (1999). Healthy people 2000 review, 1998–99. Hyattsville, MD: Public Health Service.

National Center for Health Statistics. Najjar, M. R., & Rowland, M. (1987). Anthropometric reference data. *Vital and Health Statistics* 11: (238), DHHS Pub. No. (PHS) 887–1688. Public Health Service. Washington, DC: U.S. Government Printing Office.

National Children and Youth Fitness Study I. (1985). *Journal of Physical Education, Recreation and Dance* 56 (1):43–90.

National Children and Youth Fitness Study II. (1987). *Journal of Physical Education, Recreation and Dance* 58 (9):49–96.

National Federation News. (1993). Publication of the National Federation of State High School Associations. Athletic participation survey, Kansas City, MO.

National Institute on Aging. (1993). *In search of the secrets of aging* (NIH Publication No. 93-2756). Washington, DC.

Neisser, U. (1967). *Cognitive psychology.* New York: Appleton-Century-Crofts.

Nelson, C. A. (2000). Neural plasticity and human development: The role of early experience in sculpting memory systems. *Developmental Science* 3:115–136.

Nelson, C. J. (1981). *Locomotor patterns of women over 57.* Unpublished master's thesis, Washington State University, Pullman.

Neugarten, B. L., Havighurst, R. J., & Tobin, S. S. (1968). Personality and patterns of aging. In B. L. Neugarten (Ed.), *Middle age and aging.* Chicago: University of Chicago Press.

Neumann, E., & Ammons, R. B. (1957). Acquisition and long-term retention of a simple serial perceptual motor skill. *Journal of Experimental Psychology* 53:159–161.

Newell, K. M. (1986). Constraints on the development of coordination. In M. G. Wade & H. T. A. Whiting (Eds.), *Motor development in children: Aspects of coordination and control*: 341–361. Amsterdam, The Netherlands: Martinus Nijhoff Publishers.

Nickol-Richardson, S. M., Modlesky, C. M., O'Connor, P. J., & Lewis, R. D. (2000). Premenarcheal gymnasts possess higher bone mineral density than controls. *Medicine and Science in Sports and Exercise* 32: 63–69.

Nottelmann, E. D., Susman, E. J., Blue, J. H., Inoff-Germain, G., Dorn, L. D., Loriaux, D. L., Cutler, G. B., & Chrousos, G. P. (1987). Gonadal and adrenal hormone correlates of adjustment in early adolescence. In R. M. Lerner & T. T. Foch (Eds.), *Biological-psychological interactions in early adolescence.* Hillsdale, NJ: Lawrence Erlbaum Associates.

Oberauer, K., Demmrich, A., Mayr, U., & Kliegl, R. (2001). Dissociating retention and access in working memory. *Memory and cognition* 29:18–33.

Oliver, M. (1980). Race, class, and the family's orientation to mobility through sport. *Sociological Symposium,* 30:62–86.

Oscai, L. B., Babirak, S. P., McGarr, J. A., & Spirakis, C. N. (1974). Effect of exercise on adipose tissue cellularity. *Federal Proceedings* 33:1956–1958.

Oscai, L. B., Spirakis, C. N., Wolff, C. H., & Beck, R. J. (1972). Effects of exercise and of food restriction on adipose tissue cellularity. *Journal of Lipid Research* 13:588–592.

Ostrow, A., Jones, D., & Spiker, D. (1981). Age role expectations and sex role expectations for selected sport activities. *Research Quarterly for Exercise and Sport* 52:216–227.

Overstall, P. W., Exton-Smith, A. N., Imms, F. J., & Johnson, A. L. (1977). Falls in the elderly related to postural imbalance. *British Medical Journal* 1:261–264.

Paffenbarger, R. S., Jr., Hyde, R. T., Wing, A. L., & Hsieh, C. C. (1986). Physical activity, all-cause mortality, and longevity of college alumni. *New England Journal of Medicine* 314:605–613.

Painter, M. A. (1994). Developmental sequences for hopping as assessment instruments: A generalized analysis. *Research Quarterly for Exercise and Sport* 65 (1):1–10.

Palisano, R. J., Kolobe, T. H., Haley, S. M., Lowes, L. P., & Jones, S. L. (1995). Validity of the Peabody Developmental Motor Scales as an evaluative measure of infants receiving physical therapy. *Physical Therapy* 75:939–948.

Palmer, C. F. (1989). The discriminating nature of infant's exploratory actions. *Developmental Psychology,* 25:885–893.

Panton, L. B., Graves, J. E., & Pollock, M. L. (1990). Effect of aerobic and resistance training on fractionated reaction time and speed of movement. *Journal of Gerontology* 45 (1):26–31.

Pargman, D. (1997). *Understanding sport behavior.* Upper Saddle River, NJ: Prentice Hall.

Parizkova, J., & Carter, J. E. L. (1976). Influence of physical activity on stability of somatotypes in boys. *American Journal of Physiology and Anthropology* 44:327–339.

Parten, M. (1932). Social play among preschool children. *Journal of*

Abnormal and Social Psychology 27: 243–269.

Patlak, M. (1992). The long and short of it: New medications for growth disorders. *FDA Consumer:* 30–34.

Payne, V. G. (1985). Effects of object size and experimental design on object reception by children in the first grade. *Journal of Human Movement Studies* 11:1–9.

Payne, V. G., & Isaacs, L. D. (1987). *Human motor development: A lifespan approach.* Mountain View, CA: Mayfield Publishing Company.

Payne, V. G., Morrow, J. R., Johnson, L., & Dalton, S. N. (1997). Resistance training in children and youth: A meta-analysis. *Research Quarterly for Exercise and Sport* 68 (1):80–88.

Perlmutter, M. (1983). Learning and memory through adulthood. In M. W. Riley, B. B. Hess, & K. Bond (Eds.), *Aging in society: Selected reviews of recent research.* Hillsdale, NJ: Lawrence Erlbaum Associates.

Perlmutter, M., & Hall, E. (1985). *Adult development and aging.* New York: John Wiley & Sons.

Perry, B. (1997). As quoted in Fertile minds. *Time* (February 3): 49–56.

Peters, M. (1988a). The size of the corpus callosum in males and females: Implications of a lack of allometry. *Canadian Journal of Psychology* 42 (3):313–324.

Peters, M. (1988b). Footedness: Asymmetries in foot preference and skill and neuropsychological assessment of foot movement. *Psychological Bulletin* 103 (2):179–192.

Petersen, G. (1967). *Atlas for somatotyping children.* Assen, The Netherlands: Van Gorcum.

Petlichkoff, L. M. (1996). The dropout dilemma in youth sports. In O. Bar-Or (Ed.), *The child and adolescent athlete* (pp. 418–430). Osney Mead, Oxford: Blackwell Science Ltd.

Petrofsky, J. S., & Lind, A. R. (1975). Aging, isometric strength and endurance, and cardiovascular responses to static effort. *Journal of Applied Physiology* 38:91–95.

Pettersen, L., Yonas, A., & Fisch, R. O. (1980). The development of blinking in response to impending collision in preterm, full term, and postterm infants. *Infant Behavior and Development* 3:155–165.

Piaget, J. (1952). *The origins of intelligence in children.* New York: International Universities Press. (Original work published 1936).

Piaget, J. (1963). *The origins of intelligence in children.* (M. Cook, Trans.). New York: W. W. Norton.

Piaget, J. (1985). *The equilibration of cognitive structures: The central problem of intellectual development.* Chicago: University of Chicago Press.

Pineau, A. & Streri, A. (1990). Intermodal transfer of spatial arrangement of the component parts of an object in infants aged 4–5 months. *Perception* 19:795–804.

Piper, M. C., & Darrah, J. (1994). *Motor assessment of the developing infant.* Philadelphia: W. B. Saunders.

Plude, D. J., Enns, J. T., & Brodeur, D. (1994). The development of selective attention: A life-span overview. *Acta Psychologica* 86:227–272.

Pollock, M., Wilmore, J., & Fox, S. (1978). *Health and fitness through physical activity.* New York: John Wiley & Sons.

Pontius, A. A. (1973). Neuro-Ethics of "walking" in the newborn. *Perceptual and Motor Skills* 37:235–245.

Porac, C., Coren, S., & Duncan, P. (1980). Lifespan age trends in laterality. *Journal of Gerontology* 35:715–721.

Powell, K. E., & Blair, S. N. (1994). The public health burdens of sedentary living habits: theoretical but realistic estimates. *Medical Science Sports Exercise* 26:851.

Prechtl, H., & Hopkins, B. (1986). Developmental transformations of spontaneous movements in early infancy. *Early Human Development,* 14:233–238.

Previc, F. H. (1991). A general theory concerning the prenatal origins of cerebral lateralization in humans. *Psychological Review* 98 (3):299–334.

Provins, K. A. (1992). Early infant motor asymmetries and handedness: A critical evaluation of the evidence. *Developmental Neuropsychology* 8 (4): 325–365.

Quirion, A., deCareful, D., Laurencell, L., Method, D., Vogelaere, P., & Dulac, S. (1987). The physiological response to exercise with special reference to age. *Journal of Sports Medicine and Physical Fitness* 27: 143–149.

Ramey, C. T. & Ramey, S. L. (1994). Which children benefit the most from early intervention? *Pediatrics* 94:1064–1066.

Rantanen, T., Era, P., & Heikkinen, E. (1997). Physical activity and the changes in maximal isometric strength in men and women from the age of 75 and 80 years. *Journal of American Geriatrics Society* 45:1439–1445.

Rapaport, S. (1994). Interview. *U. S. News and World Report* (November 28):94.

Reed, E. S., (1989). Chaining theories of postural development. In: Woollacott, M. H., Shumway-Cook, A. (Eds.), *Development of posture and gait across the life span:* 1–24. Columbia, SC: University of South Carolina Press.

Resnick, B. (2001). Testing a model of overall activity in older adults. *Journal of Aging and Physical Activity* 9:142–160.

Richter, C. P. (1934). The grasp reflex of the newborn infant. *American Journal of Developmental Children,* 48:327–332.

Rikli, R., & Busch, S. (1986). Motor performance of women as a function of age and physical activity level. *Journal of Gerontology* 41: 645–649.

Roach, E. G., & Kephart, N. C. (1966). *Purdue perceptual motor survey.* Columbus, OH: Merrill.

Roberton, M. A. (1977). Stability of stage categorizations across trials: Implications for the "stage theory" of overarm throw development. *Journal of Human Movement Studies* 3:49–59.

Roberton, M. A. (1978). Longitudinal evidence for developmental stages in the forceful overarm throw. *Journal of Human Movement Studies* 4: 167–175.

Roberton, M. A. (1984). Changing motor patterns during childhood. In J. R. Thomas (Ed.), *Motor development during childhood and adolescence:* 48–85. Minneapolis: Burgess.

Roberton, M. A. (1990). Interlimb timing changes in the development of hopping. North American Society for Psychology of Sport and Physical Activity abstracts.

Roberton, M. A., & Halverson, L. E. (1984). *Developing children—their changing movement.* Philadelphia: Lea & Febiger.

Roberton, M. A., Halverson, L. E., Langendorfer, S., & Williams, K.

(1979). Longitudinal changes in children's overarm throw ball velocities. *Research Quarterly for Exercise and Sport* 50:256–264.

Roberton, M. A., Williams, K., & Langendorfer, S. (1980). Prelongitudinal screening of motor development sequences. *Research Quarterly for Exercise and Sport* 51:724–731.

Robin, D. J., Berthier, N. E., & Clifton, R. K. (1996). Infant's predictive reaching for moving objects in the dark. *Developmental Psychology* 32 (5):824–835.

Rochat, P., & Goubet, N. (1995). Development of sitting and reaching in 5- to 6-month-old infants. *Infant Behavior and Development* 18:53–68.

Rogol, A. D. (1996). Delayed puberty in girls and primary and secondary amenorrhoea. In O. Bar-Or (Ed.), *The child and adolescent athlete*: 538–742. Osney Mead, Oxford: Blackwell Science Ltd.

Rook, K. S. (2000). The evolution of social relationships in later adulthood. In S. H. Qualls & N. Abeles (Eds.), *Psychology and the aging revolution*. Washington, DC: American Psychological Association.

Rose, D. J. (1997). *A multilevel approach to the study of motor control and learning*. Needham Heights, MA: Allyn & Bacon.

Rosenhall, U. & Rubin, W. (1975). Degenerative changes in the human vestibular sensory epithelia. *Acta Otolaryngol* 79:67–81.

Ross, J. G., & Gilbert, G. G. (1985). The national children and youth fitness study: A summary of findings. *Journal of Physical Education, Recreation and Dance* 56 (1):45–50.

Ross, J. G., & Pate, R. R. (1987). The national children and youth fitness study II. A summary of findings. *Journal of Physical Education, Recreation and Dance* 58 (9):51–56.

Rovee-Collier, C. (2001). Infant learning and memory. In A. Fogel & G. Bremner (Eds.), *Blackwell handbook of infant development*. London: Blackwell.

Rowland, T. W. (1996). *Developmental exercise physiology*. Champaign, IL: Human Kinetics.

Rudman, D., Feller, A. G., Nagraj, H. S., Gergans, G. A., Lalitha, P. Y., Goldberg, A. F., Schlenker, R. A., Cohn, L., Rudman, I. W., & Mattson, D. E. (1990). Effects of human growth hormone in men over 60 years old. *The New England Journal of Medicine* 323 (1):1–6.

Rudolph, R. (1982). Aspects of child health. In A. Rudolph (Ed.). *Pediatrics*. 17th ed.: 1–7. Norwalk, CT: Appleton-Century-Croft.

Sabatino, D. A. (1985). Review of Bruininks-Oseretsky test of motor proficiency. In J. V. Mitchell, Jr. (Ed.), *Ninth mental measurement yearbook*. Lincoln, NE: Buros Institute of Mental Measurements.

Saling, M., Alberts, J., Stelmach, G., & Bloedel, J. (1998). Reach-to-grasp movements during obstacle avoidance. *Experimental Brain Research* 118:251–258.

Salthouse, T. A. (1996). The processing-speed theory of adult age differences in cognition. *Psychological Review*, 103 (3):403–428.

Salvia, J. Z., & Ysseldyke, J. E. (1991). *Assessment*. 5th ed. Boston: Houghton Mifflin.

Santrock, J. W. (2002). *Life-span development*. 8th ed. Dubuque, IA: McGraw-Hill.

Satarino, W. A., Haight, T. J., Tager, I. B. (2000). Reasons given by older people for limitation or avoidance of leisure time in physical activity. *Journal of American Geriatrics Society* 48:505–512.

Schaie, K. W., & Willis, S. L. (1991). *Adult development and aging*. 3rd ed. New York: HarperCollins.

Scheibel, A. B. (1996). Structural changes in the aging brain. In J. E. Birren, R. B. Sloane, & G. D. Cohen (Eds.), *Handbook of mental health and aging*. 3rd ed.: 147–174. San Diego, CA: Academic Press.

Schieber, F. (1992). Aging and the senses. In J. E. Birren, R. B. Sloane, & G. D. Cohen (Eds.), *Handbook of mental health and aging*. 2nd ed.: 252–306. San Diego: Academic Press.

Schmidt, R., & Lee, T. (1994). *Motor control and learning*. 3rd ed. Champaign, IL: Human Kinetics.

Schmidt, R. A. (1975). A schema theory of discrete motor skill learning. *Psychological Review* 82:225–260.

Schmidt, R. A. (1977). Schema theory: Implications for movement education. *Motor Skills: Theory into Practice* 2:36–48.

Schmidt, R. A. (1988). *Motor control and learning*. 2nd ed. Champaign, IL: Human Kinetics.

Schneider, W., & Pressley, M. (1997). *Memory development between 2 and 20*. 2nd ed. Mahwah, NJ: Lawrence Erlbaum Associates.

Schultz, R., & Curnow, C. (1988). Peak performance and age among super-athletes. *Journal of Gerontology* 43:113–120.

Schultz, R., Musa, D., Staszewski, J., & Siegler, R. S. (1994). The relationship between age and major league baseball performance: Implications for development. *Psychology and Aging* 9 (2):274–286.

Schutte, J. E., Townsend, E. J., Hugg, J., Shoup, J., Molina, R. M., & Blomquist, C. G. (1984). Density of lean body mass is greater in blacks than in whites. *Journal of Applied Physiology* 56:1647–1649.

Schwartz, R. S., Shuman, W. P., Bradbury, V. L., Cain, K. C., Fellingham, G. W., Beard, J. C., Kahn, S. E., Stratton, J. R., Cerqueina, M. D., & Abrass, I. B. (1990). Body fat distribution in healthy young and older men. *Journal of Gerontology* 45 (6):181–185.

Seefeldt, V. (1972). *Developmental sequences of catching skills*. Paper presented at the American Alliance for Health, Physical Education, Recreation and Dance, Houston.

Seefeldt, V. (1974). Perceptual-motor programs. In J. H. Wilmore (Ed.), *Exercise and sports science reviews* (Vol. 2). New York: Academic Press.

Seefeldt, V., & Branta, C. F. (1984). Patterns of participation in children's sport. In J. Thomas (Ed.), *Motor development during childhood and adolescence*. Minneapolis: Burgess.

Seefeldt, V., & Haubenstricker, J. (1976). *Developmental sequences of fundamental motor skills*. Unpublished research, Michigan State University, East Lansing.

Seefeldt, V., & Haubenstricker, J. (1982). Patterns, phases, or stages: An analytical model for the study of developmental movement. In J. A. Kelso & J. E. Clark (Eds.), *The development of movement control and coordination*. New York: John Wiley & Sons.

Seils, L. (1951). The relationship between measure of physical growth and gross motor performance of primary-grade children. *Research Quarterly* 22:244–260.

Seitz, J. A. (2000). The bodily basis of thought. *New Ideas in Psychology* 18 (1):23–40.

Sekuler, R., & Blake, R. (2002). *Perception*. 4th ed. New York: Alfred A. Knopf.

Shaffer, D. R. (2002). *Developmental psychology: Childhood and adolescence*. Pacific Grove, CA: Brooks/Cole.

Shannon, C. E., & Weaver, W. (1949). *The mathematical theory of communication*. Urbana: University of Illinois Press.

Shapiro, D. C., & Schmidt, R. A. (1982). The schema theory: Recent evidence and developmental implications. In J. A. Kelso & J. Clark (Eds.), *The development of movement control and coordination*. New York: John Wiley & Sons.

Sheldon, W. H., Dupertuis, C. W., & McDermott, E. (1954). *Atlas of men: A guide for somatotyping the adult male of all ages*. New York: Harper.

Shephard, R. J. (1978). *Physical activity and aging*. Chicago: Yearbook Medical.

Shock, N. W. (1962). The physiology of aging. *Scientific American* 206 (1):100–110.

Shonkoff, J. P. & Phillips, D. A. (2000). *From Neurons to Neighborhoods: The Science of Early Childhood Development*. Washington, DC: National Academy Press.

Shumway-Cook, A., Baldwin, M., Pollisar, N., & Gruber, W. (1997). Predicting the probability of falls in community-dwelling older adults. *Physical Therapy* 77:812–819.

Shumway-Cook, A., & Woollacott, M. H. (2001). *Motor control*. Baltimore: Williams & Wilkins.

Siegler, R. S. (2001). Children's discoveries and brain-damaged patients' rediscoveries. In J. L. McClelland & R. J. Siegler (Eds.), *Mechanisms of Cognitive Development*. Mahwah, NJ: Lawrence Erlbaum Associates.

Siegler, R. S., & Crowley, K. (1991). The microgenetic method. A direct means for studying cognitive development. *American Psychologist* 46:606–620.

Singer, L. T., Hawkins, S., Huang, J., Davillier, M., & Baley, J. (2001). Developmental outcomes and environmental correlates of very low birth weight, cocaine-exposed infants. *Early Human Development* 64 (2):91–103.

Slater, A., Mattock, A., & Brown, E. (1990). Size constancy at birth: Newborn infants' responses to retinal and real size. *Journal of Experimental Child Psychology* 49:314–322.

Smith, E. L., & Serfass, R. C. (Eds.). (1981). *Exercise and aging: The scientific basis*. Hillside, NJ: Enslow.

Smoll, F. L., & Schutz, R. W. (1990). Quantifying gender differences in physical performance: A developmental perspective. *Developmental Psychology* 26 (3):360–369.

Snyder, E. E., & Spreitzer, E. A. (1983). *Social aspects of sport*. 2nd ed. Englewood Cliffs, NJ: Prentice Hall.

Soken, H. H., & Pick, A. D. (1992). Intermodal perception of happy and angry expressive behaviors by seven-month-old infants. *Child Development* 63:787–795.

Spelke, E. S. (1987). The development of intermodal perception. In P. Salapatek & L. Cohen (Eds.), *Handbook of infant perception: Vol 2. From perception to cognition*: 233–273. Orlando, FL: Academic Press.

Spirduso, W. W. (1975). Reaction and movement time as a function of age and physical activity level. *Journal of Gerontology* 30:435–440.

Sporns, O., & Edelman, G. M. (1993). Solving Bernstain's problem: A proposal for the development of coordinated movement by selection. *Child Development* 64 (4):960–981.

Sporting Goods Manufacturing Association (2002). *Sports Participation in America*. North Palm Beach, FL.

Steffen, T. M., Hacker, T. A., & Mollinger, L. (2002). Age- and gender-related test performance in community-dwelling elderly people: Six-minute walk test, Berg balance scale, timed up & go test, and gait speeds. *Physical Therapy* 82 (2):128–137.

Stine-Morrow, E. A., & Soederberg Miller, L. M. (1999). Basic Cognitive Processes. In J.C. Cavanaugh & S. K. Whitbourne (Eds.), *Gerontology: An interdisciplinary perspective*. New York: Oxford University Press.

Stoffregen, T. A. (2000). Affordances and events. *Ecological Psychology* 12:1–28.

Stone, M. J., & Kozman, A. (1996). Activity, exercise, and behavior. In J. E. Birren & K. W. Schaie (Eds.), *Handbook of the psychology of aging*. 4th ed.: 338–352. San Diego: Academic Press.

Strohmeyer, H. S., Williams, K., & Schaub-George, D. (1991). Developmental sequences for catching a small ball: A prelongitudinal screening. *Research Quarterly for Exercise and Sport* 62 (3):257–266.

Suitor, J. J., & Reavis, R. (1995). Football, fast cars, and cheerleading: Adolescent gender norms, 1978–1989. *Adolescence* 30:265–272.

Surwillo, W. W. (1977). Developmental changes in the speed of information processing. *Journal of Psychology* 97:102.

Sutherland, D. H. (1984). *Gait disorders in childhood and adolescence*. Baltimore: Williams and Wilkins.

Swanson, H. L. (1999). What develops in working memory? A life span perspective. *Developmental Psychology* 35 (4):986–1000.

Swanson, M. W., Streissguth, A. P., Sampson, P. D., & Carmichael Olson, H. (1990). Prenatal cocaine and neuromotor outcome at four months: Effect of duration of exposure. *Journal of Development and Behavioral Pediatrics* 20 (5):325–334.

Swearingen, J. J., Braden, G. E., Badgley, J. M., & Wallace, T. F. (1969). *Determination of centers of gravity in children*. Washington, DC: Federal Aviation Administration.

Takkinen, S., Suutama, T., & Ruoppila, I. (2001). More meaning by exercising? Physical activity as a predictor of a sense of meaning in life and of self-rated health and functioning in old age. *Journal of Aging and Physical Activity* 9:128–141.

Tan, L. E. (1985). Laterality and motor skills in four-year-olds. *Child Development* 56:119–124.

Tanner, J. M. (1990). *Fetus into man: Physical growth from conception to maturity*. Cambridge, MA: Harvard University Press.

Tanner, J. M., Whitehouse, R. H., Cameron, N., Marshall, W. A., Healy, M. J. R., & Goldstein, H. (1983), *Assessment of skeletal maturity and prediction of adult height*. 2nd ed. London: Academic Press.

Teeken, J. C., Adam, J. J., Paas, F. G. W., Martin, P. J. von Boxtel, Houx, P. J., & Jolles, J. (1996). Effects of age and gender on discrete and reciprocal aiming movements. *Psychology and Aging* 11 (2):195–198.

Temple, I. G., Williams, H. G., & Bateman, N. J. (1979). A test battery to assess intrasensory and intersensory development of young children. *Perceptual and Motor Skills*, 48:643–659.

Tessier-Lavigne, M., & Goodman, C. S. (1996). The molecular biology of axon guidance. *Science* 274:1123–1133.

Thelen, E. (1979). Rhythmical stereotypes in normal human infants. *Animal Behavior* 27:699–715.

Thelen, E. (1995). Motor development: A new synthesis. *American Psychologist* 50 (2):79–95.

Thelen, E. (1996). Normal infant stereotypies. In R. L. Sprague & N. M. Newell (Eds.), *Stereotyped movements: Brain and behavior relations.* Hyattsville, MD: American Psychological Association.

Thelen, E. (2000). Motor development as foundation and future of developmental psychology. *International Journal of Behavioral Development*, 24 (4):385–397.

Thelen, E., & Cooke, D. W. (1987). The relation between newborn stepping and later locomotion: A new interpretation. *Developmental Medicine and Child Neurology* 29: 380–393.

Thelen, E., Corbetta, D., & Spencer, J. P. (1996). Development of reaching during the first year: Role of movement speed. *Journal of Experimental Psychology: Human Perception and Performance* 27 (5):1059–1076.

Thelen, E., & Fisher, D. M. (1982). Newborn stepping: An explanation for a "disappearing reflex." *Developmental Psychology* 18:760.

Thelen, E., Schoner, G., Scheier, C., & Smith, L. B. (2001). The dynamics of embodiment: A field theory of infant preservation reaching. *Behavioral and Brain Sciences* 24:1–86.

Thelen, E., & Smith, L. B. (1994). *A dynamic systems approach to the development of cognition and action.* Cambridge, MA: The MIT Press.

Thelen, E., & Ulrich, B. D. (1991). Hidden skills: A dynamical systems analysis of treadmill stepping during the first year. *Monographs of Society for Research in Child Development* 56 (1), serial #223.

Thomas, J. R., Thomas, K. T., Lee, A. M., Testerman, E., & Ashy, M. (1983). Age differences in use of strategy for recall of movement in a

large-scale environment. *Research Quarterly for Exercise and Sport* 54: 264–272.

Thomas, R. J., Nelson, J. K., & Church, G. (1991). A developmental analysis of gender differences in health-related physical fitness. *Pediatric Exercise Science* 3:28–42.

Till, R. E. (1985). Verbatim and inferential memory in young and elderly adults. *Journal of Gerontology* 40:316–323.

Timiras, P. S. (1994). Aging of the skeleton, joints and muscles. In: Timiras P. S., (Ed.), *Physiological basis of aging and geriatrics.* 2nd ed. Ann Arbor, MI: CRS.

Tough, S., Newburn-Cook, C., Johnston, D., Svenson, L., Rose, S., & Belik, J. (2002). Delayed childbearing and its impact on population rate changes in lower birth weight, multiple birth, and preterm delivery. *Pediatrics* 109 (3):399-403.

Toupet, M., Gagey, P. M., & Heuschen, S. (1992). Vestibular patients and aging subjects lose use of visual input and expend more energy in static postural control. In B. Vellas, M. Toupet, & L. Rubenstein, et al. (Eds.) *Falls, balance and gait disorders in the elderly.* Paris: Elsevier: 183–198.

Touwen, B. C. L. (1988). Motor development: Developmental dynamics and neurological examination in infancy. In E. Meisami & P. S. Timitas (Eds.), *Handbook of human growth and developmental biology* (Vol. 1). Boca Raton, FL: CRS Press.

Tulving, E. (1985). How many memory systems are there? *American Psychologist* 40: 385–398.

Turvey, M. T. (1990). Coordination. *American Psychologist* 4: 938–953.

Ulrich, B. D., & Ulrich, D. A. (1985). The role of balancing in performance of fundamental motor skills in 3-, 4-, and 5-year-old children. In J. E. Clark & J. H. Humphrey (Eds.), *Motor development: Current selected research* (Vol. 1). Princeton, NJ: Princeton Book Co.

Ulrich, D. A. (1999). *Test of gross motor development.* Austin, TX: Pro-Ed.

U.S. National Senior Sports Organization. (1989). *U.S. senior sports records.* Baton Rouge, LA: Author.

Van der Fits, I. B. M., Klip, A. W. J., van Eykern, L. A., & Hadders-Algra, M. (1999). Postural adjustments during spontaneous and

goal-directed arm movements in the first half year of life. *Behavioural Brain Research* 106:75–90.

Van Geert, P. (1998). A dynamic systems model of basic developmental mechanisms: Piaget, Vygotsky and beyond. *Psychological Review* (October): 1–65.

Van Praag, H., Kempermann, G., & Gage, F. H. (1999). Running increases cell proliferation and neurogenesis in the adult mouse dentate gyrus. *Nature Neuroscience* 2 (3): 266–270.

Van Strien, V. (2000). Origins of human handedness. In M. Mandal, B. Bulman-Fleming, & G. Tiwari (Eds.). *Side bias: A neuropsychological perspective:* 41–62. Dordrecht, The Netherlands: Klumer Academic Publishers.

Vereijken, B. (1991). The dynamics of skill acquisition. Unpublished dissertation, Free University, The Netherlands.

Wagner, S., Winner, E., Cicchetti, D., & Gardner, H. (1981). "Metaphorical" mapping in human infants. *Child Development* 52:728–731.

Wallis, C. (1996). The most intimate bond. *Time* (March 25): 60–64.

Walsh, R. P. (1983). Age differences in learning and memory. In D. S. Woodruff & J. E. Birren (Eds.), *Aging: Scientific perspectives and social issues.* 2nd ed. Pacific Grove, CA: Brooks/Cole.

Wang, X., Zuckerman, B., Kaufman, G., Pearson, C., Wang, G., Chen, C., Wise, P., Bauchner, H., & Xu, X. (2000). *Maternal cigarette smoking, genetic susceptibility, and birthweight.* Paper presented at the joint meeting of the Pediatric Academic Societies and the American Academy of Pediatrics, Boston.

Warren, M. P. (1980). The effects of exercise on pubertal progression and reproductive function in girls. *Journal of Clinical Endocrinology and Metabolism* 51:1150–1156.

Weiss, M. R. (1993). Psychological effects of intensive sport participation on children and youth: Self-esteem and motivation. In B. R. Cahill & A. J. Pearl (Eds.), *Intensive participation in children's sports:* 39–69. Champaign, IL: Human Kinetics.

Weiss, M. R., & Barber, H. (1996). Socialization influences of collegiate male athletes: A tale of two decades. *Sex Role* 33:129–140.

Weiss, M. R., Ebbeck, V., & Wiese-Bjornstal, D. M. (1993). Developmental and psychological factors related to children's observational learning of physical skills. *Pediatric Exercise Science* 5:301–317.

Weiss, M. R., & Knoppers, A. (1982). The influence of socializing agents on female collegiate volley players. *Journal of Sport Psychology* 4:267–279.

Weiss, M. R., & Sisley, B. (1984). Where have all the coaches gone? *Sociology of Sport Journal* 1 (4): 322–347.

Welford, A. (1984). Between bodily changes and performance: Some possible reasons for slowing with age. *Experimental Aging Research* 10:73–88.

Welford, A. T. (1977). Motor performance. In J. E. Birren & K. W. Schaie (Eds.), *Handbook of the psychology of aging*. New York: Van Nostrand Reinhold.

Wellman, B. L. (1937). Motor achievements in preschool children. *Childhood Education* 13:311–316.

Weltman, A. (1989). Weight training in prepubertal children: Physiologic benefit and potential damage. In O. Bar-Or (Ed.), *Advances in pediatric sport science* (Vol. 3). Champaign, IL: Human Kinetics.

Whitbourne, S. K. (1985). *The aging body: Physiological changes and psychological consequences*. New York: Springer-Verlag.

Wickens, C. D., & Benel, D. C. R. (1982). The development of time-sharing skills. In J. A. S. Kelso & J. E. Clark (Eds.), *The development of movement control and co-ordination*. New York: John Wiley & Sons.

Wickstrom, R. L. (1983). *Fundamental motor patterns*. 3rd ed. Philadelphia: Lea & Febiger.

Wild, M. (1938). The behavior pattern of throwing and some observations concerning its course of development in children. *Research Quarterly* 9:20–24.

Wilkinson, R. T., & Allison, S. (1989). Age and simple reaction time: Decade differences for 5,325 subjects. *Journal of Gerontology* 44 (2): 29–35.

Williams, H., & Breihan, S. (1979). Motor control tasks for young children. Unpublished manuscript, University of Toledo.

Williams, H., Temple, I., & Bateman, J. (1978). Perceptual-motor and cognitive learning in young children. *Psychology of motor behavior and sport II*. Champaign, IL: Human Kinetics.

Williams, H. G. (1983). *Perceptual and motor development*. Englewood Cliffs: Prentice Hall.

Williams, H. G. (1990). Aging and eye-hand coordination. In H. G. Williams (Ed.), *Development of eye-hand coordination*. Columbia: University of South Carolina Press.

Williams, H. G., & Greene, L. S. (1990). *Williams–Greene Test of Physical/Motor Function*. Laboratory report from the Motor Development/Motor Control Laboratory, Department of Exercise Science, University of South Carolina, Columbia.

Williams, K., Haywood, K., & Van Sant, A. (1990). Movement characteristics of older adult throwers. In J. E. Clark & J. H. Humphery (Eds.), *Advances in motor development research* (Vol. 3): 29–44. New York: AMS Press.

Williams, K., Haywood, K., & Van Sant, A. (1991). Throwing patterns of older adults: A follow-up investigation. *International Journal of Aging and Human Development* 33: 279–294.

Willmott, M. (1986). The effect of vinyl floor surface and carpeted floor surface upon walking in elderly hospital inpatients. *Age and Ageing* 15:119–120.

Wilmore, J. H., & Costill, D. L. (1999). *Physiology of Sport and Exercise*. 2nd ed. Champaign, IL: Human Kinetics.

Winter, D. A., Patla, A. E., Frank, J. S., & Walt, S. E. (1990). Biomechanical walking pattern changes in the fit and healthy elderly. *Physical Therapy* 70:340–347.

Witelson, S. F., & Kigar, D. L. (1988). Anatomical development of the corpus callosum in humans: A review with references to sex and cognition. In Molfese, D. L. & S. J. Segalowitz (Eds.), *Brain lateralization in children*. New York: The Guilford Press.

Wodrich, D. L. (1997). *Children's psychological testing: A guide for non-psychologists*. 3rd ed. Baltimore: Paul H. Brooks.

Woollacott, M. (1993). Age-related change in posture and movement. *The Journals of Gerontology* 48: 56–60.

Wulf, G. (1991). The effect of type of practice on motor learning in children. *Applied Cognitive Psychology* 5:123–124.

Wyke, B. (1975). The neurological basis of movement. In K. S. Hold (Ed.), *Clinics in Developmental Medicine* (No. 55). London: William Heinemann.

Yan, J. H., Thomas, J. R., Stelmach, G. E., & Thomas, K. T. (2000). Developmental features of rapid aiming arm movements across the lifespan. *Journal of Motor Behavior* 32 (2): 121–140.

Yan, J. H., Thomas, J. R., & Thomas, K. T. (1998). Children's age moderates the effect of practice variability: A quantitative review. *Research Quarterly for Exercise and Sport* 69 (2): 210–215.

Yekta, A. A., Pickwell, L. D., & Jenkins, T. C. A. (1989). Binocular vision, age and symptoms. *Ophthalmic and Physiological Optics* 9:115–120.

Zauner, C. W., Maksud, M. G., & Melichna, J. (1989). Physiological considerations in training young athletes. *Sports Medicine* 8 (1):15–31.

Zelazo, N. A., Zelazo, P. R., Cohen, K. M., & Zelazo, P. D. (1993). Specificity of practice effects on elementary neuromotor patterns. *Developmental Psychology* 29 (4):686–691.

Ziviani, J. (1983). Qualitative changes in dynamic tripod grip between seven and fourteen years of age. *Developmental Medicine and Child Neurology* 25:778–782.

Index

Page references followed by *fig* indicates an illustrated figure; followed by *t* indicates a table.

AAHPERD (American Alliance for Health, Physical Education, Recreation and Dance), 414
Accommodation, 24–25
Action, 29
Activity-dependent development, 48
Activity theory, 436
Adaptation
  as assimilation/accommodation balance, 25
  defining, 7–8
Adolescence
  age/gender-related motor performance changes in, 334–338
  body fat throughout, 94–100
  described, 14
  growth/development characteristics of, 333–334
  motor performance changes in, 338–339*fig*, 340*fig*–347, 341*fig*, 342*fig*, 343*fig*
  motor skill refinement in, 347–353, 348*fig*, 350*t*, 351*fig*
  pubescent growth spurt during, 70, 72–73*fig*
  self-esteem during, 432–434
  See also Puberty
Adolescence sociocultural influences
  coaches and teachers, 430–431
  described, 424
  family, 425*fig*–427
  gender-role expectations and stereotyping, 431–432
  peer relations, 427–430, 428*fig*
  possible influences of race, 434
  self-esteem, 432–434
Adolph, K., 203, 204
Adrenal glands, 160*fig*, 162
Adrian, M. J., 288, 378, 408
Adulthood
  described, 14
  peak motor performance during early, 358–365

regression during late, 12–13, 16–17, 365–383
Adults
  assessment instruments for older, 413–416, 414*t*
  comparing visual system of newborn and, 174*fig*
  developmental continuum of motor behavior in, 357
  primary sociocultural influences during, 435–437*fig*
  summary of gait changes in older, 379*t*
  summary of physiological differences between adults and, 132*t*
Aerobic power, 118–119
Afferent neurons, 42
Affordances
  challenging infant to develop skills, 28*fig*
  defining, 7
  environmental context of development and, 203
African-Americans
  athletic performance of, 364–365*t*
  sociocultural influences on motor development of, 434
Age
  average scores on bent-knee sit-ups by, 131*fig*
  basis for motor performance changes related to, 334–338
  biological, 102
  BMR as function of, 127*fig*
  body composition change as function of, 98*fig*
  changes in grip strength with, 359*fig*
  chronological vs. physiological, 367
  dental, sexual, skeletal, 103–105*fig*
  male/female world records and changes with, 369*fig*
  maternal, 143

mean performances for masters-level swimming events and, 370*fig*
  morphological, 102–103
  peak performance of selected events and, 363*t*
  processing speed related to, 234*fig*
  reaction time/movement time as function of, 223*fig*, 361*fig*, 373*fig*
  red blood cell values in relation to, 126*fig*
  relationship of exercise tolerance with, 360*fig*
  resting heart rate and, 122*t*
  VO$_2$max (maximal oxygen uptake) as function of, 119*fig*, 359*fig*
Age-related stereotyping, 436
Aging
  biological theories of advanced, 365–367
  BMR changes and, 134
  body mass changes with, 101
  cardiorespiratory function changes and, 133–134
  changes of physique with, 82
  decline in VO$_2$max and, 118
  defining, 9, 365
  flexibility changes and, 135–136*fig*, 375–376
  hypothetical curve on physiological function of males and, 133*fig*
  information processing changes with, 232–236*t*
  muscular strength changes and, 134–135
  neurological changes with, 60–62*t*, 371–372
  perception changes with, 199–202*t*
  regression of abilities with advanced, 12–13, 16–17, 365–383

skeletal changes due to, 89–91, 90*fig*

skeletal tissue/body fat changes and, 376–377

summary of changes after peak maturity, 137*t*

summary of physical growth changes with, 102*t*

summary of selected physiological changes with, 136*t*

theories of advanced, 23

AIMS (Alberta Infant Motor Scale), 300–400*fig*

Alcohol, prenatal development and, 146–147

Alertness, 211–212

Allison, M. T., 432

Alzheimer's disease, 61

American Academy of Pediatrics, 157, 350

Ames, E. W., 17

Ammons, R. B., 221

Androgens, 72

Annett, M., 280, 321

Annett's Right-Shift Theory, 280, 328–329

A-not-B error, 176

Anthrop, J., 432

Anthropometry, 66–68

Apgar scale, 245, 395, 398*t*

Apgar, V. A., 396

Arneil, G. C., 247

Assessment

basic terminology of, 390–391

comprehensive physical-motor, 389*t*

considerations for proper, 393–394

product-oriented/process-oriented, 391

purposes of, 391–393

Assessment battery, 394

Assessment instruments

considerations in selection of, 393–394

fitness assessment, 416*t*

infant assessment, 398–403

newborn assessment, 245, 395, 395–398, 396*t*, 397*t*

older persons assessment, 413–415, 414*t*

other commonly used, 411–413, 412*t*

overview of, 394–395

process-oriented, 407–411, 409*t*–410*t*

summary on selected, 415*t*

up to school-age populations assessment, 403–411, 404*t*, 405*t*, 407*t*, 409*t*, 410*t*

Assimilation, 24–25

Athletes

African-American, 364–365*t*

interscholastic sport, 349–352, 350*t*

youth sport participation, 347–349, 348*fig*

See also Sports

ATP (adenosine triphosphate), 118

Attention

aging and changes in, 232

alertness and, 211–212

described, 211

divided, 212–213

selective, 213–215

Auditory-kinesthetic integration, 198–199

Auditory perception, 193–195, 200

Auditory system, 194

Autonomic system, 41–42

Babinski reflex, 251, 252*fig*

Babkin reflex, 251

Balance

biological regression and, 372–375

children pursuing cognitive, 24

quantitative changes in, 347

selected abilities, 191*t*

vestibular awareness and, 190–192

Ball bouncing, 316–318, 346–347

Bandura, A., 23

Banks, M. S., 174

Bar-Or, O., 126

Barr, H. M., 147

Bartlett, D., 225

Basal ganglia, 41

Basic information-processing model, 211*fig*

Baumgartner, T. A., 416

Bayley II, 322

Bayley, N., 17

Bayley Scales of Infant Development, 398–399*t*

Behavior schema, 24

Benel, D.C.R., 213

Bernstein, N., 30, 228

Bertenthal, B. I., 232, 275

Berthier, N. E., 176

Biacromial (shoulder) width

measuring, 80*fig*

values of, 80*fig*

Bicristal breadth (hip width)

measuring, 80*fig*

values of, 80*fig*

Bimanual control, 325–326

BINS (Bayley Infant Neurodevelopmental Screener), 398–399

Biodynamics, 30

Biological age, 102

Biological systems theory

described, 22, 29

developmental biodynamics, 29–31

information-processing view of, 29

Biology context, 13

Biomechanics, 287

Birren, J. E., 366

Blair, S. N., 382

Blake, R., 177, 180

Blood characteristics

blood pressure, 125–126

blood volume, 124–125

red blood cells content, 125, 126*fig*

Blood pressure, 125–126

Blood volume, 124–125

BMAT-R (Basic Motor Ability Tests-Revised), 404–405*t*

BMI (body mass index), 95–96*fig*, 97*fig*

BMR (basal metabolic rate)

aging and changes in, 134

described, 126–127*fig*

Body awareness, 186–187

Body composition

body fat growth and, 97–100

change as function of age, 98*fig*

cross age for boys/girls, 99*fig*

described, 92–97

skeletal muscle tissue growth and, 100–101

Body fat

biological regression and, 376–377

critical-weight theory on menarche and, 155–156

growth through lifecycle, 97–100

measuring, 94–97

Body mass

body composition and, 92–101

body weight and, 91–92*fig*
changes with aging, 101
defining, 91
postnatal development, 152–153
skeletal muscle tissue growth, 100–101
Body proportions
changes in ratio of sitting height to stature, 76–78
changes relative to the head, 74–76, 75*fig*, 76*t*, 77*fig*, 78*fig*
changes in shoulder/hip ratio, 78–81*fig*
postnatal development, 153
Body weight
for boys/age percentile (2 to 20 years), 93*fig*
development of, 91–92
distance curves for, 92*fig*
for girls/age percentile (2 to 20 years), 94*fig*
ratio of strength index to, 129*fig*
Bone formation, 88*fig*–89
Bosch, A., 365
BOT (Bruininks-Oseretsky Test of Motor Proficiency), 406–407*t*
Botwinick, J., 232
Bouchard, C., 82, 107, 152, 159
Bower, T. G. R., 258
Boys
average age/sexual development in, 104*fig*
BMI/age percentiles (2 to 20 years) in, 96*fig*
body composition across age for, 99*fig*
head circumference for ages (birth to 36 months), 77*fig*
hormonal influence during puberty and, 72–73*fig*
physical development and motor performance of, 108–109
stature/age percentiles (2 to 20 years), 86*fig*
weight/age percentile (2 to 20 years), 93*fig*
X-ray showing skeletal maturity in, 105*fig*
See also Gender-related differences; Men
Brain, the
changes in major structures of, 58–59

critical period of brain wiring, 50–51
effects of experience on development of, 51–52
lateral dominance of limb control and, 59*fig*
lateralization and corpus callosum, 59–60
myelination, 53–55, 54*fig*
overview of, 39–41
summary of developmental events, 56*t*
Brain growth spurt, 48
Brain (hemispheric) lateralization, 59–60
Brain stem, 40–41
Branta, C. F., 348
Brazelton Behavioral Assessment Scale, 245, 395–398, 397*t*
Breihan, S. K., 347
Broca's area, 41
Broekhoff, J. C., 152
Bronfenbrenner's ecological systems theory, 25, 26, 27*fig*, 423–424
Busch, S., 375

Cadopi, M., 217
Cardiac output, 123
Cardiorespiratory development
blood characteristics, 124–126*fig*
BMR (basal metabolic rate), 126–127*fig*, 134
cardiorespiratory system, 114–124*fig*
early growth and, 115–117
postnatal development, 158
summary of changes with aging, 136*t*
Cardiorespiratory function
biological regression/ performance of, 368–369
changes with aging, 133–134
Cardiorespiratory system
aerobic and anaerobic powers of, 118–121
aging and changes in function, 133–134
basic structure and structure of, 114–117
cardiac output and stroke volume of, 123
heart rate and, 121–123
vital capacity and pulmonary ventilation, 123–124*fig*

Carson, L., 227
Case history, 20
Case-Smith, J., 230
Catching
developmental characteristics, 307–308
developmental sequence for, 309*t*–310*t*
development of, 304, 306
immature patterns of, 308*fig*
mature two-hand pattern of, 309*fig*
movement pattern descriptions, 306–307
quantitative changes in, 344
CDC (Centers for Disease Control and Prevention), 31, 67, 143, 149, 150
Cell body (soma), 42
Cell death, 55–56
Cell proliferation process, 47–48
Cellular clock theories, 366
Cellular garbage/mutation theories, 366–367
Cephalocaudal development, 8–9
Cerebellum, 41
Cerebral cortex, 41
Cerebral lobe development, 58–59
Cerella, J., 235
Change
age/gender-related quantitative motor performance, 334–338
developmental, 4–5
developmental/motor development specialist goals regarding, 5
methods for studying fundamental motor skill, 287–289
multidisciplinary approach to study of behavioral, 5
neurological, 39–63
quantitative motor performance, 338–347
See also Development; Regression
Childhood
body fat throughout, 94–100
described, 14
early and latter divisions of, 14
play activities during, 427–429, 428*fig*
See also Early childhood; Infancy; Later childhood
Childhood sociocultural influences
coaches and teachers, 430–431

described, 424
family, 425*fig*–427
gender-role expectations and
  stereotyping, 431–432
peer relations, 427–430, 428*fig*
possible influences of race, 434
self-esteem, 432–434
Children
  gender-role
    expectations/stereotyping of,
    431–432
  malnutrition in, 150–151
  play activities by, 427–429,
    428*fig*
  postnatal development of,
    151–159
  selected fine visual-motor char-
    acteristics of, 183*t*
  self-esteem of, 432–434
  summary of physiological dif-
    ferences between adults and,
    132*t*
Chromosomes, 37
Chronological age, 367
Chronosystem, 26
Chugani, H. T., 50
Chunking process, 216
Clarke, H. H., 131
Clark, J. E., 271, 272
Clifton, R. K., 198
Climbing, 318–320, 319*fig*
CNS (central nervous system)
  anatomy of the, 40*fig*
  the brain, 39–41
  changes in major brain struc-
    tures of, 58–59
  neurons and, 42–43*fig*, 52–53
  prenatal development of, 69
  sequence of early development,
    46–60
  spinal cord, 39
Coaches, 430–431
Coakley, J. J., 430
Cochlea, 194
Cognition/programming relation-
  ship, 225
Cognitive-development view,
  24–25
Cohort effects, 19
Coincident timing, 182
Component approach, 288–289
Composite approach, 288
Conception, 68, 71*t*
Confronting the visual cliff, 180*fig*
Conjoined twins, 231*fig*–232

Construction of norms, 392
Construction/self-help skills,
  322*fig*
Contextual learning, 218–219
Continuity view, 9
Contributing views
  cognitive-developmental view,
    24–25
  learning-behavioral view, 23–24
  maturation view, 23
Cooper, J. M., 288, 408
Coordinative structures, 30, 228
Corballis, M. C., 280
Corpus callosum, 60
Correlational method, 21
Correlations, 393
Corso, J. F., 201
Costill (1999 after Wilmore), 369
Craik, R., 378
Cratty, B. J., 346
Crawling/creeping locomotion,
  265, 266*fig*, 267
Crawling reflex, 255*fig*
Criterion-referenced standards,
  390–391
Critical periods
  described, 11
  in early brain development,
    52
  in neuronal development,
    50–51, 56–57*fig*
Critical-weight theory, 155–156
Cross-lateral climbing pattern,
  318–319*fig*
Cross-linkage theory, 366
Cross-sectional design, 18–19,
  20*fig*
Culture, 421–422
Cummings, M. F., 180
Curnow, C., 361

David, K., 306
DDST (Denver Developmental
  Screening Test), 403–404*t*
Deach, D., 315
Deach's four stages of kicking,
  315, 316*fig*
Dendrite, 42
Dendritic development, 49*fig*
Dental age, 103
Denver Developmental Screening
  Test, 322
Department of Education, 31
Depth perception, 178–180
Determining status, 392

Development
  contributing view of, 23–25
  defining, 8
  general terminology relating to,
    6–9
  information process as
    approach to understanding,
    167, 210
  movement-based approaches
    to, 204–206
  observations (assumptions)
    about, 9–13
  physical growth and, 66–74*t*
  role of environmental/biology
    context in, 11, 13
  sociocultural influences on,
    421–439
  theoretical view of, 22–23
  See also Change; Growth
Developmental biodynamics,
  29–31
Developmental contextualism
  Bronfenbrenner's ecological
    systems theory, 25, 26, 27*fig*,
    423–424
  ecological task analysis (Con-
    strains) model [ETA model],
    27–28
  Gibson's ecological perspective,
    25, 26–27, 202–204
  overview of, 25–26
Developmental continuum
  described, 14–15
  early childhood motor behav-
    ior, 285
  early movement behavior, 243
  motor behavior in adult years,
    357
  motor behavior during later
    childhood/adolescence, 333
  phases of, 15–17
Developmentally appropriate
  school programs, 352–353
Developmental motor pattern, 287
Developmental psychology
  biological systems theory,
    29–31
  cognitive-developmental view
    of, 24–25
  environmental context theory,
    25–28
  learning-behavioral view of,
    23–24
  maturation view of, 23
  theoretical views of, 22–23

Developmental systems perspective, 4, 22

Developmental theories of motor control
approach of, 227–228
coordinative structures, 228
dynamic systems, 228–229
neuronal group selection, 229–232

Development assumptions
aging and regression of abilities, 12–13, 16–17, 365–383
critical/sensitive periods in development, 11
development aided by stimulation, 11–12
development as continual process, 9–11
environmental context role in development, 11, 13
motor skill development as dynamic phenomenon, 12
plasticity in development, 12
study of development as holistic process, 11

Diagnosis/screening, 392
Diastolic blood pressure, 125–126
Diencephalon, 40–41
Differentiation, 49–51, 202
Direct instruction, 422–423
Directional awareness, 188–190
Directionality, 189–190
Discontinuity view, 9–10
Disease/prenatal development relationship, 145–146
Dishabituation, 217

Distance curves
body weight, 92fig
change in height, 67fig
stature, 85fig

Divided attention, 212–213
DNA (deoxyribonucleic acid), 37
Down syndrome, 143, 144
Drawing and writing, 322–325, 323fig
Dribbling, 316–318, 317fig, 346–347
Drugs/chemical substances and prenatal development relationship, 146–147
DSFMSI (Developmental Sequence of Fundamental Motor Skills Inventory), 411
Dupertuis, C. W., 81

Dynamic system research
described, 30–31
on reflex behavior, 258
on walking, 271–273
Dynamic systems, 228–229
Dynamic systems theory, 30

Early childhood
described, 14
fine motor manipulative behavior, 320–326
functional (motor) asymmetries, 326–330
fundamental motor skill development, 286–289
movement patterns during, 289–320
play activities during, 427–429, 428fig
up to school-age populations assessment instruments, 403–411, 404t, 405t, 407t, 409t, 410t
See also Childhood

Early movement behavior
reflexive behavior, 244–259
rudimentary behavior, 261–281
spontaneous movements (stereotypies), 259–261fig, 275fig
See also Movement

Eckert, H. M., 17, 277, 337, 374
Eclectic theoretical perspective, 31
Ecological systems theory, 25, 26, 27fig, 423–424
Ecological Task Analysis (Constraints) Model, 25, 27–28
Edelman, G. M., 230
Efferent neurons, 42
Einkauf, D. K., 135
Eisenburg, R. B., 194
Eklund, R. C., 434
Elderly assessment instruments, 413–415, 414t
Embodiment, 176
Embryonic period, 69
Emotional state of mother, 145

Environmental contexts
defining, 7
ecological systems theory on development in, 25, 26, 27fig, 423–424
Gibson's ecological perspective on, 25, 26–27, 202–204
role in development, 11, 13

See also External (environmental) factors
Environmental Context Theory, 22
Environment element, 28
Equilibrium. See Balance
Era, P., 374
Erikson, E. H., 10
Espenschade, A., 17, 338, 340
Estrogen, 72–73t
Evaluation, 390
Exercise tolerance/age relationship, 360fig
Exosystem, 26

Experience
defining, 7
development and contextual, 24
early brain development and, 51–52

Experimental method, 20

External (environmental) factors
brain development and, 52
developmental outcome and role of, 47fig
fetus affected by, 142
prenatal development and, 145–149fig
See also Environmental contexts

Extrapyramidal system, 44
Eye preference, 329–330

Fagard, J., 276
Family beliefs/attitudes, 425fig–427
Farrell, S. W., 382
Fetal alcohol syndrome, 146–147

Fetal period
body fat growth during, 97–98
environmental factors and, 142
general body form changes during, 71fig
growth/development of heart during, 116
physical development during, 69–70
See also Prenatal development

Fetal position, 145
Fetal skeleton, 88fig
Field of vision, 180–181
Figure-ground perception, 178

Fine motor manipulative behavior
bimanual control, 325–326
construction and self-help skills, 322fig
described, 320

drawing and writing, 322–325, 323*fig*
finger differentiation, 320–321
manual control and speed, 321*fig*
Finger differentiation, 320–321
Fisher, D. M., 258
Fisk, P. M., 235
Fitness assessment instruments, 416*t*
Fitt's Law, 224, 235
Flexibility
  aging and changes in, 135–136*fig*, 375–376
  average scores on bent-knee sit-ups by age, 131*fig*
  described, 130–131
  sit-and-reach test measuring, 131–132*fig*
FMPAI (Fundamental Movement Pattern Assessment Instrument), 410*t*–411
Footedness, 328–329
Forfar, J. O., 247
Free-radical theory, 366
From Neurons to Neighborhoods (National Academies), 205–206
Functional (motor) asymmetries
  described, 326–327
  eye preference, 329–330
  footedness, 328–329
  handedness, 327–328
Fundamental motor skill development
  basic terminology, 286–287
  methods for studying change, 287–289
  movement patterns (process characteristics), 289–320
Fundamental movement phase, 16
Fundamental movement skill, 286

Gait changes, 379*t*
Galaburda, A. S., 281
Galloping, 299–300
Gender-related differences
  BMR as function of sex, 127*fig*
  expected height increase per year, 84*t*
  hormonal influence during puberty and, 72–73*fig*
  late childhood/adolescence and increasing, 334
  quantitative motor performance changes and, 334–338

selected anatomical, 74*t*
selected biological, 336*t*
skeletal development, 89
VO₂max (maximal oxygen uptake) and, 120*t*
See also Boys; Girls; Men; Women
Gender-role conflict, 432
Gender-role expectations, 431–432
Gender roles, 431
Gender-role stereotyping, 431
Gene, 37
Geneotype, 38
General information-processing (perceptual-motor) model, 171*fig*
Genetic abnormalities, 144–145
Genetic theories, 366
Germinal period, 68
Geschwind, N., 281
Gesell, A., 17, 23
GH (growth hormone), 72, 159–161
Gibson, E. J., 26, 197, 202, 230
Gibson, J. J., 26, 202
Gibson's ecological perspective, 25, 26–27, 202–204
Gidoni, E. A., 259
Girls
  average age/sexual development in, 104*fig*
  BMI/age percentiles (2 to 20 years) in, 97*fig*
  body composition across age for, 99*fig*
  head circumference during infancy, 78*fig*
  hormonal influence during puberty and, 72–73*fig*
  menarche in, 70, 72, 103, 107*fig*, 155–156
  physical development and motor performance of, 108–109
  stature age percentiles (2 to 20 years), 87*fig*
  weight/age percentile (2 to 20 years), 94*fig*
  X-ray showing skeletal maturity in, 105*fig*
  See also Gender-related differences; Women
Glands
  adrenal, 160*fig*, 162
  other glandular functions, 162–163

pancreas, 160*fig*, 161
pituitary, 159–161, 160*fig*
thyroid, 160*fig*, 161
GMP (generalized motor program), 225, 226
Goldfield, E., 231
Gonads, 72–73*fig*, 160*fig*, 162
Gould, D., 434
Graspability, 203
Grasping reflex, 245, 248, 250*fig*
Grasping techniques, 277*fig*
Greenspan, E., 427
Greulich, W. W., 105
Growth
  adolescent growth spurt, 72–73*fig*
  defining, 8
  heart development, 115–117
  later childhood, 333–334
  psychological function and, 358–359*fig*, 360*fig*–361*fig*, 368*fig*
  See also Development; Physical growth/development
Growth cone, 50
Growth curve, 67
Growth/refinement phase, 16
Guyton, A. C., 39

Habituation, 217
Hadders-Algra, M., 230
Hale, S., 223
Hall, 288
Halverson, L. E., 17, 292, 298, 303
Handedness, 327–328
Harris, O., 434
Haubenstricker, J., 301, 335, 342
Head
  average circumference of, 76*t*
  body proportions relative to, 74–76, 76*t*
  circumference for boys during infancy, 77*fig*
  circumference for girls during infancy, 78*fig*
  measuring circumference of, 75*fig*
  postural control of, 262, 263*fig*, 264
Heart
  blood flow direction and, 115*fig*
  cardiac output and stroke volume, 123

growth/development of, 115–117
Heart rate
    age and resting, 122*t*
    overview of, 121–123
Height
    distance curves for, 67*fig*, 85*fig*
    expected increase per year, 84*t*
    measuring sitting, 79*fig*
    ratios of stature to sitting, 76–78, 79*fig*
    stature for girls/age percentiles (2 to 20 years), 87*fig*
    stature for males/age percentiles (2 to 20 years), 86*fig*
    structural development and, 82–86*fig*
    velocity curves for, 67–68*fig*, 85*fig*
    See also Physical growth/development
Heikkinen, E., 374
Hepper, P. G., 281
Heredity
    defining, 7, 37
    genotype/phenotype and, 38
    genes, chromosomes, DNA and, 37
    physical attributes and estimated genetic contribution, 38*t*
Hick's Law, 222–223
Hippocrates, 17
Hirata, K., 362
Hopping, 298–299*fig*, 345–346
Hormonal activity
    adolescent growth spurt and, 72–73*fig*
    aging and, 367
    described, 159
    GH (growth hormone), 72, 159–161
    glands and, 159–162, 160*fig*
    other glandular functions and, 162–163
Hormonal theories, 367
Hughes Basic Gross Motor Assessment, 411
Hunt, L., 434
Hypothalamus, 40–41

Ille, A., 217
Immune system theories, 367
Inbar, O., 121

Individual family member influence, 426
Infancy
    affordances challenges to development skill, 28*fig*
    described, 13
    early motor asymmetries in, 281
    head circumference for boys during, 77*fig*
    head circumference for girls during, 78*fig*
    importance of reflexes in development, 244–246
    measuring recumbent length in infants, 83*fig*
    recording kinematics during reaching, 19*fig*
    Rovee-Collier's investigation of memory during, 218*fig*–219
    visual system of, 174*fig*–177, 175*fig*
    See also Childhood
Infant assessment instruments
    Alberta Infant Motor Scale (AIMS), 399–400*fig*, 401
    Bayley Scales of Infant Development, 398–399*t*
    Posture and Fine Motor Assessment of Infants (PFMAI), 401*fig*–402
    Test of Infant Motor Performance (TIMP), 402–403
    Toddler and Infant Motor Evaluation (TIME), 402
Infection/prenatal development relationship, 145–146
Information processing
    attention and, 211–215, 232
    auditory perception and, 193–195, 200
    basic model of, 211*fig*
    changing with aging, 232–236*t*
    described, 167, 210
    kinesthetic perception and, 184–193, 200–201
    memory and, 215–222, 232–233
    movement time and speed of, 222–224, 223*fig*, 234–235, 361*fig*, 373*fig*
    perception and, 170–171
    perception changes with aging and, 199–202*t*
    programming, 224–232, 235

tactile perception and, 195–196
    visual perception and, 172–184*t*, 199–200
    See also Motor control
Information-processing view, 29
In-line skating, 351*fig*
Integration, 49–51
Intermodal perception, 196
Internal (maternal) factors, 143–144
Interneurons, 42
Interscholastic sports, 349–352, 350*t*
Interviews, data gathering using, 20–21

Jacquet, A. Y., 276
Johnson, R., 345
Journal of the American Medical Association, 382
Jumping
    biological regression and, 378–379
    developmental characteristics, 295, 297*fig*–298
    development of, 293–294
    general sequence patterns of, 293*t*
    movement pattern descriptions, 294–295*fig*, 296–297*fig*
    quantitative changes in, 342*fig*–343*fig*
    standing long, 296
    vertical, 294, 296*fig*

Kail, R., 223
Kavale, K., 205
Kellogg, R., 324
Kelso, J.A.S., 30, 229
Keogh, J., 106, 185, 193, 341, 346
Kicking
    developmental characteristics, 315–316*fig*
    development of, 313–315
    movement pattern descriptions, 315
    quantitative changes in, 343
Kinematics, 287
Kinematics of infant reaching, 19*fig*
Kinesiology, 288
Kinesthesis, 184
Kinesthetic acuity, 185
Kinesthetic memory, 185

Kinesthetic perception
   changes with aging, 200–201
   described, 184
   development of, 185–193
   structure and function of system, 184–185
Kinesthetic perception development
   body awareness and, 186–187
   directional awareness, 188–190
   overview of, 185–186
   rhythmic (temporal) awareness, 192–193
   spatial awareness, 187–188
   vestibular awareness, 190–192
Kinetics, 287–288
Klinefelter's syndrome, 145
Knobloch, H., 325
Knowledge/metamemory relationship, 221–222, 233
Knudson, D., 304
Kreutzfeldt, J., 375
Kugler, P. N., 30
Kwashiorkor, 150

Labyrinthine righting reflex, 252–253fig
Landreth, C., 277
Larroque, B., 147
Lateral dominance, 59fig, 280
Laterality, 188–189
Lateral preference, 188, 280
Later childhood
   age/gender-related quantitative motor performance changes in, 334–338
   described, 14
   growth/development characteristics of, 333–334
   motor skill refinement, 347–353, 348fig, 350t, 351fig
   quantitative motor performance changes, 338–339fig, 340fig–347, 341fig, 342fig, 343fig
   See also Childhood
LBW (low birth weight), 148–149fig
Leap, 293
Learning
   defining, 7
   inferred from motor performance, 8
   observational (modeling), 23–24, 423

recall memory and contextual, 218–219
   See also Socialization
Learning-behavioral view, 23–24
Ledebt, A., 272
Lee, T. D., 211, 225
Left-right maturational gradient programming, 280
Lerner, R. M., 25
Life-span development periods
   adolescence (from 12 to 18 years), 14
   adulthood (18 years and older), 14
   childhood (from 2 to 12 years), 14
   infancy (from birth to 2 years), 13
   prenatal (conception to birth), 13
Life-span perspective
   on life-span development periods, 13–14
   theoretical basis of, 5
Lipfuscin, 366–367
Lockman, J. J., 30
Locomotion (rudimentary), 265, 266fig, 267–273
Locomotor reflexes, 246–247, 255–257fig
Locomotor skills, 285–286
Londeree, B. R., 123
Longevity, 381–382
Longitudinal design, 19, 20fig
Long-term memory
   abilities of, 220–221
   changes with aging, 233
   overview of, 217

McArdle, W. D., 38, 133
McCarthy Scales of Children's Abilities, 413
McDermott, E., 81
MacNeilage, P. R., 329
Macrosystem, 26
Magill, R. A., 211
Maksud, M. G., 152
Malina, R. M., 82, 107, 152, 159
Malnutrition, 150–151
Manipulation
   bimanual control and, 325–326
   defining, 273, 320
   drawing and writing, 322–325, 323fig

finger differentiation and, 320–321
   manual control speed and, 321fig
   selected construction/self-help achievements, 322fig
Manipulative skills, 286
Manis, F. R., 213
Manual control
   defining, 273–274
   rudimentary, 273fig–279
   speed of manipulation and, 321fig
Marker, K., 155
Marking time climbing pattern, 318, 319fig
Material age, 143
Matson, P. D., 205
Maturation
   defining, 7
   summary of aging changes after peak, 137t
   See also Sexual maturation
Maturation theory, 23
Mature movement pattern, 287
Maturity estimates
   defining, 102
   dental, sexual, skeletal age, 103–105fig
   morphological age, 102–103
Maturity variations, 106–108
Maximal oxygen uptake. See VO₂max (maximal oxygen uptake)
Measurement, 390
Medulla, 40
Melichna, J., 152
Meltzoff, A. N., 197
Memory
   abilities of, 217–222
   aging and changes in, 232–233
   described, 215
   relationship to motor response, 216fig
   structures of, 215–217
Memory processing abilities, 217–219
Memory span technique, 216–217
Men
   distance curves for stature, 85fig
   expected height increase per year, 84t
   hypothetical curve on physiological function over life span, 133fig

typical velocity curves, 85*fig*
world records and changes with age, 369*fig*
See also Boys; Gender-related differences
Menarche
 critical-weight theory on, 155–156
 onset of, 70, 72, 103
 secular trend for, 107*fig*
Mesosystem, 26
Metamemory, 221–222, 233
Microgenetic design, 19–20
Microsystem, 26
Milani-Comparetti, A., 259
Modeling (observational learning), 23–24, 423
Moeschberger, M. L., 123
Molnar, G., 259
Moore, M. K., 197
Morgan, M. J., 280
Moro reflex, 245, 246, 248, 249*fig*
Morphological age, 102–103
Morrison, C., 304
Motivation of individuals, 393
Motoneurons, 42
Motor area, 41
Motor asymmetries
 described, 279–280
 early infant, 281
 functional, 326–330
 theoretical views of, 280–281
Motor behavior
 defining, 8
 peak motor performance, 358–365
 regression, 12–13, 16–17, 365–383
Motor control
 defining, 8
 developmental theories of, 227–232
 memory systems and response of, 216*fig*
 See also Information processing
Motor development
 careers in, 31–32
 general terminology related to, 8–9
 primary determinants of, 6*fig*
 research in, 17–21*t*
 rudimentary behavior and, 261–281
 study of, 5
Motor developmental specialists, 5

Motor development careers, 31–32
Motor development research
 benefits of, 17–18
 described, 17
 design methods of, 18–21*t*, 20*fig*
 dynamic systems, 30–31
Motor learning, defining, 8
Motor pathways, 44, 45*fig*
Motor performance
 bases for age/gender-related quantitative changes in, 334–338
 comparison of average fitness scores, 363*t*
 learning inferred from, 8
 physical development and implications for, 108–109
 quantitative changes in, 338–347
 regression of, 12–13, 16–17, 365–383
 See also Peak motor performance
Motor skill refinement
 interscholastic sports, 349–352, 350*t*
 school physical education and, 352–353
 youth sport participation and, 347–349, 348*fig*
Motor skills development
 dynamic phenomenon of, 12
 refinement of, 347–353, 348*fig*, 350*t*, 351*fig*
Motor system properties, 31
Motor unit, 44*fig*
Movement
 Gibson's ecological perspective on role of, 203
 locomotor, nonlocomotor, manipulative skill, 285–286
 perception of, 181–182
 rudimentary behavior and, 261–281
 spontaneous (stereotypies), 259–261*fig*, 275*fig*
 theoretical views of voluntary, 257–259
 See also Early movement behavior
Movement-based approaches, 204–206
Movement patterns
 ball bouncing and dribbling, 316–318, 317*fig*, 346–347

catching, 304, 306–308*fig*, 309*fig*–310*fig*, 344
climbing, 318–320, 319*fig*
described, 386–387
development of mature and sport skill, 287
galloping, sliding, and skipping, 299–301*fig*, 300*fig*
hopping, 298–299*fig*, 345–346
jumping, 293*t*–298, 295*fig*, 296*fig*, 297*fig*, 342*fig*–343*fig*, 378–379
kicking, 313–316*fig*, 343
running, 289–292*t*, 290*fig*, 378–380*fig*
striking, 310–313*fig*, 312*fig*, 314*t*, 345, 380–381
throwing, 301–304*fig*, 303*t*, 305*t*–306*t*, 340–342, 341*fig*, 380–381
walking, 266*fig*–268*fig*, 269–273, 270*fig*, 377–378
Movement time, 222–224, 223*fig*, 234–235, 361*fig*, 373*fig*
Mozart Effect theory, 205, 206
Multidisciplinary approach, study of behavioral change using, 5
Muscular endurance, 130
Muscular strength
 aging and changes in, 134–135
 biological regression and, 370–371
 development of, 127–130, 156–157
 index of right/left grip of arm, 128*fig*
 ratio of body weight to, 129*fig*
Myelin, 45, 53–55
Myelination
 estimated timeline of process, 54*fig*
 overview of, 53–55
Myogenic behavior, 55

NASPE (National Association for Sport and Physical Education), 353
National Academies, 205
National Institute on Aging, 366
National Institutes of Health, 31
National Science Foundation, 31
Naturalistic observation, 20
nature-nurture relationship, 37
Nelson, C. J., 379
Nerve conduction velocity, 44–45

Nervous system
  CNS (central nervous system),
    39–41, 40*fig*, 42–43*fig*, 69
  early development changes of,
    46–60
  impulse conduction in, 44–46
  motor pathways of, 44, 45*fig*
  neurological changes with
    aging, 60–62*t*
  neuromuscular (motor) unit
    and, 44*fig*
  neurons and, 42–43*fig*
  PNS (peripheral nervous sys-
    tem), 39, 41–42, 43
  sequence of early development,
    46–60
Neumann, E., 221
Neurofibrillary tangles, 61
Neurogenic behavior, 55
Neurological changes
  aging and, 60–62*t*, 371–372
  basic structure and function,
    39–46, 40*fig*
  early development, 46–60
Neuromuscular (motor) unit, 44*fig*
Neuronal connection
  development, 49–51
Neuronal group selection, 30,
  229–232
Neurons
  described, 42–43*fig*
  development of after birth,
    52–53
  early development processes of,
    48
Newborn assessment tools
  Apgar score, 245, 395, 396*t*
  Brazelton Behavioral Assess-
    ment Scale, 245, 395–398,
    397*t*
Newell, K. M., 28, 261
Nodes of Ranvier, 43*fig*, 45
Nonlocomotor (stability) skills,
  286
Norm-referenced standards, 390
Norms
  construction of, 392
  defining, 422
Nutrition
  maternal, 143–144
  postnatal development and,
    149–151

Objectivity, 393
Object permanence, 175*fig*–176

Object positioning changes, 277*fig*
Observational learning (modeling),
  23–24
Older persons assessment instru-
  ments, 413–415, 414*t*
Ossification, 69, 87–88
Osteoarthritis, 136
Osteoporosis, 91, 136, 374
Overarm throwing. *See* Throwing
Overexclusive mode, 214
Overstall, P. W., 374

Palisano, R. J., 406
Palmar grasp, 245, 323
Palmar-mandibular reflex, 251
Pancreas, 160*fig*, 161
Parachute reflexes, 253–255, 254*fig*
Parathyroid glands, 162
Parental beliefs/attitudes,
  425*fig*–427
Parizkova longitudinal study of
  change, 154
Pasamanick, B., 325
PBC (Performance Base Curricu-
  lum), 412–413
PDMS-2 (Peabody Development
  Motor Scales II), 405–406
Peak motor performance
  age for selected events, 363*t*
  attainment of, 358
  considerations of race,
    364–365*t*
  described, 16
  growth and physiological func-
    tion, 358–359*fig*,
    360*fig*–361*fig*, 368*fig*
  motor performance characteris-
    tics of, 361–363*t*, 364
  See also Motor performance
Peer relations, 427–430, 428*fig*
Peers, 430
Percentile norms, 390
Perception
  auditory, 193–195, 200
  changes with aging, 199–202*t*
  defining, 170
  developmental biodynamics
    and, 29
  kinesthetic, 184–193, 200–201
  tactile, 195–196
  visual, 172–184*t*, 199–200
Perception of movement, 181–182
Perceptual constancy, 176–177
Perceptual integration
  auditory-kinesthetic, 198–199

overview of, 196–197
  visual-auditory, 198
  visual-kinesthetic, 197
Perceptual-motor (general
  information-processing) model,
  171*fig*
Performance standards, 392
Performer (biological factors),
  28
Peripheral vision, 180–181
Perry, B., 51
PFMAI (Posture and Fine Motor
  Assessment of Infants),
  401*fig*–402
Phase, 10
Phenotype, 38
Phillips, S. J., 271, 272
Physical activity
  biological regression and,
    381–383
  postnatal development and,
    151–159
Physical anthropology, 66–68
Physical education program,
  352–353
Physical growth/development
  body mass, 91–101, 152–153
  body proportions and physique,
    74–82, 153
  cephalocaudal and proximodis-
    tal patterns of, 66
  implications for motor
    performance, 108–109
  maturity estimates and,
    102–105*fig*
  maturity variations, 106–108
  physical anthropology/anthro-
    pometry and, 66–68
  physique, 81–82
  postnatal, 152–159
  prenatal, 68–70, 71*t*
  structural development, 82–91
  summary of physical growth
    changes with aging, 102*t*
  typical distance curves for
    height changes, 67*fig*
  See also Change; Growth;
    Height
Physical-motor assessment, 389*t*
Physiological age, 367
Physiological function
  for active/sedentary persons
    across life span, 368*fig*
  changes in grip strength with
    age, 359*fig*

changes in VO₂max with age and, 119*fig*, 359*fig*
hypothetical curve over life span of men, 133*fig*
peak of, 358–360
reaction time/movement time as function of age, 223*fig*, 361*fig*, 373*fig*
relationship of age to exercise tolerance, 360*fig*
Physique
changes with aging, 82
changes/development of, 81–82
postnatal development, 153
Piaget, J., 10, 24–25, 175, 225, 427
Piaget's theory of cognitive development, 24–25
Pick, A. D., 198
Pincer grasp, 276
Pituitary gland, 159–161, 160*fig*
PKU (phenylketonuria), 144
Placement assessment, 392
Plantar grasp reflex, 251
Plasticity, 12
Play activities, 427–429, 428*fig*
Plude, D. J., 232
PNS (peripheral nervous system)
described, 39, 41–42
Schwann cells in, 43
Postnatal development
important factors in, 149–150
nutrition and, 150–151
physical activity and, 151–159
Postural control
described, 190, 192*fig*, 262
head and upper trunk, 262, 263*fig*, 264
rolling (turning), 264
sitting, 264
standing, 264
Postural reflexes, 246, 252–255
Powell, K. E., 382
Power grip (palmar grasp), 245, 323
Prediction, 393
Prehension, 273
Prelongitudinal screening, 289
Premotor cortex, 41
Prenatal development
body form changes of developing fetus, 71*fig*
body weight, 91
external (environmental) factors, 145–149*fig*

internal (maternal) factors, 143–145
physical, 68–70, 71*t*
principles of teratogenic effects and, 142–143
See also Fetal period
Prenatal period, described, 13
Presbycusis, 200
Preshyopia, 199
Preterm birth, 148, 149*fig*
Previc, F. H., 329
Primary degenerative dementia, aging and, 61
Primitive reflexes, 245, 246, 248–252*fig*
Process characteristics, 288
Processing speed, 222–224, 234*fig*–235
Process-oriented assessment, 391
Process-oriented assessment instruments
Developmental Sequence of Fundamental Motor Skills Inventory (DSFMSI), 411
Fundamental Movement Pattern Assessment Instrument (FMPAI), 410*t*–411
overview of, 407–408
Test of Gross Motor Development (TGMD-2), 408–409*t*
Product-oriented assessment, 391
Product performance, 333
Product values, 288
Program content assessment, 392
Program evaluation, 392
Programmed theories, 366
Programming
aging and changes in, 235
developmental theories of motor control and, 227–232
overview of, 224–226
schema theory, 226–227
Protection mechanisms, 245
Proximodistal development, 9
Pseudo thumb opposition, 276
Psychological Testing (Kaplan and Saccuzzo), 394
Psychomotor slowing, 16–17, 371
Puberty
hormonal influence during, 72–73*fig*
pubescent growth spurt during, 70, 72–73*fig*
See also Adolescence
Pull-up reflex, 253*fig*

Pulmonary ventilation
described, 123–124
values at maximal exercise, 135*fig*
Pyle, S. L., 105
Pyramidal motor pathways, 45*fig*
Pyramidal system, 44
Pyramidal tract, 54–55

Quantitative motor performance changes
age/gender-related, 334–338
balance, 347
ball bouncing and dribbling, 346–347
catching, 344
hopping, 345–346
jumping, 342–343*fig*
kicking, 343
running speed, 338–339*fig*
striking, 345
throwing, 340*fig*–342, 341*fig*

Race
motor development and possible influence of, 434
peak performance and considerations of, 364–365
selected characteristics of African-American athletes, 365*t*
Radiation, prenatal development and, 148
Ramey, C., 52
Rarick, G. L., 17
Reaction time (RT), 212, 222–223*fig*, 361*fig*
Readiness, 7
Recall memory, 218–219
Red blood cells
content of, 125
mean values in relation to age, 126*fig*
Reflexes
approximate timetable of selected, 247*t*
defining, 244
early development of, 55
important in infant development, 244–246
types of, 246–257*fig*
Reflexive behavior
described, 244
infant development and, 244–246

theoretical views of voluntary
movement and, 257–259
Reflexive/spontaneous movement
phase, 15
Regression
advanced aging and ability,
12–13
balance and, 372–375
biological theories of advanced
aging and, 365–367
described, 16–17
flexibility, 375–376
motor behavior, 17
motor performance and biological, 368–377, 369*fig*, 370*fig*,
373*fig*
muscular strength, 370–371
neural function, 371–372
physical activity/longevity,
381–383
running and jumping,
378–380*fig*
throwing and striking, 380–381
walking, 377–378
See also Change
Reliability, 393
Research. *See* Dynamic system
research; Motor development
research
Respiratory (ventilatory) system
aerobic power and, 118–119
anaerobic power and, 119–121
basic structure of, 116*fig*
growth/development of, 117
vital capacity and pulmonary
ventilation, 123–124*fig*, 135*fig*
Rhythmic (temporal) awareness,
192–193
Richter, C. P., 250
Right-Shift Theory, 280, 328–329
Rikli, R., 374
Riticular formation, 41
RNA (ribonucleic acid), 37
Roberton, M. A., 17, 292, 298,
303
Roberton, S. R., 289
Robin, D. J., 278
Rogers, W., 235
Rogol, A. D., 156
Rolling (turning), 264
Rooting (search) reflex, 245, 248
Ross, A. O., 214
Rovee-Collier, C., 218
RT (reaction time), 212,
222–223*fig*, 361*fig*

Rudimentary behavior
locomotion, 265, 266*fig*,
267–273
manual control, 273*t*–279
motor asymmetries, 279–281
overview of, 261–262
postural control, 262, 263*fig*,
264
Rudimentary locomotion
crawling and creeping, 265,
266*fig*, 267
described, 265
walking, 266*fig*, 267–268*fig*,
269–273, 270*fig*, 271*t*
Rudimentary manual control
basic grasping techniques/
object positioning, 277*fig*
general sequence of, 273*t*
goal-directed behavior,
274–278
non-goal-directed behavior,
274
use of visual information,
278–279
Rudimentary phase, 16
Running
biological regression and,
378–380*fig*
developmental characteristics,
291–292*t*
development of, 289
initial attempts/mature pattern
of, 290*fig*–291
movement pattern descriptions,
289–291
Running speed, 338–339*fig*

Saccadic eye movements, 181
Salapatek, P., 174
Saltatory conduction, 45–46
Salthouse, T. A., 223
Salvia, J., 394
Schaie, K. W., 366
Schema, 24, 225
Schema theory, 226–227
Schmidt, R. A., 211, 221, 225, 227
School-age (up to) assessment
populations
Basic Motor Ability Tests-
Revised (BMAT-R), 404–405*t*
Bruininks-Oseretsky Test of
Motor Proficiency (BOT),
406–407*t*
Denver Developmental Screen-
ing Test (DDST), 403–404*t*

Peabody Development Motor
Scales II (PDMS-2), 405–406
School physical education,
352–353
Schultz, R., 361
Schwann cells, 43, 45
Secular trend, 107
Seefeldt, V., 307, 348
Seils, L., 345
Sekuler, R., 177, 180
Selective attention, 213–215
Self-efficacy, 436–437
Self-esteem, 432–434
Senile plaques, 61
Sensation, 170–171
Sensitive periods
described, 11
teratogenic effects and prenatal,
143
Sequential design, 20
Sexual age, 103
Sexual maturation
average age of, 104*fig*
gonads and, 72–73*fig*, 160*fig*,
162
menarche and, 70, 72, 103,
107*fig*, 155
postnatal development,
155–156
See also Maturation
SGMA report (2002), 349
Shaping, 423
Shapiro, D. C., 227
Sheldon, W. H., 81
Shephard, G. M., 366
Shephard, R. J., 133
Short-term memory. *See* Working
memory
Shoulder/hip ratio
changes in, 78–81*fig*
measuring shoulder and hip
width, 80*fig*
Shumway-Cook, A., 191, 269, 374,
378
Sibling influence, 426
Sickle-cell anemia, 144
SIGMA (Ohio State University
Scale of Intra-Gross Motor As-
sessment), 412*t*–413
Sit-and-reach test, 131–132*fig*
Sitting height
changes in ratio of stature to,
76–78
measuring, 79*fig*
ratios to stature to, 79*fig*

Sitting postural control, 264
Skeletal age, 103–105*fig*
Skeletal growth
    changes with aging, 89–91, 90*fig*
    changes/development of, 86–89, 87*fig*, 88*fig*
    postnatal development, 154–155
Skeletal muscle tissue
    biological regression and, 376–377
    growth of, 100–101
Skill-related fitness, 158–159
Skipping, 300–301*fig*
Sliding, 300*fig*
Smith, L. B., 229
Smoking/prenatal development relationship, 146
Social class, 422, 426–427
Socialization
    basic terminology of, 421–422
    processes and agents of, 422–423
    See also Learning
Socializing agent, 423
Social learning theory, 24
Social role, 422
Sociocultural influences
    during adulthood, 435–437*fig*
    basic terminology of, 421–422
    during childhood and adolescence, 424–434
    socializing processes and agents, 422–424
Soken, H. H., 198
Somatotype classifications, 81–82
Spatial awareness, 187–188
Spatial orientation, 177–178
Speed-accuracy trade-off, 224
Spinal cord, 39
Spirduso, W. W., 133
Spontaneous movements (stereotypies), 259–261*fig*, 275*fig*
Sporns, O., 230
Sports
    determinants of children's involvement in informal/organized, 430
    gender-role conflict and, 432
    influence of coaches and teachers, 430–431
    interscholastic, 349–352, 350*t*
    mean performances for masters-level swimming events/age, 370*fig*

school physical education, 352–353
    skill-related fitness and, 158–159
    Title IX and, 348, 432
    world records and changes with age, 369*fig*
    youth sport participation, 347–349, 348*fig*, 433–434
    See also Athletes
Sport skill movements, 287
Sport skill phase, 16
Sprague, R. L., 261
Stages, 10
Standardized tests, 21
Standing long jump, 296
Standing postural control, 264
Stature (standing height)
    for girls/age percentiles (2 to 20 years), 87*fig*
    for males/age percentiles (2 to 20 years), 86*fig*
    measuring, 83*fig*
    postnatal development, 152
    ratio of sitting height to, 76–78, 79*fig*
Status determination, 392
Stepping reflex, 255–256*fig*
Stereotyping, 259–261*fig*, 275*fig*
    age-related, 436
    gender-role, 431
Steroid-producing glands, 162
Stimulation
    brain development and early, 52
    development aided by positive, 11–12
Storandt, M., 232
Striking
    biological regression and, 380–381
    developmental characteristics, 313
    developmental sequence for, 314*t*
    development of, 310–311
    immature and mature patterns of, 312*fig*, 313*fig*
    movement pattern descriptions, 311–313
    quantitative changes in, 345
Stroke volume, 123
Structural development
    changes with aging, 89–91
    height, 82–86*fig*
    skeletal growth, 86–89

Structured observation, 20
Sucking reflex, 245
Sugden, D., 106, 185, 193, 341
Surwillo, W. W., 223
Swanson, H. L., 220
Swimming event performances/age, 370*fig*
Swimming reflex, 256–257*fig*
Synapse, 42
Synergies, 30
Systolic blood pressure, 125, 126

Tactile perception, 195–196
Tanner, J. M., 58, 105, 159
Teachers, 430–431
Teratogenic effects, 142–143
TGMD-2 (Test of Gross Motor Development), 408–409*t*
Thalamus, 40
Thelen, E., 6, 17, 30, 229, 259, 260, 271, 272
Thomas, R. J., 334
Throwing
    biological regression and, 380–381
    developmental sequence of overarm, 305*t*–306*t*
    development of overarm, 301–302
    mature overarm pattern of, 304*fig*
    quantitative changes in, 340*fig*–342, 341*fig*
    Wild's four developmental stages of, 302–303*t*
Thyroid gland, 160*fig*, 161
Till, R. E., 233
TIME (Toddler and Infant Motor Evaluation), 402
TIMP (Test of Infant Motor Performance), 402–403
Title IX, 348, 432
Tonic neck reflex, 250–251*fig*
Total (whole) body approach, 288
Toupet, M., 374
Tulving, E., 215
Turner's syndrome, 145
Turvey, M. T., 30

Ulrich, B. D., 271
Underwater (hydrostatic) weighing, 94–95
U.S. National Senior Olympics, 379

Validity, 393
Van der Fits, I. B. M., 274
Van Strien, 280
Velocity curves
　height, 67–68*fig*
　typical male/female, 85*fig*
Vertical jump, 294, 296*fig*
Vestibular awareness, 190–192
Visual cliff, 180*fig*
Visual functions
　coincident timing, 182
　depth perception, 178–180
　field of vision, 180–181
　figure-ground perception, 178
　object permanence, 175*fig*–176
　perception of movement,
　　181–182
　perceptual constancy, 176–177
　spatial orientation, 177–178
　visual acuity, 173–175
　visual-motor coordination,
　　182–183*t*
Visual-kinesthetic integration, 197
Visual perception
　changes with aging, 199–200
　described, 172
　developmental change in visual
　　functions, 173–183
　developmental change in visual
　　structures, 173
　summary of visual milestones,
　　184*t*
　visual process and, 172
Vital capacity, 123–124*fig*
VO$_2$max (maximal oxygen uptake)
　aerobic power and, 118
　aging and decline in, 133

anaerobic power and, 119–121
　as function of age, 119*fig*,
　　359*fig*
　gender differences in, 120*t*
　sedentary persons and rate of
　　decline in, 369
Von Hofsten, C., 275

Walker, A. S., 197
Walking
　biological regression and
　　changing patterns of,
　　377–378
　change in arm position when,
　　270*fig*
　developmental characteristics of
　　gait length/speed of, 271*t*
　developmental characteristics
　　of, 269–271
　dynamic systems research on,
　　271–273
　initial (immature) patterns of,
　　268*fig*–269
　overview of development, 267
　sequence of, 266*fig*
Warren, M. P., 156
Wear-and-tear theories, 366
Weiss, M. R., 24
Welford, A. T., 234, 235
Wellman, B. L., 346
"White Men Can't Run"
　(Burfoot), 364
Wickens, C. D., 213
Wickstrom, R. L., 286, 287, 302
Wiegand, R. L., 227
Wild, M., 17, 302
Wild's four developmental stages
　of throwing, 302–303*t*

Williams-Greene Test, 414*t*–415
Williams, H. G., 181, 200, 344,
　345, 347, 371, 372
Williams, K., 298, 380
Willmott, M., 378
Wilmore, J. H., 369
Windows of opportunity. *See* Crit-
　ical periods
Wolff's Law, 154
Women
　distance curves for stature,
　　85*fig*
　expected height increase per
　　year, 84*t*
　loss of bone density in, 90*fig*
　typical velocity curves, 85*fig*
　world records and changes with
　　age, 369*fig*
　See also Gender-related differ-
　　ences; Girls
Woollacott, M. H., 28, 191, 269,
　378
Working memory
　abilities of, 219–220
　changes with aging, 232–233
　overview of, 216–217
Writing and drawing, 322–325,
　323*fig*

Yekta, A. A., 200
Youth sport participation
　motor skill refinement through,
　　347–349
　self-esteem and, 433–434
　soccer portion of, 348*fig*
Ysseldyke, J. E., 394

Zauner, C. W., 152

Credits

Chapter 1

Figure 1.4: Courtesy of Dr. Daniela Corbetta, Infant Motor Development Laboratory, Purdue University. **Figure 1.6:** From Claire B. Kopp and Joanne B. Krakow, *The Child*, (pg. 648), © 1982 by Addison-Wesley Publishing Company, Inc. Reprinted by permission of the publisher. **Figure 1.7:** © David Young-Wolff/PhotoEdit.

Chapter 2

Figure 2.1: From L. L. Langley, I. R. Telford and J. B. Christensen, *Dynamic Anatomy and Physiology*, 3rd edition. Copyright © 1969 McGraw-Hill, Inc., New York, NY. Reprinted by permission. **Figure 2.2:** From John W. Hole, *Human Anatomy and Physiology*, third edition. Copyright © 1984 Wm. C. Brown Communications, Inc., Dubuque, Iowa. All Rights Reserved. Reprinted by permission. **Figure 2.3:** From George H. Sage, *Motor Learning and Control*, Copyright © 1984 Wm. C. Brown Communications, Inc., Dubuque, Iowa. All Rights Reserved. Reprinted by permission. **Figure 2.4:** From L. L. Langley, I. R. Telford and J. B. Christensen, *Dynamic Anatomy and Physiology*, 3rd edition. Copyright © 1969 McGraw-Hill, Inc., New York, NY. Reprinted by permission. **Figure 2.5:** © Lennart Nilsson/*A Child Is Born*, Dell Publishing. **Figure 2.6:** From J. L. Conel (1939–1963), *Postnatal Development of the Human Cerebral Cortex*, Vol. I–VI. Copyright © Harvard University Press, Cambridge, MA. Reprinted by permission. **Figure 2.8:** Adapted from Rorke & Riggs, 1969; Dekaban, 1970; Yakolev & Lecours, 1976. Reprinted by permission of Blackwell Scientific Publications, Oxford, England.

Chapter 3

Figure 3.1: From J. M. Tanner, *Fetus Into Man*, Copyright © 1978 by J. M. Tanner. Reprinted by permission of Harvard University Press, Cambridge, MA. **Figure 3.2:** From R. M. Malina, *Growth and Development: The First Twenty Years*, Copyright © 1975 Burgess Publishing Company, Minneapolis, MN. Reprinted by permission. **Figure 3.3:** From John W. Santrock, *Life-Span Development*, 2nd edition. Copyright © 1986 Wm. C. Brown Communications, Inc., Dubuque, Iowa. All Rights Reserved. Reprinted by permission. **Figure 3.5:** From John W. Santrock, *Children*, 4th edition. Copyright © 1989 Wm. C. Brown Communications, Inc., Dubuque, Iowa. All Rights Reserved. Reprinted by permission. **Figures 3.7 and 3.8:** From National Center for Health Statistics, 2000. **Figures 3.12 and 3.13:** From National Center for Health Statistics, 1983. **Figure 3.16:** From J. M. Tanner, *Fetus Into Man*, Copyright © 1978 by J. M. Tanner. Reprinted by permission of Harvard University Press, Cambridge, MA. **Figure 3.17:** From National Center for Health Statistics, 1973 and 1979. **Figures 3.18, 3.19:** From National Center for Health Statistics, 2000. **Figure 3.20:** © Carolina Biological Supply Company. **Figure 3.22:** From "Exercise and Osteoporosis" by H. J. Montoye. In *Exercise and Osteoporosis*, by H. M. Eckert and H. J. Montoye (Eds.), 1984. Champaign, IL: Human Kinetics. Copyright 1984 by the American Academy of Physical Education. Reprinted by permission. **Figure 3.23:** From "Natural Factors that Affect the Shape and Strength of the Aging Human Femur" by R. Poss, 1992, *Clinical Orthopaedics*, 274, pp. 195–196. Copyright 1992 by J. B. Lippincott Co. Reprinted by permission. **Figure 3.24:** From National Center for Health Statistics, 1973 and 1979. **Figures 3.25, 3.26:** From National Center for Health Statistics, 2000. **Figure 3.27 and 3.28:** From National Center for Health Statistics, 2000. **Figure 3.29:** From G. A. Brooks and T. D. Fahey, *Exercise Physiology: Human Bioenergetics and Its Applications*. Copyright © 1985 Macmillan Publishing Company, New York, NY. **Figure 3.30:** From *Growth, Maturation, and Physical Activity* (p. 97) by R. M. Malina and C. Bouchard, 1991, Champaign, IL: Human Kinetics. Copyright 1991 by Robert M. Malina and Claude Bouchard. Reprinted by permission. **Figures 3.33 and 3.34:** From S. I. Pyle, *A Radiographic Standard of Reference for the Growing Hand and Wrist* © Year Book Medical Publishers, Chicago, IL, 1971. **Figure 3.35:** From A. F. Roche, "Secular Trends in Stature, Weight, and Maturation" in *Monographs of the Society for Research in Child Development*, 44, Serial No. 179,

1977. Copyright © 1977 The Society for Research in Child Development, Inc., Chicago, Il. Reprinted by permission.

Chapter 4

Figure 4.1: From Ross M. Durham, *Human Physiology*, Copyright 1989 Wm. C. Brown Communications, Inc., Dubuque, Iowa. All Rights Reserved. Reprinted by permission. **Figure 4.2:** From Arthur C. Guyton, *Textbook of Medical Physiology*, 7th edition. Copyright © 1986 W. B. Saunders Company, Orlando, FL. Reprinted by permission. **Figure 4.3:** Reprinted with the permission of Simon & Schuster from the Macmillan college text: *Fitness, Health, and Work Capacity* by Leonard A. Larson. Copyright © 1974 by Macmillan Publishing Company, Inc. **Figure 4.4:** From Oded Bar-Or, *Pediatric Sports Medicine for the Practitioner: From Physiologic Principles to Clinical Applications.* Copyright © 1983 Springer-Verlag, New York. Reprinted by permission. **Figure 4.5:** From B. G. Ferris, M. D. Whittenberger, and J. R. Gallagher in *Pediatrics*, 9:659–670, Copyright © 1952; and B. G. Ferris and C. W. Smith in *Pediatrics*, 12:341–352, Copyright © 1953. Reproduced by permission of The American Academy of Pediatrics, Elk Grove Village, IL. **Figure 4.6:** Figure adapted from E. R. Mugrage and M. I. Andresen, "Values for Red Blood Cells of Average Infant and Children," 1936, 51:775–791; and "Red Blood Cell Values in Adolescence," 1938, 56:997–1003 in *American Journal of Diseases of Children*. Copyright 1936/38, American Medical Association, Chicago, IL. Reprinted by permission. **Figure 4.7:** From Altman and Dittmer, "Basal Metabolic Rate as a Function of Age and Sex" in *Metabolism*, 1968. Reprinted by permission of Federation of American Societies for Experimental Biology, Bethesda, MD. **Figure 4.8:** From H. M. Eckert, *Motor Development*, 3rd edition. Copyright © 1987 Benchmark Press, Indianapolis, IN. Reprinted by permission. **Figure 4.9:** From H. M. Eckert, *Motor Development*, 3rd edition. Copyright © 1987 Benchmark Press, Indianapolis, IN. Reprinted by permission. **Figure 4.12:** From E. L. Smith and R. C. Serfass (Eds.), *Exercise and Aging: The Scientific Basis.* Copyright © 1981 Enslow Publishers, Hillside, NJ. Reprinted by permission. **Figure 4.13:** From *Textbook of Work Physiology* (p. 232) by P. O. Astrand and K. Rodahl, 1986, New York: McGraw-Hill. **Figure 4.14:** From *Changes in Spinal Mobility with Increasing Age in Women*, by D. K. Einkauf, M. L. Gohdes, G. M. Jensen, and M. J. Jewell, 1987. *Physi-*

cal Therapy, 67, p. 374. Copyright 1987 by the American Physical Therapy Association. Reprinted by permission.

Chapter 5

Figure 5.1: © John Chiasson/Gamma Liaison/Getty Images.

Chapter 6

Figure 6.3: © George Zimbel/Monkmeyer Press. **Figure 6.4:** © William Vandivert. **Figure 6.6:** Used with permission from Karen E. Adolph.

Chapter 7

Figure 7.2: From *Motor Control and Learning: A Behavioral Emphasis*, 2d edition, page 91, by Richard A. Schmidt, 1988, Champaign, IL: Human Kinetics. Copyright © 1988 by Richard A. Schmidt. Reprinted by permission. **Figure 7.3:** Courtesy of Carolyn Rovee-Collier, Rutgers University. **Figure 7.4:** From J. Hodgkins, "Influence of Age on the Speed of Reaction and Movement in Females" in *Journal of Gerontology*, 17, 385–389. Copyright © 1962 Gerontology Society of America. Reprinted by permission. **Figure 7.5:** © Steve Wewerka/Impact Visuals. **Figure 7.6:** From "Causes of Slowing of Performance With Age" by A. T. Welford, 1977. *Interdisciplinary Topics in Gerontology*, 11, p. 46. Copyright 1977 by S. Karger AG, Basel. Reprinted by permission.

Chapter 8

Figure 8.1: Courtesy of Mead Johnson Nutritional Group. **Figure 8.2:** © Petit Format/J. Da Cunha/PhotoResearchers, Inc. **Figure 8.4:** © Laura Dwight/PhotoEdit. **Figure 8.9:** Courtesy of Mead Johnson and Company. **Figure 8.10:** © William McCauley/CORBIS. **Figure 8.13a:** © Michael Newman/PhotoEdit. **Figure 8.13b:** © Rick Gomez/CORBIS. **Figure 8.13c:** © Laurence Monneret/Getty Images.**Figure 8.16:** From Experiment by Thelen and Ulrich. Reprinted by permission of Esther Thelen. **Figure 8.19:** Courtesy of Dr. Esther Thelen, Infant Motor Development Laboratory, Indiana University.

Chapter 9

Figure 9.20: From Marian Annett, "The Growth of Manual Preference and Speed" in the *British Journal of Psychology*, 61:545–558, fig. 1 page 549. Copyright © 1970 The British Psychological Society, East Finchley, London. Reprinted by permission.

Chapter 10

Figure 10.1: From *Science and Medicine of Exercise and Sport*, 2nd edition by Warren K. Johnson and Elsworth R. Buskirk. Copyright © 1974 by Warren K. Johnson and Elsworth R. Buskirk. Reprinted by permission of HarperCollins Publishers, Inc.
Figure 10.3: From *Science and Medicine of Exercise and Sport*, 2nd edition by Warren K. Johnson and Elsworth R. Buskirk. Copyright © 1974 by Warren K. Johnson and Elsworth R. Buskirk. Reprinted by permission of HarperCollins Publishers, Inc.
Figure 10.4: From Jerry R. Thomas, *Motor Development During Childhood & Adolescence*, 1984, MacMillan Publishing. Data from L. Halverson, M. A. Roberton, and S. Langendorfer, "Development of the Overarm Throw Movement and Ball Velocity Changes by 7th Grade" in *Research Quarterly for Exercise & Sport*, 1982, vol. 53. Reprinted by permission of Jerry R. Thomas. **Figure 10.5:** From *Science and Medicine of Exercise and Sport*, 2nd edition by Warren K. Johnson and Elsworth R. Buskirk. Copyright © 1974 by Warren K. Johnson and Elsworth R. Buskirk. Reprinted by permission of HarperCollins Publishers, Inc. **Figure 10.6:** From *Science and Medicine of Exercise and Sport*, 2nd edition by Warren K. Johnson and Elsworth R. Buskirk. Copyright © 1974 by Warren K. Johnson and Elsworth R. Buskirk. Reprinted by permission of HarperCollins Publishers, Inc.
Figure 10.7: © Bob Daemmrich/The Image Works.
Figure 10.8: © George Shelley/CORBIS.

Chapter 11

Figure 11.4: From J. Hodgkins, "Influence of Age on the Speed of Reaction and Movement in Females" in *Journal of Gerontology*, 17, 385–389. Copyright © 1962 Gerontology Society of America. Reprinted by permission. **Figure 11.5:** From E. L. Smith and R. C. Serfass (Eds.), *Exercise and Aging: The Scientific Basis*. Copyright © 1981 Enslow Publishers, Hillside, NJ. Reprinted by permission. **Figure 11.8:** From W. D. McArdle, et al., *Exercise Physiology*, 2nd edition, 1986, as drawn from the data of 2d W. W. Spirduso, 1975. Reprinted by permission of W. W. Spirduso.
Figure 11.9: © David Madison/Getty Images.

Chapter 12

Figure 12.2: © Dorling Kindersley.

Chapter 13

Figure 13.1: © Warren Morgan/CORBIS.
Figure 13.2: © Bluestone Productions/Getty Images. **Figure 13.3:** © Yellow Dog Productions/Getty Images.